A Teacher's Guide to Including Students with Disabilities in Regular Physical Education

by

Martin E. Block, Ph.D.

Assistant Professor
Program Area of Health and Physical Education
Department of Human Services
Curry School of Education
The University of Virginia
Charlottesville

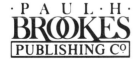

·P A U L·H·
BROOKES
PUBLISHING C?

Baltimore · London · Toronto · Sydney

Paul H. Brookes Publishing Co.
P.O. Box 10624
Baltimore, Maryland 21285-0624

Typeset by Brushwood Graphics, Baltimore, Maryland.
Manufactured in the United States of America by
The Maple Press Company, York, Pennsylvania.

Library of Congress Cataloging-in-Publication Data

Block, Martin E., 1958–
A teacher's guide to including students with disabilities in regular physical educa-
   tion / by Martin E. Block.
      p.   cm.
   Includes bibliographical references (p.   ) and index.
   ISBN 1-55766-156-1
   1. Physical education for handicapped persons. 2. Mainstreaming in education.
I. Title.
GV445.B56   1994
371.9′04486—dc20   93-38428
                                                                        CIP

British Library Cataloguing-in-Publication data are available from the British Library.

A Teacher's Guide to Including Students with Disabilities in Regular Physical Education

Contents

Foreword

Martin E. Block takes a quantum leap forward in the operationalization of contemporary adapted physical activity in this guide to including students with disabilities in regular physical education. *Adapted physical activity* today is defined as cross-disciplinary theory and practice related to life-span physical activity of individuals whose uniqueness of function, structure, or appearance necessitates ecological changes in attitudes, knowledge, and skills to ensure appropriate adaptation, equal access, and inclusion. This new definition emphasizes the reciprocal, interactive roles of physical and special educators, parents, siblings, peers, paraprofessionals, and others in changing the ecology of schools and communities to empower children and youth with disabilities to become the best they can be.

Dr. Block is the first physical educator to develop a textbook specifically and exclusively on inclusion. He defines *inclusion* as "the practice of educating all students, including students with disabilities, in regular education and regular classes" (p. 16). This book thus emphasizes the part of the least restrictive environment (LRE) philosophy of the Individuals with Disabilities Education Act of 1990 (IDEA) (PL 101-476) that has received the least attention: how to provide supports and assistance to ensure success in the regular physical education setting. The content is thus relevant to professionals who espouse either the LRE or the regular education initiative (REI) or inclusion philosophy.

Dr. Block opens 9 of his 10 chapters with anecdotal accounts of real children with disabilities: *Shameka*, a sixth grader with mental retardation; *Juan*, a fourth grader with spastic, diplegic cerebral palsy; *Lee*, a 15-year-old with mental retardation and cerebral palsy; *David*, a ninth grader with a severe visual impairment; *Ming*, a second grader with spina bifida who uses long leg braces and crutches; *Bill*, a seventh grader who is visually impaired and uses braille; *Rasheed*, a 10th grader with mental retardation who cannot speak; *Jacob*, a third grader with muscular dystrophy; *Kristen*, a seventh grader with athetoid cerebral palsy; *José*, an 11th grader who is blind; *Nick*, a 3-year-old with cerebral palsy; *Sue*, a third grader with impaired vision and paralysis resulting from an automobile accident; and *Ahmed*, a 10th grader with mental retardation and a seizure disorder. The names of these students reflect the cross-cultural inclusiveness of content as readers learn to think about individual needs based on joint assessment of the student and his or her ecosystem or environment, rather than the outdated approach of characteristics of conditions still presented in many textbooks.

Dr. Block's approach is practical, proactive, and futuristic. Section I of the text focuses on philosophy, beliefs, and attitudes in relation to physical education, inclusion, and team assessment and programming. Block's conceptualization of the Physical Education Inclusion Team (PEIT) is particularly excellent in that it emphasizes collaborative teamwork and support of all school personnel as requisites for the operationalization of inclusion philosophy in the regular physical education setting. Section II of the text describes program planning, assessment, and general and specific instructional and curricular strategies. Section III presents case studies of implementation with three different age groups: 1) preschool, 2) elementary school, and 3) middle and high school. The organization of content is exemplary, progressing from basic understanding to comprehensive explanation of skills to application/generalization of skills in varied settings.

Each chapter includes numerous illustrations and tables that enhance, supplement, and synthesize ideas in the text. For example, Tables 2.1 and 2.2 summarize benefits of inclusion to students with disabilities, to professional staff, and to students without disabilities. Table 4.1 presents a seven-step model for including children with disabilities in regular physical education. Many of the tables in this book offer task analyses and illustrative sections of individualized education programs (IEPs). Virtually everything is present in this text to guide schools and parents who want to make inclusion work. Strategies to help physical educators explain supports to administrators and seek assistance in shaping an ecology conducive to inclusion are also provided.

Adapted physical activity as a profession and an emerging discipline is changing rapidly, as are special education and related services areas. Today's authorities emphasize that adapted physical activity is not a specific placement but a philosophy of services, strategies, and processes that can occur in any setting. Much has been written about the advantages and disadvantages of separate settings versus inclusive settings, the failure of schools to provide a continuum of least restrictive environments in physical education, and problems involved in inclusion. Many physical educators are attempting to make sense out of perceived chaos and impossible challenges. Dr. Block emerges as a strong, courageous pioneer who is willing and able to show the way. He explains clearly the cooperative and supportive conditions and practices that are required for successful inclusion.

Dr. Block dares to dream, to challenge old ways, and to suggest what some may see as radical school reform. This innovative, outstanding new textbook will enable undergraduate and graduate students, professionals, parents, and others to think, believe, and act in ways consistent with the ethos of democracy and participatory, caring, cooperative infrastructures.

Claudine Sherrill, Ed.D.
Texas Woman's University
Author of Adapted Physical Activity,
Recreation, and Sport: Crossdisciplinary
and Lifespan

Preface

An ever increasing number of students with disabilities are being included in regular classrooms in their neighborhood schools. In turn, more of these students are being included in regular physical education classes (Jansma & Decker, 1990). Unfortunately, many regular physical educators are ill-prepared to provide individualized, appropriate physical education programs for students with disabilities. Regular physical educators often have very little preservice training in adapted physical education and have little or no practical experience working with students with disabilities (DiRocco, 1978; Lavay & DePaepe, 1987). What often results are frustrated, resentful physical educators who have negative attitudes toward including students with disabilities in their regular physical education programs (e.g., Aloia, Knutson, Minner, & Von Seggern, 1980). In addition, physical educators often provide inappropriate physical education for students with disabilities (DePaepe, 1984; Grosse, 1991). In some schools, students with disabilities are given mundane jobs such as scorekeeper or are excused from physical education altogether (Morreau & Eichstaedt, 1983).

Although there are many excellent published texts on adapted physical education that can help regular physical educators, none of these works specifically addresses the challenges and rewards of including students with disabilities in regular physical education. Therefore, the purpose of this book is to outline a systematic process as well as to provide specific strategies for safely, successfully, and appropriately including students with disabilities in regular physical education programs. This book is a guide for practitioners (both special education professionals and regular physical educators) that contains numerous practical examples and real-life applications.

The book is divided into three sections. Section I, which introduces the reader to terminology related to physical education, inclusion, and the collaborative team, includes three chapters. Chapter 1 should be particularly helpful to special education professionals and administrators who might not be familiar with legal mandates for physical education or what the term *physical education* encompasses. Chapter 2 should be particularly helpful to regular educators and adapted physical education specialists who may not be familiar with the terminology, history, concepts, and rationale of inclusion. Chapter 3 introduces the concept of a Physical Education Inclusion Team (PEIT). In addition, Chapter 3 reviews the role of parents, peers, the regular physical educator, and special education professionals in developing and implementing an inclusive physical education program. The chapter concludes with an example of a PEIT meeting.

The four chapters in Section II present a systematic, practical model for including students with disabilities in regular physical education. Utilizing an ecological approach to program planning, Chapter 4 outlines a systematic process for developing and implementing an inclusive physical education program with an emphasis on preplanning and training support personnel. Chapter 5 presents ways in which the ecological approach can be used to functionally assess students with disabilities and thus facilitate inclusion. This chapter emphasizes nontraditional assessment procedures referenced to real-life situations (i.e., ecological approach), as opposed to traditional norm-referenced assessments, and includes many new and easy-to-use checklists developed specifically to facilitate inclusion. Section II concludes with two chapters that present strategies for accommodating students with disabilities in regular physical education. Chapter 6 focuses on instructional and curricular modifications, including models for adapting individual skills and group games. Chapter 7 discusses modifications for students with specific deficits such as problems with balance or strength, or specific disabilities such as mental retardation or hearing impairments. In addition, specific modifications to selected individual and team sports are presented. The goal of these modifications is to ensure that students with disabilities can work on their individual goals and objectives while participating with their peers without disabilities in regular physical education safely, successfully, and meaningfully.

Section III, which contains three chapters, presents detailed case studies of how students with disabilities in different age groups can be included in regular physical education. Chapter 8 relates a case story showing how preschool students can be included in a regular, preschool movement program, including regular childcare centers, a community-based motor development program, and regular kindergarten physical education. Chapter 9 shows how elementary school students can be included in regular physical education. Finally, Chapter 10 relates a case story showing how middle school or high school students can be included in regular physical education. All three chapters apply information from the model and strategies previously described in this book to demonstrate how the process works.

Although this book is intended to be as comprehensive as possible, it is not intended to be a "cookbook" of solutions for including students with disabilities in regular physical education. Rather, the information is designed to make regular physical educators, as well as other team members, become more aware of ways to meaningfully include students with disabilities in regular physical education. Physical educators ultimately must decide which strategies will work in their settings and which will not. It is hoped that the reader will begin to develop his or her own ideas regarding the best way to include students with disabilities in regular physical education.

Finally, it should be noted that this book does not promote inclusion because of moral or philosophical reasons. Although the practices advocated in this work are grounded firmly in the belief that including students with disabilities in regular physical education is the just route to take, it is also the honest view of the author that, with support, virtually all students with disabilities, including students with significant disabilities, can be better served in inclusive physical education programs. All that is required is a systematic approach to developing and implementing individually prescribed programs within the regular setting. This book provides such a systematic approach.

REFERENCES

Aloia, G., Knutson, R., Minner, S.J., & Von Seggern, M. (1980). Physical education teachers' initial perception of handicapped children. *Mental Retardation, 18,* 85–87.

DePaepe, J.L. (1984). Mainstreaming malpractice. *Physical Educator, 41,* 51–56.

DiRocco, P. (1978). Preparing for the mainstreamed environment: A necessary addition to preservice curriculums. *Journal of Health, Physical Education, Recreation and Dance, 49*(1), 24–25.

Grosse, S. (1991). Is the mainstream always a better place to be? *Palaestra, 7*(2), 40–49.

Jansma, P., & Decker, J. (1990). *Project LRE/PE: Least restrictive environment usage in physical education.* Washington, DC: Department of Education, Office of Special Education.

Lavay, B., & DePaepe, J. (1987). The harbinger helper: Why mainstreaming in physical education doesn't always work. *Journal of Health, Physical Education, Recreation, and Dance, 58*(7), 98–103.

Morreau, L.E., & Eichstaedt, C.B. (1983). Least restrictive programming and placement in physical education. *American Corrective Therapy Journal, 37*(1), 7–17.

Acknowledgments

There are several people I would like to thank for their assistance in the development and completion of this book. First, I would like to thank my wife Vickie and daughter Samantha, the two most important people in my life, who have always brought me joy and kept me going whenever the challenge of writing this book became overwhelming.

Special thanks to all of the educators who contributed the "voices from the field" statements that appear at the beginning of each chapter in this book. They and other professionals like them who are successfully including students with disabilities in regular physical education have provided me with the practical, realistic ideas that can be found throughout the book.

Several people reviewed early versions of select chapters from the book. These people include Anne Boyce, Vonnie Colvin, Marcy Guddemi, Eileen Kelly, Luke Kelly, Sherril Moon, Katie Stanton, and my wife Vickie. Thanks go to them for providing terrific constructive feedback. Thanks also are owed to my students from both The University of Virginia and Northern Illinois University, as well as to the professionals in both regular and adapted physical education and special education who have humored me with hours of lively discussions on inclusion.

I am honored and extremely appreciative to have Claudine Sherrill as the author of the foreword to this book. I have always enjoyed reading her papers and books as well as discussing ideas with her. In keeping with the philosophy of "not re-creating the wheel," many of her wonderful ideas on including students with disabilities in regular physical education can be found throughout this text.

All of the people at Paul H. Brookes Publishing Co. have been wonderful to work with. So many of the textbooks and references I use come from Brookes Publishing, and I am thrilled to be a member of this outstanding team. I would especially like to thank Theresa Donnelly for her expert editing, advice, discussions, and gentle reminders that helped me see this project to completion.

Finally, I would like to thank all the students both with and without disabilities as well as their regular and adapted physical education teachers who allowed me to observe their programs and discussed the practical matters of inclusion with me. This book is the direct result of these observations and candid discussions. These students and teachers are proof that inclusive physical education works!

> *This book is dedicated to the memory of my mother, Helen Block. Her enthusiasm for life and caring ways inspired everyone who had the good fortune to meet her. I can only hope to have as positive an influence on the people I meet and teach as she had on me.*

INTRODUCTION

Chapter 1

What Is Physical Education?

We should realize that special educators and regular educators alike are wearing a new hat. We are being guided into an arena that brings change for everyone. Change is difficult, but in the end we must consider who will benefit. I was recently consulting with an elementary physical education teacher concerning the inclusion of a student with spina bifida in his program. As he was struggling with how to adapt his program, he drew a square and said, "This is what I teach. The students are either on the inside or the outside. Although I care about these kids, we can only adapt so much." In response, I drew a larger square and said, "I like to think of it as, "This is what I teach and all my students are on the inside, benefiting from my instruction."

—Robynn Rome

Do you remember physical education when you were in school? For good or bad, your personal physical education experiences no doubt helped to shape your view of physical education. If you had physical education teachers who had long-term goals in mind, who used a variety of motivating activities to help students achieve these long-term goals, who organized the environment so that every student was successful and active, and who really tried to teach and instruct rather than merely supervise, then you probably have a very positive view of physical education. However, if you had a teacher whose program focused on playing games rather than working on skills and concepts, who used tired activities over and over again, who did not seem to care if students improved or acquired motor and fitness skills, who made students stand in line forever waiting their turn, and who allowed the same lesser-skilled students to constantly be picked last, to be ridiculed by peers, and to fail, then you probably have a negative view of physical education. Your view will be even more negative if you were one of the lesser-skilled students.

Unfortunately, many of us have previous physical education experiences that have led us to think of physical education as a time where children play games and socialize—a glorified recess. Thus, it seems perfectly logical that parents and professionals alike consider physical education a great place to include students with disabilities since "they just play games and have fun in physical education anyway." However, physical education is much more than just glorified recess or Little League. Sherrill (1993) noted that physical education should be considered an "academic subject" just like math and reading. Good physical education programs are instructional in nature and provide a planned sequence of activities every day that help students improve their motor skills, physical fitness, cognitive skills related to movement and sports, and feelings of self-

Robynn Rome is an APE specialist, High Plains Educational Cooperative, Ulysses, Kansas.

worth. In addition, good physical education programs are fun, challenging, and motivating for all students, not just skilled students.

BENEFITS OF PHYSICAL EDUCATION

Students who participate in *quality* physical education programs receive a variety of benefits including the development of: 1) a variety of motor skills and abilities related to lifetime leisure skills, 2) improved understanding of the importance of maintaining a healthy lifestyle, 3) improved understanding and appreciation of movement and the human body, 4) improved knowledge of the rules and strategies of particular games and sports, and 5) improved self-confidence and self-worth as they relate to physical education and recreation activities (Graham, Holt-Hale, & Parker, 1993; NASPE, 1992; Sherrill, 1993). (See NASPE's detailed definition of a physically educated person in Table 1.1.)

The benefits of physical education described above are even more important for students with disabilities. Many students with disabilities have more free time than their peers without disabili-

Table 1.1. National Association for Sport and Physical Education (NASPE) definition of a physically educated person

The Physically Educated Person . . .
HAS Learned Skills Necessary to Perform a Variety of Physical Activities
1. . . . moves using concepts of body awareness, space awareness, effort, and relationships.
2. . . . demonstrates competence in a variety of manipulative, locomotor, and nonlocomotor skills.
3. . . . demonstrates competence in combinations of manipulative, locomotor, and nonlocomotor skills performed individually and with others.
4. . . . demonstrates competence in many different forms of physical activity.
5. . . . demonstrates proficiency in a few forms of physical activity.
6. . . . has learned how to learn new skills.

IS Physically Fit
7. . . . assesses, achieves, and maintains physical fitness.
8. . . . designs safe, personal fitness programs in accordance with principles of training and conditioning.

DOES Participate Regularly in Physical Activity
9. . . . participates in health enhancing physical activity at least three times a week.
10. . . . selects and regularly participates in lifetime physical activities.

KNOWS the Implications of and the Benefits from Involvement in Physical Activities
11. . . . identifies the benefits, costs, and obligations associated with regular participation in physical activity.
12. . . . recognizes the risk and safety factors associated with regular participation in physical activity.
13. . . . applies concepts and principles to the development of motor skills.
14. . . . understands that wellness involves more than being physically fit.
15. . . . knows the rules, strategies, and appropriate behaviors for selected physical activities.
16. . . . recognizes that participation in physical activity can lead to multicultural and international understanding.
17. . . . understands that physical activity provides the opportunity for enjoyment, self-expression, and communication.

VALUES Physical Activity and Its Contributions to a Healthful Lifestyle
18. . . . appreciates the relationships with others that result from participation in physical activity.
19. . . . respects the role that regular physical activity plays in the pursuit of lifelong health and well-being.
20. . . . cherishes the feelings that result from regular participation in physical activity.

From National Association for Sport and Physical Education Outcomes Committee. (1992). Definition and outcomes of the physically educated person. In *Outcomes of quality physical education programs* (p. 7). Reston, VA: NASPE; reprinted by permission.

ties (e.g., in the past, students with disabilities have had limited opportunities to participate in after-school clubs or community programs) (Dattilo, 1991). In addition, most individuals with disabilities have limited recreation skills that greatly restrict their abilities to participate in community activities and interact with peers who do not have disabilities. Extra free time coupled with limited recreation skills often leads to a sedentary lifestyle that in turn can lead to health and social problems. Quality physical education programs can help students with disabilities acquire critical lifetime leisure skills including appropriate behaviors and an appreciation for continued participation in active recreational pursuits.

LEGAL DEFINITION OF PHYSICAL EDUCATION

While the previous discussion reviewed the general perception of physical education as well as professional views of physical education, there is actually a legal definition of physical education that is included in Public Law (PL) 101-476—Individuals with Disabilities Education Act (IDEA). IDEA, which was originally authorized in 1975 as Public Law 94-142—Education for All Handicapped Children Act—provides specific guidelines and practices for educating students with disabilities (Sherrill, 1993). (See Table 1.2 for a brief chronology of PL 101-476.) The term *handicapped child* was used in the original law. With the reauthorization of this law as Individuals with Disabilities Education Act (IDEA), current terminology is *child with disability*. Not only did legislators define physical education, but physical education was considered so important that they

Table 1.2.   Chronology of PL 101-476, Individuals with Disabilities Education Act (IDEA)

Year	Act	Description
1975	PL 94-142 Education for All Handicapped Children Act of 1975 (EHA)	Landmark legislation that provided free and appropriate education, including physical education, for all eligible children ages 3–21. EHA is currently known as Part B in the current Individuals with Disabilities Education Act (IDEA).
1983	PL 98-189 EHA Amendments of 1983	Increased funding and provided *incentives* for states to develop and implement an early intervention system to serve children with disabilities from birth to age 5. States were not mandated to provide services to children birth to age 3 at this point.
1986	PL 99-457 EHA Amendments of 1986	*Required* states to provide services to eligible preschoolers ages 3–5 years or lose some federal funding. Also, Part H of 99-457 (still referred to as Part H in IDEA) commissioned funds to states to develop and implement a comprehensive, multidisciplinary, interagency program of early intervention services for infants and toddlers with disabilities (birth to age 2) and their families.
1990	PL 101-476 EHA Amendments of 1990 (Changed name to IDEA)	Renamed EHA as Individuals with Disabilities Education Act (IDEA) (all reference to *handicap* in previous is replaced with term *disability*). Major changes included new definitions of attention deficit hyperactivity disorder and traumatic brain injury, and created new eligibility category for autistic condition. Reemphasized least restrictive environment with focus on training regular education personnel and the use of assistive technology. Added new term, Transition Services, which emphasized a coordinated effort to help students age 16 and older (age 14 for students with severe disabilities) acquire skills needed to move from school to postschool activities. As such, social services, recreation therapy, and rehabilitation counseling reemphasized.

Adapted from Cowden & Eason (1991).

made it the only curricular area that was specifically placed within the definition of special education:

> The term special education means specially designed instruction, at no cost to the parent, to meet the unique needs of a handicapped child including classroom instruction, INSTRUCTION IN PHYSICAL EDUCATION (emphasis added), home instruction, and instruction in hospitals and institutions. (*Federal Register*, August 23, 1977, p. 42480)

Physical education services were further defined in the law as follows:

> (a) **General**. Physical education services, specifically designed as necessary, must be made available to every handicapped child receiving a free appropriate public education.
> (b) **Regular physical education**. Each handicapped child must be afforded the opportunity to participate in the regular physical education program available to non-handicapped children unless:
>   (1) the child is enrolled full time in a separate facility; or
>   (2) the child needs specially designed physical education, as prescribed in the child's individualized education program.
> (c) **Special physical education**. If specially designed physical education is prescribed in a child's individualized education program, the public agency responsible for the education of that child shall provide the services directly, or make arrangements for it to be provided through other public or private programs.
> (d) **Education in separate facilities**. The public agency responsible for the education of a handicapped child who is enrolled in a separate facility shall insure that the child receives appropriate physical education services in compliance with paragraphs (a) and (c) of this section. (*Federal Register*, August 23, 1977, p. 42489)

Comments from the Report of the House of Representatives on the original PL 94-142 reinforced the importance of physical education:

> specifically included physical education within the definition of special education to make clear that the Committee expects such services, specially designed where necessary, to be provided as an integral part of the educational program for every handicapped child. (*Federal Register*, August 23, 1977, p. 42489)

Clearly, this law defines physical education as an important, direct service that should be a part of all students' educational programs. Contrast this with the law's stipulation regarding related services such as physical, occupational, and recreation therapy:

> transportation and such developmental, corrective, and other supportive services as are required to assist a handicapped child benefit from special education (shall be provided). (*Federal Register*, August 23, 1977, p. 42479)

These services are provided only to those students who need extra support to benefit from special education. Because physical education is included in the definition of special education and related services are provided to assist students who need extra support to benefit from special education, related services can be viewed as support given to students to help them benefit from physical education! All students should receive physical education services, while only those students who need extra support to benefit from special education require related services. Related services (including physical, occupational, or recreation therapy) *cannot* be considered a substitute for the physical education requirement; nor can recess, unstructured free time, or training in sedentary recreation activities (e.g., board and card games) be considered as appropriate substitutes for physical education.

COMPONENTS OF PHYSICAL EDUCATION

While it is clear that physical education should be viewed as an important part of a student's overall education program, what exactly is physical education? Physical education is defined in IDEA as:

the development of physical and motor fitness, fundamental motor skills and patterns, and skills in aquatics, dance, and individual and group games and sports (including intramural and lifetime sports). The term includes special physical education, adapted physical education, movement education, and motor development. (Federal Register, August 23, 1977, p 42480)

The following provides a more detailed examination of each component contained within the definition of physical education:

Physical and motor fitness refers to development of both health-related and skill-related fitness. Health-related fitness focuses on factors pertaining to a healthy lifestyle and the prevention of disease related to a sedentary lifestyle (Graham et al., 1993; Hastad & Lacy, 1989). Hastad and Lacy (1989, p. 178) provided the following definitions of the specific components of health-related fitness:

- *Cardiovascular efficiency* (aerobic endurance)—ability to exercise the entire body for extended periods of time without undue fatigue. Moving (e.g., riding a bike, walking, jogging) without stopping for extended periods of time retains or increases cardiovascular efficiency.
- *Muscular strength*—ability of muscles to exert force (e.g., to lift heavy objects). Lifting weights or other objects that are more than one lifts in activities of daily living increases muscular strength.
- *Muscular endurance*—ability of muscles to exert force over an extended period of time. Lifting weights or heavy objects repeatedly retains or increases muscular endurance.
- *Flexibility*—range of motion available in the musculature (i.e., muscles, tendons, and ligaments). Stretching activities help musculature retain or increase elasticity.
- *Body composition*—refers to the amount of body fat a person carries. A fit person has a relatively low percentage of body fat. Performing aerobic and strength activities as well as following a reasonable diet helps retain or decrease percentage of body fat.

Skill-related fitness refers to specific fitness components associated with successful performance in motor activities and sports (Graham et al., 1993; Hastad & Lacy, 1989). Hastad and Lacy (1989, p. 1248) provided the following definitions of the specific components of skill-related fitness:

- *Agility*—ability to rapidly and accurately change the position of the body in space. Quickly changing positions in wrestling or avoiding a tackler in football are examples of agility.
- *Balance*—the maintenance of equilibrium while stationary (static balance) or moving (dynamic balance). Performing a head stand or maintaining balance while swinging a golf club are examples of static balance, and walking a balance beam or running in a football game without falling are examples of dynamic balance.
- *Coordination*—ability to simultaneously perform multiple motor tasks smoothly and accurately. Hitting a tennis ball, using a smooth throwing pattern when pitching a ball, or dribbling a soccer ball are examples of athletic skills that require coordination.
- *Reaction time*—difference between the stimulation (seeing, hearing, feeling something) and the response (moving) to the stimulation. A sprinter's response to the starting gun or a racquetball player's reaction to a hard-hit ball are examples of activities that require short reaction time.
- *Speed*—ability to perform a movement in a short period of time. A batter running to first base or a basketball player dribbling a ball quickly down the court are examples of activities that require speed.

Fundamental motor skills and patterns refers to the development of basic motor skills that form the foundation for more advanced, specific movements used in individual and team sports and activities (Gabbard, 1992; Graham et al., 1993; Wickstrom, 1983). Each fundamental motor skill has a distinct pattern or structure that defines the movement. Fundamental movement patterns are usually divided into locomotor and manipulative patterns. Locomotor patterns are movements used by individuals to travel from one place to another, while manipulative patterns are used to propel balls away from the body or receive balls. Table 1.3 provides more detailed description of the most common fundamental locomotor and manipulative patterns as described by Graham et al. (1993) and Wickstrom (1983).

Aquatics refers to activities conducted in the water. Activities that can be conducted in the water include: 1) swimming, which involves moving independently in the water using various strokes; 2) water exercises, which work on the development of health-related fitness; and 3) hydrotherapy, which involves using the water environment to work on specific therapeutic goals such as walking, relaxing, and maintaining/increasing range of motion (Priest, 1990).

Rhythm and dance refers to the ability to repeat an action or movement with regularity and in time to a particular pattern (Kirchner, 1992). Rhythm involves three major components: 1) tempo (speed), 2) pattern (even or uneven beats), and 3) accent (emphasis) (Kirchner, 1992).

Table 1.3.   Description of fundamental locomotor and manipulative patterns[a]

Walking:	Standing upright with eyes forward, swing one leg forward while swinging the opposite arm forward. Then swing the other leg forward and the other arm forward.
Running:	Standing upright with eyes forward, bend arms at elbow. Push off and swing one leg forward while swinging opposite arm forward. Then swing the other leg forward and the other arm forward.
Jumping:	Standing upright with eyes forward and feet shoulder-width apart, bend legs at knee and bring both arms behind body. Simultaneously, lean forward, swing arm forward, and forcefully straighten out legs.
Galloping:	Standing upright with eyes forward, start with one leg forward of the other. Slide the back leg toward the front leg, and then step forward with the front leg. Pump arms either together or alternating.
Hopping:	Stand upright with one leg bent so that the foot is off the ground. Bend the support leg at the knee while bringing both arms back behind the body. Simultaneously, lean forward, swing arms forward, and forcefully straighten out support leg.
Skipping:	Alternate hopping on one foot, then stepping onto the other foot, and then hopping with that foot. Hop-step on one foot followed by hop-step on opposite foot.
Throwing:	Propelling a small ball away from the body using one hand. Skillful throwing is initiated by a forward step with opposite leg, followed by hip and trunk rotation, and concluded with a whipping arm action.
Catching:	Receiving and controlling a ball that is tossed or kicked to student. Skillful catching is noted by extending arms to meet the ball, retracting hands upon contact with ball, and using hands to catch ball rather than trapping ball against body.
Striking (bat):	Propelling a ball away from body by hitting ball with a long-handled implement. Skillful, two-handed striking consists of stepping forward, followed by quick hip, trunk, and arm rotation, swinging horizontally, and whipping arms forward in a forceful follow-through.
Striking (racquet):	Propelling ball away from body by hitting ball with a racquet. Skillful, one-handed striking consists of stepping forward, followed by quick hip, trunk, and arm rotation, swinging horizontally, and whipping arm forward in a forceful follow-through.
Kicking:	Propelling ball away from body by using foot to impart force on ball. Skillful kicking consists of planting support leg next to ball, bring kicking leg back by flexing knee, forcefully swinging leg forward to contact ball, then continuing to swing leg forward in forceful follow-through.
Punting:	Propelling ball away from body using foot to impart force on ball. Punting is different from kicking in that the ball is held and then dropped by student, and the ball is kicked before ball touches the ground.

[a]Locomotor patterns also can include pushing a manual wheelchair/controlling an electric wheelchair.

Table 1.4. Popular individual sports

Archery	Gymnastics	Scuba Diving
Badminton	Hiking	Shooting
Boccie	Horseback Riding	Skiing
Bowling	Horseshoes	Swimming
Croquet	Hunting	Table Tennis
Cycling	Ice Skating	Tennis
Darts	Martial Arts	Track and Field
Fencing	Racquetball	Water Skiing
Golf	Roller Skating	Weight Training

Dance refers to a combination of movement and rhythm where movement qualities, movement components, and rhythmic movements are purposefully integrated into a progression with a beginning, middle, and end (Krebs, 1990). Dance can include basic rhythmic activities and action songs for young children to traditional dances (e.g., ballroom, folk, square), aerobic dances, and modern dances (creative dance) for older children and adults (Krebs, 1990).

Individual sports includes culturally popular sports that involve one player or teams of no more than two players. Popular individual sports in America are listed in Table 1.4. Activities within each sport can include working on skills, playing lead-up games (simpler or modified forms of traditional sports that help students acquire game skills and concepts), playing recreational games, or playing competitive games. In addition, many of the sports listed above are considered lifetime leisure activities since they can be played by individuals across the life span.

Team sports includes culturally popular sports that involve three or more players per side. Popular team sports in America are listed in Table 1.5. As is the case with individual sports, activities in each team sport can include working on skills, playing lead-up or modified games, playing recreational games, or playing competitive games. It is interesting to note that some team sports (e.g., football, baseball) are not considered lifetime leisure activities because most individuals do not participate in these activities after middle age. However, team sports such as volleyball and softball are often played by older adults and thus should be considered lifetime leisure activities.

OBJECTIVES OF PHYSICAL EDUCATION

The components of physical education help define the types of activities that should be included in a comprehensive physical education program. However, presenting activities without purpose or focus is not what physical education is about. Good physical education programs use these activities to promote global physical education objectives that facilitate psychomotor (motor and fitness performance), cognitive (intellectual skills), and affective development (feelings, opinions, attitudes, beliefs, values, interests, and desires) (Sherrill, 1993). Pangrazi and Dauer (1992) outlined

Table 1.5. Popular team sports

Baseball	Rugby
Basketball	Soccer
Field Hockey	Softball
Floor Hockey	Team Handball
Football	Volleyball
Lacrosse	

several physical education objectives which, when taken together, define the purpose of physical education. These objectives include:

1. *A physical education program should help each student become competent in a variety of body management and physical skills.* These skills include: a) body management (ability to move the body through various circumstances and environments); b) rhythmic ability (move with a certain regularity or timing); c) fundamental skills (locomotor and manipulative patterns); and d) specialized skills (individual and team sports).

2. *A physical education program should provide all students with the opportunity to develop and maintain a level of health-related physical fitness commensurate with individual needs. Allied to this objective is giving students an understanding of how to develop and maintain an adequate fitness level throughout life.* Students should not only be exposed to activities that promote health-related fitness, they should also learn how to develop and maintain physical fitness throughout life. For example, all students, including students with disabilities, should learn how to perform activities that promote cardiovascular efficiency such as jogging at a steady speed, brisk walking, riding a bicycle, or pushing a wheelchair. Students also should learn how to regulate the intensity (getting heart rate up to a training level), duration (how long to exercise to gain cardiovascular benefits), and frequency (how often to exercise to gain cardiovascular benefits).

3. *Each student should enjoy a broad experience in movement activities, leading to an understanding of movement and the underlying principles involved.* This objective refers to participation and training in a variety of movement activities. Participation in a variety of movement activities enables students to learn not only how to move but how to become skillful movers and apply various movement patterns to various settings. For example, students with disabilities should not only learn the most skillful way to throw and catch but learn how to use these basic skills in a variety of situations including lead-up and traditional sports such as softball or basketball.

4. *The physical education environment should be such that students acquire knowledge of desirable social standards and ethical concepts.* Social objectives that can be enhanced in physical education include cooperation, appropriate levels of competition, tolerance for varying abilities, and general good citizenship and fair play. Situations can be set up in which cooperation and teamwork are needed or in which one team loses and members learn how to be "good sports."

5. *Each student should develop a desirable self-concept through relevant physical education experiences.* Self-concept refers to how a child feels about his or her ability. Part of self-concept is associated with physical abilities and physical fitness. In addition, success in physical education can promote positive self-concepts in children who have difficulty in other aspects of school. Thus, physical education programs should be success-based by modifying activities to meet the needs of each student based on his or her unique abilities. For example, a shooting station in basketball might include baskets set at different heights, students using different-sized balls, or allowing students to shoot from various distances.

6. *Through physical education, each student should acquire personal values that encourage living a full and productive life.* This includes opportunities that promote enjoyment in participation in physical activity, healthly lifestyles and stress reduction, and trying their best in all activities. Again, developing success-based programs in which students learn skills that are geared to meet their individual needs will promote student enjoyment and enhance the likelihood that the students will want to continue to participate in physical activity throughout their lives.

7. *Through physical education, students must acquire knowledge of safety skills and habits, and develop an awareness of safety with respect to themselves and others.* Students should learn good safety habits, which can prevent serious injury, such as wearing protective gear, using a buddy system in the water, and warming up prior to participation.

8. *Through physical education, students should learn physical skills that allow them to partici- pate in and derive enjoyment from wholesome recreational activities throughout their life- times.* Upon graduation from physical education, students should have competency in at least two or three lifetime recreation activities in which they could participate throughout their adult years. Ideally, some of these recreational competencies would include activities that promote health-related fitness such as aerobic dancing, weight training, or swimming. This may be the most important objective of physical education for all students, including students with disabilities; that is, helping students acquire the skills needed to participate as indepen- dently and successfully as possible in lifetime leisure skills.

WHAT IS ADAPTED PHYSICAL EDUCATION?

Legislators who created IDEA believed that students with disabilities could benefit from physical education and that physical education services, modified when necessary, should be a part of all students' educational programs. Many students with disabilities can participate in regular physi- cal education without the need for modifications to the regular program. However, some students with disabilities will have difficulty safely and successfully participating in and benefiting from regular physical education without modifications or support. Various adaptations will be neces- sary if these students can be expected to truly benefit from regular physical education. When students with disabilities need extra support to benefit from regular physical education, or when these students need a special physical education program as an alternative to regular physical education, they qualify for *adapted physical education.*

Adapted physical education is a subdiscipline of physical education with an emphasis on physical education for students with disabilities. The term *adapted physical education* generally refers to school-based programs for students age 3–21, while a more global term, *adapted physi- cal activity*, refers to programs across the life span including postschool programs (Sherrill, 1993). Since this book focuses on school-age students, the term *adapted physical education* will be used throughout.

Various definitions of adapted physical education have been developed over the past 20 years (e.g., Auxter & Pyfer, 1989; Dunn & Fait, 1989; Sherrill, 1993). However, the definition devel- oped by Dunn and Fait (1989) seems to be most appropriate for this text. They defined adapted physical education as follows:

> Adapted physical education programs are those that have the same objectives as the regular physi- cal education program, but in which adjustments are made in the regular offerings to meet the needs and abilities of exceptional students. (Dunn & Fait, 1989, p. 4)

Note that both regular and adapted physical education share the same objectives as outlined above. In addition, the components of physical education as defined in IDEA should be included in a comprehensive adapted physical education program. The major difference between regular and adapted physical education is that in the latter "adjustments" or adaptations are made to the regular offerings to ensure safe, successful, and beneficial participation. Simple adaptations such as asking a peer to provide assistance, modifying the equipment and rules of games, or providing alternative activities under the guidance of a trained adapted physical education specialist do little to disrupt the learning environment while creating a productive and enjoyable physical education experience for all students. It is important to realize that adaptations, including specific therapeutic activities, can be implemented within the regular physical education setting. For example, a high school–age student with cerebral palsy who uses a wheelchair can work on special stretching exercises during regular physical education while his peers perform their warm-up activities. Similarly, this student can work on individual goals such as pushing his wheelchair forward and developing the ability to play cerebral palsy soccer (an official sport of the National Cerebral Palsy Athletic Association) while his peers practice their running and soccer skills. This student may require special equipment such as a wheelchair and a larger ball as well as extra assistance in the form of a peer tutor, volunteer, or paraprofessional. However, the student can easily be accommodated in the regular program and still receive an appropriate, individualized physical education program designed to meet his unique needs.

While the objectives of adapted and regular physical education are the same, how these objectives are prioritized will vary from individual to individual in adapted physical education. For example, while all students should work on health-related physical fitness, maintenance of low levels of health-related physical fitness might be a priority goal for a student with muscular dystrophy or cystic fibrosis while such a fitness goal may be a lesser priority for physically fit students without disabilities. Similarly, motor skill development might be a priority for a student with a learning disability or cerebral palsy while social/affective development might be a priority for a student with a behavior disorder. Health-related physical fitness, motor skill development, and social development are important goals for all students in physical education, but each of these goals takes on different levels of importance for different students. Since activities that promote physical fitness, motor skill development, and social development are offered to some extent or another in regular physical education, it is relatively easy to accommodate students with disabilities who have these goals as priorities within regular physical education.

DEVELOPMENTALLY APPROPRIATE
PROGRAMMING IN PHYSICAL EDUCATION

Physical education is comprised of several different components designed to promote certain global objectives (i.e., to be physically educated), and it is important that all students receive training in all of these components if these objectives are to be achieved. Yet, should young children learn how to play team sports or participate in intricate dances? Should older students and young adults participate in simple rhythm activities and activities that promote fundamental motor skill development? The answer is no. Students should be exposed to all of the above physical education components, but these should be presented across the life span of the student. The term *developmentally appropriate* refers to presenting activities that are geared to a student's developmental status, previous movement experiences, fitness and skill level, body size, and age (Council on Physical Education for Children, 1992). Developmentally appropriate practices suggest that programming as well as instruction should be different for preschool-age children compared to elementary-age students compared to secondary level students. Wessel and Kelly (1986) outlined major content areas for regular physical education activities broken down by grade level. (See Table 1.6.) Note that younger children are presented activities that promote development of motor skills and movement competencies, while older students are learning to apply these skills and competencies to culturally popular sports and lifetime leisure/fitness activities. Most physical educators understand what is appropriate for younger students and what is appropriate for older students. However, this understanding is often lost when it comes to students with disabilities. Oftentimes, physical educators present activities based on a student's *developmental* rather than *chronological age*. Unfortunately, such an approach may result in students with disabilities graduating from school with a smattering of developmental skills such as the ability to throw a ball or

Table 1.6. Major content areas for regular physical education by grade level

Lower elementary school (K–3rd grade)	Upper elementary/middle school (4th–7th grade)	High school (8th–12th grade)
Locomotor patterns • run • skip • jump • slide • gallop • leap • hop • climb	**Locomotor patterns for sports** • locomotor patterns used in sports • combine two or more locomotor patterns • locomotor patterns used in dance	**Locomotor sports** • track events • special sports applications of locomotor patterns • locomotor patterns used in dance • locomotor patterns used in leisure activities
Manipulative patterns • throw • catch • kick • strike	**Manipulative patterns for sports** • throw • volley • catch • dribble • kick • punt • strike	**Ball sports** • basketball, soccer, softball, volleyball, etc. • bowling, golf, tennis, racquetball, etc.
Body management • body awareness • body control • space awareness • effort concepts	**Body management for sports** • gymnastics • body management skills applied to sports	**Body management for sports** • body management skills applied to sports
Health and fitness • endurance, strength, and flexibility to perform locomotor and manipulative skills	**Health and fitness** • cardiorespiratory endurance • muscular strength and endurance • flexibility	**Health and fitness** • personal conditioning • lifetime leisure exercises • introduction to body composition concepts
Rhythm and dance • moving to a beat • expressing self through movement • singing games • applying effort concepts	**Dance** • folk • modern • interpretive • aerobic	**Dance** • folk • modern • interpretive • aerobic and social
Low organized games • relays and tag games • games with partners • games with a small group	**Lead-up games to sports** • lead-up games to team sports	**Modified and regulation sports** • modified sport activities • regulation sports

Adapted from Wessel, J.A., & Kelly, L. (1986). *Achievement-based curriculum development in physical education.* Philadelphia: Lea & Febiger; reprinted with permission.

walk on a balance beam but no real ability to participate in lifetime leisure skills such as bowling, golf, weight training, or aerobic dance. It is critical that students with disabilities, including students with significant disabilities, be exposed to chronological age–appropriate activities that will lead to the development of functional skills that they can use when they graduate from school (see Block, 1992, for a more in-depth discussion of helping students acquire lifetime leisure skills).

SUMMARY

The purpose of this chapter was to define physical education and introduce the concepts which comprise a comprehensive physical education program. Physical education is considered a direct service in PL 101-476, Individuals with Disabilities Education Act (IDEA), which means that all students, including students with disabilities, are required to receive physical education. In addition, specialized physical education services, which can be provided in integrated or separate settings, should be provided to any student with disabilities who needs such services.

Physical education consists of a diverse program of activities including motor skills, physical fitness, and individual and team sports. These activities should be presented in such a way that they facilitate the achievement of global physical education objectives which include motor skill competency, social and cognitive development, and healthy self-concept. How much time and emphasis a particular student spends working on a particular component (as well as how these skills will be presented) will vary based on several factors such as a student's age, abilities, and interests.

Chapter 2

What Is Inclusion?

It was quite a struggle convincing our regular physical education staff to include students with disabilities into their programs. A lot had to do with negative attitudes and lack of information. Our high school physical education teachers were particularly reluctant to include students who used wheelchairs in regular physical education. They were worried that including these students would somehow detract from what they had developed over the years. Gradually, the teachers became more comfortable with the students, and they have not only accepted these students but actually look forward to having them in the class!

—Jill Heenan

Shameka is a sixth grader who has mental retardation and has attended a special school for students with significant disabilities for the past 6 years. However, this special school recently closed, and Shameka was placed in her "home school," the school she would attend if she did not have a disability. Furthermore, Shameka has been placed in a regular sixth-grade class rather than a special education class, and she is considered a full member of this class rather than a student who comes in for some classes and is pulled out for others. Shameka walks to school with neighborhood friends, she now has several friends in her class with whom she sits during lunch and assemblies, and she "hangs out" with other friends during recess.

Since Shameka is at a different level of the physical education curriculum compared to her peers without disabilities and, in many cases, has different goals and objectives from her peers, support is provided through adapted equipment, adaptations to the curriculum, adaptations to instruction, and assistance from peer tutors, paraprofessionals, and education specialists. This also is true in physical education where Shameka receives support from an eighth-grade peer tutor, special equipment for various activities such as a shorter, lighter racquet for tennis and hitting a ball off a tee for softball, and special instruction that includes more feedback, more demonstrations, and more physical assistance. Still, Shameka is in regular physical education, and is perceived as a regular member of her sixth-grade class. Although her skill level is generally lower than that of most of her classmates, her classmates do not seem to mind since they all have their own particular strengths and weaknesses. She really does not stand out more than any other sixth grader in her class, because the physical educator individualized the curriculum for all students. For example, in an introductory tennis unit, students use different weight racquets, stand different distances from the net, practice different skills, and receive different levels of instruction based on their needs. Thus, the curriculum is modified for all students so that they can be successful, challenged, and meaningfully involved in the program.

Jill Heenan is an APE specialist for the School Association of Special Education in DuPage County, Roselle, Illinois.

15

While this scenario may seem too good to be true, such programs are being implemented in many schools that have adopted an "inclusion" philosophy. When done right, inclusion programs like the one described above are demonstrating that students with varying abilities who are grouped together (including students with significant disabilities) can receive an appropriate and challenging educational program. In addition, such programs foster more favorable attitudes and a better understanding of individual differences. But why the seemingly sudden shift from self-contained, special education programs to full inclusion programs? What exactly does inclusion mean? The purpose of this chapter is to review the concept of inclusion and the rationale for inclusive programs versus segregated programs. In addition, there will be a brief review of educational philosophies that have guided programming for individuals with disabilities over the past several years.

WHAT IS INCLUSION?

Inclusion is the practice of educating all students, including students with disabilities, in regular education and regular classes (Forest & Lusthaus, 1989; Stainback & Stainback, 1990). Inclusion does not mean "dumping" students with disabilities into the mainstream without proper support. Furthermore, inclusion does not mean that all students necessarily work toward or are expected to achieve the same educational goals using the same instructional methods. Rather, inclusion means providing all students with appropriate educational programs geared to their abilities and needs with supports and assistance as needed to ensure success (Stainback & Stainback, 1990; Stainback, Stainback, & Forest, 1989). The idea of providing supports in the form of adapted equipment, specialized instruction, and personnel is critical within the inclusion model (Block & Krebs, 1992; Stainback & Stainback, 1990). Regular and special education staff, separate entities in traditional educational models, work collaboratively in inclusive programs to provide appropriate and meaningful programs for all students. A school that has truly adopted an inclusive philosophy is one in which everyone belongs, is accepted, is valued, and is supported by peers, staff, and community members. Inclusive schools are not only sensitive to individual differences but actually celebrate these differences (Stainback & Stainback, 1990).

In terms of physical education, inclusion means that students with disabilities are placed in regular physical education programs from the beginning. These students are not viewed as visitors but as true members of the physical education class. In addition, these students are not considered as individuals with disabilities. Rather, each one is viewed as simply another student in the class who may learn and move differently from his or her peers. In fact, *all students* are viewed as individuals who have unique educational objectives, who may be on different levels of the physical education curriculum, who may need different challenges and different instruction to meet their unique motor and fitness needs, and who may need varying amounts of supports to ensure meaningful participation and success in all physical education activities. Inclusive physical education is a place where individual differences are not hidden or ridiculed but rather shared among students who learn to respect each other's limitations and unique abilities. Supports in the form of adapted equipment, specialized instruction, and personnel are provided to any student who needs them as well as to the regular physical educator. Regular physical educators work collaboratively with other key team members (e.g., adapted physical education specialist, therapists, parents) to provide the most appropriate, beneficial, and meaningful programs to all students.

EVOLUTION OF INCLUSION

In the first half of this century, when special education was in its infancy, students with disabilities were viewed as fundamentally different from students without disabilities. These differences led to the development of an alternative educational model for students with disabilities. This alternative model included teachers who had special training and who used special materials, equipment, and teaching methodologies. The end result was a rather elaborate dual system of education with regular education on the one hand and special education on the other (Stainback, Stainback, & Bunch, 1989). In many cases, this dual system led to the development of regular schools for students without disabilities and "special education centers" for students with disabilities. Programs for children with specific types of disabilities became so specialized that different day and residential facilities were created for children with learning disabilities, children with hearing impairments, children with visual impairments, children with mental retardation, children with emotional disturbances, and children with physical disabilities. (Many of these special schools are still in existence.)

In 1954, civil rights legislation was passed (i.e., *Brown v. Board of Education*) that asserted that separate was not equal in terms of programs and services for persons of different races. In the late 1950s and early 1960s, separate schools for African-American children were closed, and integration of public schools began. Parents of students with disabilities took notice of integration and began advocating for their children to be placed in regular schools. Slowly, students with disabilities were moved from special schools to special education classes within regular schools. In most cases, one school within the school district became the school where all children with disabilities were housed, as in a wing or annex within the regular school. Special education teachers still were viewed as somewhat "special" either due to special training or through some special capacity to work with students who had disabilities (Stainback et al., 1989a). Regular and special education personnel rarely interacted, and students with disabilities continued to receive their education away from the mainstream. The dual system continued within the confines of a regular school.

The idea of including students with disabilities in regular classrooms in their neighborhood schools (the school they would attend if they did not have disabilities) with support services was first envisioned in the mid-1970s. Many parent groups and professional organizations passed resolutions supporting the concept known as *mainstreaming*. The Council for Exceptional Children (CEC) defined mainstreaming in terms of basic themes relative to what it is and what it is not. They suggested that mainstreaming was:

1. Providing the most appropriate education for each student in the least restrictive setting
2. Placing students based on assessed educational needs rather than clinical labels
3. Providing support services to general educators so they may effectively serve children with disabilities in the regular setting
4. Uniting general and special education to help students with disabilities have equal educational opportunities

The Council noted that mainstreaming was not:

1. Wholesale return of all exceptional children to regular classes
2. Permitting children with special needs to remain in regular classes without the support services they needed
3. Ignoring the need of some children for a more specialized program than could be provided in the general education program (Council for Exceptional Children, 1975)

Similarly, lawmakers advocated placing children with disabilities in the *least restrictive environment* (LRE) when they passed PL 94-142, Education for All Handicapped Children Act, in 1975. LRE was defined by lawmakers as:

to the maximum extent appropriate, children with disabilities, including children in public and private institutions or other care facilities, are educated with children without disabilities, and that special classes, separate schooling, or other removal of children with disabilities from regular educational environments [including physical education] occur only when the nature or severity of the disability is such that education in regular classes with the use of supplementary aids and services cannot be achieved. (*Federal Register,* August, 1977, p. 42497 [*current terminology added*])

This passage suggested that the LRE for students with disabilities was one that, whenever possible, was the same environment where students without disabilities received their education. Clearly, the lawmakers advocated placing students with disabilities in regular schools and regular classrooms (including regular physical education) whenever possible (Aufsesser, 1991; Taylor, 1988; Turnbull, 1990). This passage also suggested that *appropriate* placement of students with disabilities into regular settings might necessitate the use of supplementary aids, support, and services. Without such support, the student might fail in the regular setting. In other words, it might not be the setting that is inappropriate but rather the support that is given to a student within that setting (Block & Krebs, 1992).

Unfortunately, mainstreaming has been associated with unsuccessful dumping of students with disabilities into regular education classes without support (DePaepe, 1984; Lavay & DePaepe, 1987). The term has been misused so much that it is no longer recommended by the Council for Exceptional Children. Similarly, LRE has been operationalized as having students with disabilities based in special education classes and brought into regular programs only occasionally. This resulted in students with disabilities being perceived as visitors to regular education (*them*), not members of the class (*us*) (Schnorr, 1990).

The idea of fully including students with disabilities into regular education programs was not truly taken seriously until research in the 1970s and 1980s began to show that special class placements were by and large ineffective in educating students with disabilities (e.g., Semmel, Gottlieb, & Robinson, 1979). For example, Wang, Reynolds, and Walberg (1987) suggested that traditional "pull-out" programs were limited for a variety of reasons including: 1) the system for classifying students with disabilities was not educationally sound, 2) there was virtually no evidence that suggested students with disabilities were making any educational gains simply based on special education placement, and 3) special class placement promoted isolation and stigmatization.

In 1986, Madeleine Will (then Assistant Secretary for the Office of Special Education and Rehabilitative Services, U.S. Department of Education) argued for what she called the "regular education initiative" (REI), which has become synonymous with inclusion. In her article, Educating Students with Learning Problems: A Shared Responsibility, Will (1986) argued that the present dual system of separate special and regular education was not effective for students with mild disabilities. Will suggested several changes to the current dual system, all of which were designed to serve students with disabilities appropriately in regular education. She proposed the following: 1) increased instructional time, 2) empowerment of principals to control all programs and resources at the building level, 3) provision of support systems for regular education teachers, and 4) the use of new approaches such as curriculum-based assessment, cooperative learning, and personalized curricula (Will, 1986). Proponents of REI encouraged the elimination of traditional special education classrooms in favor of a new merger between special and regular education (e.g., Stainback & Stainback, 1990; Stainback, Stainback, & Jackson, 1992).

While Will originally targeted students with mild disabilities, other professionals argued that students with severe (significant) disabilities also should receive their education in regular classrooms (e.g., Giangreco, York, & Rainforth, 1989; Snell, 1988; Snell & Eichner, 1989; Stainback & Stainback, 1990; Taylor, 1988). They noted that students with severe disabilities could learn important life skills in the regular setting without interfering with the program for students without disabilities. In addition, they pointed out that heterogeneous grouping actually could enrich both students with and without disabilities in terms of education, attitudes, and perception of others who may be different in some way (Stainback & Stainback, 1990). Students with severe disabilities who needed special services such as adapted equipment and special therapies still could receive these services, but the services would be brought into the regular setting rather than having the student brought to the special services.

Today, there are successful inclusive schools in many communities. Students with disabilities, including students with severe disabilities, attend their home schools and are full members of their regular, age-level classrooms. Rather than having a dual system of special and regular education, these inclusive schools operate under one education system. Within this one system, all students are provided educational opportunities geared to their abilities and needs. In many cases, different students have different educational objectives and utilize different methods to learn. In addition, support services are provided within the regular education setting to any student who needs them. Regular education and special education staff work together to provide each student, including the student *without disabilities*, whatever support or assistance he or she might need to reach his or her potential (Stainback & Stainback, 1990). Regular education staff feel comfortable working with students with disabilities, and special education staff feel comfortable working with students without disabilities who may need extra help. Diversity and heterogeneity are seen as a positive element of these schools that foster appreciation of individual differences.

RATIONALE FOR INCLUSION

The major purpose of inclusion is to provide opportunities for all students to develop the skills and attitudes needed to learn, live, and work together in all aspects of society (Stainback & Stainback, 1990). Individuals will only learn how to live and work together if they grow up together in an environment that supports individual differences. Inclusive schools provide such learning opportunities for both students with and without disabilities. Stainback, Stainback, and Bunch (1989) recently presented a rationale for merging regular and special education into one educational system for all students that included the following key points:

1. *Instructional needs of all students vary from individual to individual.* A student with disabilities should be viewed as just another student whose instructional needs should be individualized to optimize learning. Individualization can be implemented in an inclusive setting as easily as in a segregated setting. For example, most physical education classes are comprised of students with varying motor abilities, physical fitness, and knowledge of the rules and strategies of games. Good physical educators present activities in such a way that individual students' needs are accommodated. A student with disabilities is just another student who requires activities to be individualized to accommodate his or her unique abilities.

2. *A dual system is inefficient since there is inevitably competition and duplication of services.* Much of what takes place in separate settings takes place in regular settings. This is particularly true with the majority of activities presented in regular and adapted physical education programs. For example, most elementary-age students in regular physical education work on the development of fundamental motor patterns, perceptual motor skills, physical fitness, and simple rhythms and games. These same activities are appropriate for most elementary-age students with disabilities. Similarly, high school–age students work on individual and team sports including lifetime leisure sports and physical fitness. Again, adapted physical education programs designed for high school–age students with disabilities work on the same activities! What happens with a dual system is that two professionals are teaching the same activities at the same time, which causes conflict with gym time and equipment. A more logical and cost-effective model would be to include students with disabilities into the regular program with modifications as needed to ensure their success.

   3. *Dual systems foster inappropriate attitudes.* Students with disabilities, especially students who spend most of their time separated from peers who do not have disabilities, are viewed as "special" and different by regular education teachers and peers (e.g., Voeltz, 1980, 1982). Teachers assume that educational programs that take place in special education must be extraordinary. That is, special education staff often are viewed as "exceptional" people who have different skills and abilities compared to regular education staff and who use different equipment and materials with their students who have disabilities (equipment and materials that take years of special training to master). Similarly, students with disabilities often are viewed as more "different" than similar to students without disabilities in that they learn differently and have different interests than students who do not have disabilities. In fact, most students with disabilities are more similar to than different from their peers without disabilities. They probably enjoy watching the same television shows and listen to the same music as their peers who do not have disabilities, cheer for the same sports teams, enjoy the same recreational activities, and hate cleaning their rooms or doing their homework. Unfortunately, teachers and peers who are not exposed to students with disabilities may view them as different—people who should be pitied, teased, or feared. By combining students with and without disabilities, teachers learn that teaching students with disabilities is not that different from teaching typical students. Similarly, peers who do not have disabilities quickly learn that students with disabilities are more similar to than different from themselves (Forest & Lusthaus; 1989; Stainback, Stainback, and Bunch, 1989).

BENEFITS OF INCLUSION

In addition to the rationale for merging regular and special education, there are specific benefits available in inclusion programs that are not available in segregated settings. For example, students with disabilities have more "normal" role models and natural cues if they receive their education in the regular education setting. Such role models and natural cues often lead to more appropriate behavior (e.g., attending, waiting turn, following directions). Similarly, peers without disabilities learn to understand, tolerate, and even appreciate individual differences when integrated with students who have disabilities. For example, students without disabilities learn to accept simple rule modifications so that all students can be included, challenged, and successful. Tables 2.1 and 2.2, adapted from Snell and Eichner (1989) and Stainback and Stainback (1985, 1990), outline several benefits of including students with disabilities in regular education programs.

Table 2.1.   Benefits of inclusion to students with disabilities

---

Opportunity to learn social skills in inclusive, more natural environments (learn with natural cues and consequences; do not have to generalize to inclusive environments later in life)

More stimulating, motivating environment. (Think about the halls of a regular junior high school, the cafeteria, the recess yard, the bus-loading area. Dress, conversations, and social exchanges are characteristic of their age and location.)

Opportunity to learn appropriate social skills (refrain from stigmatizing behavior, appropriate greetings, wearing age-appropriate clothes)

Availability of age-appropriate role models who do not have disabilities

Participation in a variety of school activities suited to the student's chronological age and neighborhood (e.g., recess, lunch, assemblies, music, art, athletic events)

Potential for new friendships with peers who do not have disabilities

Better integration of parents, special education teachers, and other special education staff into regular schools allowing for new experiences, relationships, and less isolation

---

Adapted from Snell and Eichner (1989) and Stainback and Stainback (1985, 1990).

Table 2.2. Benefits of inclusion to professional staff and to students without disabilities

Special education teachers (as well as adapted physical educators) tend to have higher expectations for their students with disabilities when students are placed in inclusive environments.

Special education teachers learn what is appropriate for students without disabilities

With adult guidance, student attitudes toward persons with disabilities improve (fewer fears, teasing, stares, and negative comments).

When given guidance from adults, students without disabilities learn to appreciate individual differences (see the positive in everyone, find strengths and weaknesses in everyone).

Perspective: having acne or getting a "C" on a test is not as devastating when you see a person next to you working as hard as possible just to keep his or her head up and eyes focused.

Future parents of children with disabilities, future taxpayers, future teachers and doctors learn to face persons with disabilities with greater personal knowledge and optimism and less prejudice.

SPECIFIC PHILOSOPHIES THAT SUPPORT INCLUSION

Inclusion should not be confused with early attempts at mainstreaming. Mainstreaming tended to place students with disabilities in regular education without support. In addition, students often were expected to follow the same curriculum as students without disabilities. Inclusion philosophies suggest that each student's unique educational needs be met through adaptations to the curriculum and with the provision of supports. The following, adapted from Stainback and Stainback (1990), outlines some of the key philosophies regarding inclusion:

Adapt the Curriculum

One of the greatest misconceptions of inclusion programs is that all students must somehow fit into the existing curriculum. In many cases, the curriculum used in the regular class is not appropriate for students with disabilities. In such cases, the curriculum must somehow be adapted to meet the unique educational objectives and learning needs of the student. For example, an elementary student with cerebral palsy may have difficulty performing activities in a typical tumbling/gymnastics unit. This student still could work on balance skills, rolls, and movement concepts, but she will work on these skills differently than her peers. This student might, for example, work on simple sitting balance while her peers work on more complex sitting balances such as a V-sit (make a V with the body so that the legs and arms are up in the air and only the bottom rests on the floor). While other students work on forward and backward rolls, this student might work on independently rolling from stomach to back and then getting to a standing position. Note how all students work on the same basic physical educational objective (movement control) and learn together within the same regular physical education activities (tumbling unit), but some students are evaluated using different curriculum objectives.

In some cases, the curriculum may not seem to match the needs of a particular student at all. In such cases, different parts of the curriculum might be presented at different times for different students. For example, a middle school student who is blind may not need to work on lacrosse, an activity found in many physical education curriculums in the mid-Atlantic and northeast part of the United States. This student might be given opportunities to feel the equipment and learn the rules of lacrosse, but during most of the lacrosse unit this student works on the softball/beep baseball skills of throwing, striking with a bat, and retrieving beep balls (balls that emit a beeping noise to aid students with visual impairments). Softball is part of the middle school curriculum, but it is offered at a different time of year. Still, the basic skills of lacrosse are catching with lacrosse stick, tossing with lacrosse stick, and advancing the ball by tossing or running. Softball also includes skills such as catching (with hands), tossing (throwing), and advancing the ball (striking). Thus, this student works on similar educational objectives (catching, tossing, advancing a ball), but in a way that is more beneficial to him. In addition, this student can work on these skills within the regular physical education class. (See chap. 6 and chap. 7, this volume, for more information on adapting the curriculum.)

Integrate Personnel and Resources

Another misconception about inclusion is that students with disabilities will be "dumped" into regular programs without support. As noted earlier, the inclusion philosophy directs supports to follow the student into the mainstream. Supports include specialized equipment, special instruction, and personnel such as volunteers, teacher assistants, and education specialists. In fact, support that would have been given to the student when he or she was in a segregated program should follow the student into the inclusive program. For example, the student in the example above who is blind should have beep balls and sound devices in any activity that uses balls. Such equipment can be obtained free from various associations serving persons who are blind. (The student's vision therapist can assist the regular physical educator in procuring this equipment.) In addition, the student's orientation and mobility specialist might come into regular physical education once or twice a week to assist the student in moving around the physical education environment. Other students might have special equipment such as walkers, standers, mats, or bolsters that should be brought to regular physical education. If these students had peer tutors or teacher assistants working with them in segregated physical education, then these supports should be provided for them in inclusive programs.

Utilize Natural Proportions

One of the reasons that early attempts at mainstreaming in physical education often failed was that entire special education classes (up to 10 students) were placed in one regular physical education class. Such a situation was doomed for failure right from the start since no physical educator could adequately meet the needs of all his or her students without disabilities plus another 10 students with unique needs. Inclusion philosophy suggests that students with disabilities be placed following the principle of *natural proportions*. Natural proportions basically means that the normal distribution of persons with and without disabilities be maintained when placing students in regular classes. Incidence of disability suggests that perhaps 10%–15% of the school-age population has some type of disability, the greatest numbers with high incidence disabilities such as learning disabilities, emotional disabilities, and mental retardation and fewer with low incidence disabilities such as cerebral palsy, hearing impairments, or visual impairments. Such numbers translate to two to three students with disabilities (usually mild disabilities) placed in each class, with an occasional class having a student with a low incidence type of disability. Therefore, only two to three students with disabilities should be placed in any one physical education class at a time. Such a situation is much more manageable for the regular physical educator, especially when students with more significant disabilities come to physical education with extra support personnel.

Based In, Not Confined To

Including students with disabilities means that students are *based in* regular physical education, not *confined to* regular physical education (Block, in press; Brown et al., 1991). *Based in* means that students are welcomed by students without disabilities and the regular physical educator and are considered full members of the class. However, meaningful amounts of time may be spent elsewhere, such as in other physical education environments within the school or in community-based recreation environments. Younger students and students whose IEP objectives match the regular curriculum tend to spend more time in regular physical education. Older students (those in transition from school to post-school settings) and students whose IEP objectives do not match the regular curriculum spend more time in other settings.

For example, a 7-year-old student with cerebral palsy is working on walking with a walker in various directions, at various speeds, and around various obstacles. Since the regular physical education program in second grade involves learning locomotor patterns and movement concepts, this student can spend the majority of her time in regular physical education. Even when the class is working on other activities such as tumbling, this student can work on her walking skills by walking around the mats while other students roll across the mats. She could even take a few turns rolling in order to work on general body control. On occasion, she also goes in the hallway with a teacher assistant to work on walking up stairs that lead to another floor in the school (stairs that she has trouble climbing).

In another class, an 18-year-old student with mental retardation is working on bowling, hitting a golf ball at a driving range, weight training, and riding a stationary bike. When the regular physical education class is engaged in fitness, golf, and bowling units, this student can be included with modifications to accommodate his unique needs. However, if this student is going to be able to make a smooth transition to community recreation in 3 years (when he graduates at age 21), he will need to spend meaningful amounts of time in community-based recreation settings such as a local bowling alley, a local driving range, and a local health club. Therefore, this student goes to these community recreation sites when the class is engaged in activities that do not match his IEP objectives (e.g., when the class is doing wrestling or basketball). To continue to promote meaningful interactions with peers who do not have disabilities, the special education teacher who accompanies this student in the community includes two students without disabilities (two different students each day) who go to these community recreation sites with the student with mental retardation. In addition, all class members know that everyone spends varying amounts of time in community recreation. Thus, peers without disabilities participate with the student with mental retardation as a buddy, not as a helper. However, they also provide natural supports as needed (e.g., helping student tie shoes, helping student remember when his turn is, helping student keep score).

GENERAL PHILOSOPHIES THAT SUPPORT INCLUSIVE PROGRAMS

There are many general philosophies that have been proposed by special education and adapted physical education professionals regarding educational content and best teaching practices for students with disabilities (e.g., Block, 1992; Brown et al., 1979; Moon & Bunker, 1987). These philosophies should guide any program for students with disabilities, especially programs that include students with disabilities in regular education settings. These philosophies include the following: chronological age appropriateness, functionality, community-based programming, choice making, and partial participation. The following reviews each of these philosophies with specific reference to how these philosophies can be incorporated into inclusive programs.

Chronological Age Appropriateness

Chronological age appropriateness refers to gearing activities, expectations, interactions, and materials toward a student's chronological age rather than toward his or her developmental or functional age. That is, a student who is 16 years old should be taught skills that are typically used by other 16-year-olds regardless of the student's abilities. A student's particular functional abilities will be important when deciding *how* to present individually chronological age–appropriate activities. As Block (1992) noted, it is important to consider a person's functional abilities when determining *how* to instruct students, but the decision on *what* to teach should be based on a student's chronological age.

The easiest way to determine if a skill is age-appropriate is to find out what students without disabilities and of the same age do. In terms of physical education, an examination of the regular physical education curriculum for that age group would reveal what other students that age are doing in physical education. (See Table 1.6 for an example of a physical education curriculum by grade level.) For example, physical education activities for most kindergarten through third-grade students include locomotor patterns, ball skill patterns, body awareness and control activities, and simple games including relays, tag, and dodgeball. For high school students, physical education activities focus more on individual and team sports and physical fitness. Thus, a 7-year-old student with mental retardation and cerebral palsy resulting in functional abilities of a 12-month-old should still be presented activities that would be normal for 7-year-olds (i.e., locomotion, ball skills, body awareness and control, and games). These activities will have to be modified to meet her unique abilities. In addition, some activities that are determined to be nonfunctional for this particular student might be eliminated. (See next section on functionality.) For example, if this student uses a wheelchair for mobility, then traditional locomotor patterns may be replaced by wheelchair mobility activities.

Why is it important to present chronological age–appropriate skills rather than skills geared to a student's functional abilities? As noted earlier, three of the major goals of physical education are to: 1) help students acquire the skills needed to maintain a healthy lifestyle, 2) participate in lifetime leisure activities in the community, and 3) develop appropriate social skills so that students can interact with peers during recess and community recreation activities. The best way to ensure that these goals are met is to present activities that match the student's chronological age. For example, presenting gross motor activities such as creeping, crawling, and rolling or simple fine motor activities such as putting-in and taking-out to a 16-year-old student with a significant disability may match his or her developmental status. However, these activities do not help this student maintain physical fitness, acquire lifetime leisure skills, or interact with other 16-year-olds. That is, when the student graduates from school, what lifetime leisure skills will he or she be able to participate in? Rolling races? Creeping around a track? Will the student have the skills needed to maintain physical fitness? Will the student have had opportunities to interact with same-age peers in preparation for inclusive community recreation programs? Very few (if any) high school–age students regularly participate in rolling, creeping, or crawling or putting-in/taking-out, so there would be very little opportunity to interact with same-age peers. On the other hand, what if this student participated in chronological age–appropriate activities such as team sports (presented with modifications as needed to meet the student's unique abilities) and individual sports such as aerobic dance, swimming, bowling, and weight training (again, modified to meet the student's unique abilities)? These chronological age–appropriate activities are directly related to skills the student would need to participate in lifetime leisure skills. Similarly, these activities promote physical fitness and afford opportunities for interactions with peers who do not have disabilities since these are activities that most high school students participate in during physical education and after-school recreation.

Determining if an activity is chronological age appropriate is fairly easy, particularly if the student with disabilities attends a chronological age–appropriate regular school (i.e., a school that serves students without disabilities of the same age). First, you should examine the regular physical education curriculum to determine what other students that age do throughout the year. (See chap. 4, this volume, for more detail.) For example, you can quickly find out from the regular physical educator what physical education activities are planned for fourth-grade students during the year. A fourth-grade student with disabilities should probably participate in many of these same activities. The difference will be how many of these activities the student will participate in and how these activities are presented. The second aspect of age-appropriateness is determining the activities same-age students who do not have disabilities engage in during recess and in their neighborhood. These recreation activities can be determined by talking with same-age students without disabilities or by observing same-age students playing during recess and in their neighborhood. Generally, you would probably find that swinging and climbing on playground equipment is popular for preschool children and children up to about third grade. After that, most upper-level elementary-age students begin to play team sports such as kickball, dodgeball, tag, and soccer. High school–age students tend to participate in community recreation activities such as bowling, roller skating, miniature golf, and community sports programs. Once you know what same-age peers without disabilities do for recreation, you can begin to prioritize which age-appropriate activities to present to students with disabilities.

In terms of inclusion, age appropriate programming is probably easiest to implement when students with disabilities are placed in regular physical education classes with same-age peers. After all, age-appropriate should be referenced to what same-age students do in regular physical education. While physical educators running segregated programs have to guess what same-age students without disabilities do, physical educators who place their students with disabilities in regular physical education will immediately see what is age appropriate and age inappropriate. Similarly, students with disabilities will have numerous age-appropriate models in terms of what to wear, how to behave, and what to do.

Functionality

The term *functionality* refers to skills that are most often used by all persons in a variety of "real life" settings now (in school, in the neighborhood, at home) and in the future (at home, at work, and in the community). That is, functional skills are those skills that are critical for an individual to be as independent as possible in activities that are important for him or her today and in the future. By contrast, nonfunctional skills are those skills that are rarely used by individuals during the course of a typical day or will not be needed later in life. For example, dressing is a functional skill since it is a skill that is used every day, and learning how to put a circuit board together is functional for older students who will soon be going to work. However, zipping up a zipper on a fine-motor dressing board or placing pegs in a pegboard are nonfunctional since these are not skills needed on a regular basis.

In terms of physical education/recreation, a functional skill is one that is important now or in the future for the student so that he or she can independently participate in lifetime leisure skills and maintain fitness and health. For example, walking or pushing one's wheelchair is a functional skill that is needed on a daily basis. Similarly, bowling or tennis are functional skills for older students since these students may participate in these activities on a regular basis in the community upon graduation. However, tossing a bean bag to a clown target is not functional for these older students, because such a skill is not something that the student will be doing on a regular basis upon graduation.

It should become apparent that functionality must be directly tied to the concept of age appropriateness. For example, tossing a bean bag to a clown target or playing tag may be very functional for a preschool child or a young elementary-age student but not for a high school student. Similarly, bowling and tennis are functional for high school–age students and adults but not appropriate for young children. Thus, functional must be defined in terms of what is important for students at a particular age. Similarly, functional must be referenced to the community where the student lives and plays. While bowling may be functional for an 18-year-old student, it is not functional if the community where the student lives has no bowling alleys. Similarly, cross-country skiing is a great functional skill if you live in the northeast or in the Rockies, but it is not functional if you live in Florida or Texas. Again, functional is defined as something that is used or will be used by the student on a regular basis.

Not all physical education activities are necessarily functional for particular students. How then do you determine if a particular physical education/recreation skill is functional? Since age appropriateness is tied so closely to functionality, one way to determine if a skill is functional is to observe same-age peers to see what they do on a regular basis. Activities that peers do on a regular basis are probably functional skills. For example, while wrestling is part of most middle school physical education curricula, very few students participate in wrestling on a regular basis. On the other hand, soccer and softball are much more popular with middle school–age students, and you would probably see many middle school–age students playing soccer or softball during recess and in their neighborhoods after school. Observing preschoolers and young elementary-age students would reveal that playing on playground equipment, in sandboxes, and riding tricycles and Big Wheels are functional activities. Similarly, you should examine what community activities are available and popular and thus functional.

In terms of inclusion, the best way to determine if an activity is functional is to have the student placed in regular physical education and participate in recess with peers who do not have disabilities to see what is most important to these students. Thus, inclusion programs actually facilitate the implementation of functional programs. However, as noted above, all activities that take place in regular physical education are not necessarily functional for a particular student. For example, field hockey and wrestling may be taught in middle and high school physical education, but for a student with spina bifida who uses a wheelchair for mobility, these activities may not be very functional. Rather, this student may have wheelchair tennis and basketball, swimming, and weight training targeted as functional skills. Thus, this student may in fact do different activities than her peers in order to participate in truly functional activities. Still, peers without disabilities can be pulled from regular physical education to participate in these activities with this student in order to provide opportunities for interactions with peers who do not have disabilities. (See chap. 4, this volume, for more detail on programming decisions.)

Community-Based Programming

As noted previously, inclusion means *based in*, not *confined to*. As such, some time may be spent outside the regular classroom in other school sites or in community-based activities. The term *community-based programming* refers to teaching chronological age–appropriate, functional skills in the natural environment. That is, teach skills in *real* environments rather than *artificial* environments. For preschool students, the natural setting tends to be regular childcare centers and local playgrounds. For elementary-age students, the natural setting tends to be regular physical education, the playground during recess, and the neighborhood. For high school–age students, the natural setting is regular physical education and community recreation facilities such as local bowling alleys, swimming pools, health clubs, tennis courts, golf courses, and community sports leagues. For example, if a high school student is being taught how to bowl in an effort to help him acquire the skills needed to bowl independently some day, then bowling should be taught at the bowling facility where this student will most likely bowl upon graduation. Similarly, if a goal for an elementary-age student is to learn how to climb the school's playground equipment during recess, then this student should be taught this skill during recess.

The rationale behind teaching skills in the community is based on research on generalization. Many students with disabilities, particularly students with mental retardation, autism, or learning disabilities, have difficulty generalizing skills learned in one environment to other environments. What happens is that the student learns a skill in one environment, perhaps a quiet hallway or in an empty gymnasium, but cannot demonstrate the learned skill in different, more stimulating environments. For example, a physical education teacher wants Maria, a second grader with autistic tendencies, to learn how to play dodgeball during regular physical education and during recess. The physical educator decides that regular physical education and recess are too stimulating for Maria, so she teaches dodgeball skills to Maria first thing in the morning in the gymnasium when no other students are present. After 4 weeks, Maria has learned how to move away from balls rolled toward her and to roll balls toward her teacher when her teacher stands in the circle. The physical educator now thinks that Maria is ready to play dodgeball during regular physical education and recess. Of course, dodgeball during physical education, while somewhat controlled by the teacher, is a noisy, active affair with children yelling and jumping around with excitement. Recess outside is even more stimulating with no adult supervision. Although Maria did learn the basic skills of dodgeball in the quiet gymnasium, she cannot handle all the stimulation of the game as it is played in regular physical education or recess. Maria just shakes her hands in front of her face, jumps up and down, runs around the gym, and hits her head. Even when the teacher slows the game down and tries to give Maria the ball, she just pushes the ball away. Unfortunately, Maria was unable to generalize the skills learned in one environment to another even though the basic skills were the same. Maria's teacher must now reteach dodgeball skills to Maria in the regular setting (including recess) if she expects Maria to learn not only the skills of dodgeball but how to handle the stimulation of a real game. Maria's teacher would have saved 4 weeks of teaching time if she had started with Maria in the regular setting rather than teaching her the skill in the sterile setting.

Community-based programming for middle and high school–age students often means leaving school grounds to go to a local recreation facility. David, a student with spastic, quadriplegic cerebral palsy who uses an electric wheelchair, along with two or three peers who do not have disabilities, might go to a a local YMCA to receive practice and instruction in swimming and weight lifting. David will learn swimming and weight lifting skills in the environment where he will eventually use these skills upon graduation. In addition, he will learn important ancillary skills that he will need to be successful at the YMCA such as how to check in, how to find the locker room, pool, and weight room, how to use the locker room, how to use the specific weight-lifting equipment at the YMCA, and how to interact with staff and other other YMCA members. He would not be able to learn these ancillary skills if he received all of his instruction at school.

Teaching skills in natural environments does not mean that a student cannot be taught in isolation on occasion. However, the majority of training should take place in the setting where the student will eventually use the skill. For example, Maria could go to regular physical education and recess to practice dodge ball skills 3 days per week, and 2 days per week she could practice specific rolling and dodging skills in a less stimulating setting (perhaps the gymnasium with only three or four peers who do not have disabilities playing). Similarly, David could practice weight lifting at the school's weight room 2 days per week, then go to the YMCA 2 days per week.

As noted earlier, functionality is directly related to age appropriateness and the availability of facilities in the community. By running a community-based program from the beginning, you will have a better idea of what recreation facilities and programs are available in the community and thus appropriate to teach your students with disabilities (and, for that matter, your students without disabilities!).

In terms of inclusion, community-based instruction for younger students should be regular physical education. Thus, inclusive programs in which students with disabilities participate in regular physical education facilitate learning skills in natural environments. For older students, part of their program might include traveling to community-based recreation facilities. The student can still have opportunities to interact with peers without disabilities if these peers travel with the student to community recreation facilities.

Choice Making

Physical educators usually dictate the activities that comprise the physical education curriculum. They also make most of the decisions regarding what equipment to use, how to use it, when to use it, and with whom to use it. In addition, adapted physical education specialists and special education professionals associated with the student with disabilities often make decisions regarding what activities and skills to prioritize. Decisions may involve choosing certain activities over others, using certain types of adaptations, playing certain positions in games, and making modifications to games. While the decisions these professionals make are often appropriate, the student with disabilities is rarely asked his or her opinion.

Choice making refers to giving students a chance to participate in the decisions regarding what skills they want to work on during physical education and how they want to work on these skills. This does not mean relinquishing all decisions to the student with disabilities. Rather, choice making refers to allowing the student to participate in the decision process. After all, who knows more about his or her particular needs than the student with disabilities!

Decisions can vary from choosing specific activities to choosing specific pieces of equipment. For example, a student can choose between two lifetime leisure skills (tennis versus golf) based on his or her interests. Similarly, a student can choose a short bat versus a longer bat in a game of softball, can tell the pitcher where to toss the ball (or have the ball placed on a tee), tell the teacher what position he or she feels comfortable playing, and who he or she would like for a partner for assistance. Again, a student should not be granted every desire. The student is just another voice in the process, and professionals should listen carefully to the requests. Professionals also should consider such factors as safety and chance for success when listening to the student make choices. If they feel that a particular choice is inappropriate, they should explain this to the student and give other, more appropriate, choices.

Obviously, the ability to make choices is related to a person's cognitive ability. Students with physical or sensory impairments or learning disabilities usually can make appropriate choices. This is particularly true for students with physical disabilities and visual impairments who can assist the regular physical educator in making appropriate adaptations to activities and games. But even students with mental retardation can make choices. For example, all bats can be laid out on the ground so that the student with mental retardation can look and feel each bat and then choose one that he or she likes. Similarly, a student can be encouraged to point to or reach for a student he or she prefers to be his or her partner. Students who have difficulty communicating can indicate through smiles, cries, or physical positioning if they prefer certain activities or pieces of equipment. Again, the key is to allow the student to participate in the decision process. Allowing the student to have choices makes for a more motivated, better-behaved participant!

In terms of inclusion, a student should be given the choice as to when he or she wishes to be included and when he or she wants to work in smaller groups. For example, a student with spina bifida may wish to be included in softball, volleyball, soccer, and basketball in regular middle school physical education. However, this student may wish to work on other activities when the class is doing gymnastics. Maybe this student can do aerobic dance, work out in the weight room, or practice tennis or basketball with other students. The student should be allowed to participate in deciding on which alternative activity he or she would like to work.

Partial Participation

Many students with disabilities will not be able to participate in regular physical education activities independently. However, with assistance, the use of adapted equipment, and changes to the game, all students can participate in all activities. Providing assistance and adaptations to students with disabilities so that they can participate in age-appropriate, functional activities in natural environments is called *partial participation*. The student is encouraged to do as much of the skill as possible, then, whatever the student cannot do is supplemented through physical assistance or adapted equipment. For example, a high school student who is blind might be able to swing a bat independently during a softball game. However, the student cannot hit a pitched ball, so he or she is allowed to hit a ball off a tee. In addition, first base is placed a little closer to the student, and a peer calls the student's name so that the student knows in which direction to run. With these simple modifications, the student can now participate (at least partially) in a regular softball game during physical education.

Partial participation includes a variety of supports. For some students, support can be in the form of physical assistance by a peer tutor or teacher assistant. For example, a peer tutor can help the student move from station to station, perform various skills, and provide instructional cues and feedback. Other students may need support in the form of adapted equipment. For example, a student who uses a wheelchair may need a shorter basket in which to shoot during a basketball unit, or a student who is blind may need auditory cues on the target to know where to throw. Finally, support can be in the form of modified rules to traditional games. For example, a student can be allowed five free dribbles and a free pass in a game of basketball to account for his or her limited coordination. Similarly, a student could be allowed to let the ball bounce three times before hitting it over the net in a game of tennis or racquetball. The goal is to allow the student to be as independent as possible, but also to provide the student with support so that he or she can complete the skill and participate in the activity. When implemented properly, partial participation should allow virtually all students with disabilities to participate in age-appropriate, functional activities in natural settings.

Partial participation allows students with disabilities to participate in all functional, regular physical education activities. All that is needed is the provision of support in the form of physical assistance, adapted equipment, and/or rule changes. One of the main reasons why some professionals feel that students with disabilities should be segregated is that they can receive more individualized instruction in segregated programs. In essence, partial participation is providing individualized instruction in the regular setting; thus, there is no need for segregation.

SUMMARY

There is a growing shift from segregated special education programs to a merger between regular and special education. As always, the bottom line in any educational program for students with disabilities is to provide quality programming that is designed to meet each student's individual needs. With proper preparation and support, quality programming can take place in inclusive settings. Benefits to both participants with and without disabilities provide an additional incentive to include students in regular programs. In addition, following specific philosophies of inclusion as well as general philosophies of chronological age appropriateness, functionality, community-based instruction, choice making, and partial participation can facilitate the inclusion of students with disabilities in regular physical education.

Chapter 3

A Team Approach to Including Students with Disabilities in Regular Physical Education

I teach students with relatively mild disabilities in my regular elementary physical education classes. My instruction mainly focuses on skill development, and typically I find a tremendous variation in skill levels in my students without disabilities. To accommodate this typical range, I try to individualize goals and instruction through the use of progressions and developmental sequences. Since I already individualize for students without disabilities, it has not been that difficult for me to provide an individualized program for students with disabilities. I also believe that inclusion is important to the child's self-esteem. For example, I provide special accommodations to students with disabilities during fitness testing, and I also encourage students to do their best and not worry about how their scores compared to other students. I find that students with disabilities will try harder and show improved self-concept when they are given reasonable accommodations and encouragement. Finally, we utilize a team approach in which special education teachers, classroom teachers, and specialists (i.e., physical education, art, music) work together to make the best possible situation for students with disabilities.

—Betsy Beals

Juan is a fourth grader who is fully included in a regular fourth-grade class at Johnson Elementary School. Juan has spastic, diplegic cerebral palsy and uses a manual wheelchair for mobility. In addition, Juan has difficulty with speech, so he uses a communication board that has pictures and symbols to which he points. He also is considered legally blind and has mental retardation. As a full member of his fourth-grade class, Juan attends regular physical education with his classmates who do not have disabilities.

As one can imagine, Mrs. Jackson, the regular physical educator at Johnson Elementary, had no idea what to do (or what *not* to do) with Juan in regular physical education. Like most regular physical educators, Mrs. Jackson had taken one class in adapted physical education when she did her undergraduate training 10 years ago. In addition, she had attended some workshops on inclusion through the school system. Still, she had no idea what to do with Juan. Should Juan participate in the same activities as his classmates or should he do different activities? If he should do

---

Betsy Beals is a regular physical educator at Northwoods Elementary School in Cary, North Carolina.

different activities, what activities should he do? Are there things he should not do because of his disability? How do I communicate with him, and how do I give him instruction? Will he break if I touch him?

Fortunately, Mrs. Jackson knew that there was a team of experts available to help her with Juan. Juan's physical therapist talked to Mrs. Jackson about what cerebral palsy is, detailed Juan's specific type of cerebral palsy, and provided information regarding what activities Juan could and could not do. In addition, she showed Mrs. Jackson the best positions for Juan for throwing, catching, and striking a ball, and moving his wheelchair. (She gave Mrs. Jackson pictures of Juan in these positions to refer to as needed.) As it turned out, the physical therapist planned on assisting Juan in regular physical education once a week, so she would be available to provide information on a regular basis.

Next, Juan's speech therapist explained Juan's speech problems and his system of communication. She explained how Juan communicated with his picture board. In addition, she explained Juan's receptive language abilities, that is, how well he understood what others were saying to him. She provided suggestions to Mrs. Jackson regarding how to instruct Juan using a multisensory approach including simple verbal cues, physical prompting, and physical assistance.

Juan's vision therapist discussed Juan's visual impairment and his visual abilities with Mrs. Jackson. Although Juan was legally blind, he did have quite a bit of residual vision that he should be encouraged to use. The vision therapist showed Mrs. Jackson where to stand when talking to or demonstrating skills to Juan so that he could use his residual vision. She also gave Mrs. Jackson several ideas of how to enhance the visual stimuli in the environment, such as giving Juan bright-colored balls, larger targets, and having Juan's partner wear a bright-colored pinny or vest.

Finally, Juan's special education teacher and parents discussed Juan's personality, interests, likes and dislikes, and general temperament. Juan's parents noted that Juan particularly liked a neighborhood boy named Bill who was in his class. In addition, Juan's parents explained what recreation activities they liked to participate in and how they tried to include Juan in these activities. For example, the family often goes to the park to have picnics, throw a frisbee, and play softball. Juan enjoyed these activities when they were adapted to his abilities, and Juan's parents explained how they made adaptations. Similarly, the special education teacher explained how she instructs Juan and makes modifications to meet his needs. In addition, she explained how hard Juan tries to do all activities and how he seems to appreciate the chance to participate with his peers in a variety of activities.

Suddenly, Mrs. Jackson wasn't as worried about Juan. She now knows much more about his disability, his abilities, his personality, and how to work with him. In fact, Mrs. Jackson is rather excited about having Juan in her class and figuring out ways to best include him in her program! With the assistance of Juan's physical therapist, Mrs. Jackson evaluated Juan's abilities in physical education referenced to the fourth-grade curriculum, to the skills he would need in his neighborhood and during recess, and to lead-up skills related to lifetime leisure skills in which Juan would most likely participate upon graduation. The results of this assessment were then shared with the collaborative team (including Juan's parents), and a formal individualized physical education plan was developed.

The scenario outlined above describes how parents and a variety of professionals can be invaluable resources to regular educators and adapted physical education specialist attempting to include students with disabilities in regular physical education. Together, all persons who work with a student with disabilities (including the regular physical educator) are members of the student's *collaborative team*. Most school districts employ a variety of professionals and specialists who can participate on collaborative teams. Even districts that do not employ a full complement of specialists have access to these professionals at least on a consultative basis. The purpose of this chapter is to describe the concept of collaborative teams as well as to detail the role of key professionals who often participate in collaborative teams. Specific reference to how team members can facilitate inclusion is provided.

COLLABORATIVE TEAM

All students are required to have an individualized education program (IEP) that specifies in writing all aspects of their educational program. The concept of an IEP was specifically developed to guarantee that students would receive all the necessary services and the best educational program possible. Many professionals are involved in the development and implementation of a student's IEP. In fact, the Individuals with Disabilities Education Act of 1990 (IDEA) mandates that a student's IEP be developed by a team that includes the student (when appropriate), the student's parents, the student's teachers and therapists, and a representative from the local education agency (PL 101-476, Sec. 1401, 20). While IEP teams are designed to encourage teamwork and interaction among team members, some team members choose to work in isolation from other professionals. For example, a speech therapist might work on teaching a student to use a communication book in her speech room, but she does not necessarily share this information with the special education teacher, parents, or other professionals. Such an isolationist approach limits the carryover and generalization of skill development.

Fortunately, most professionals are interested in working cooperatively and collaboratively with other professionals during the development and implementation of a student's IEP. Such a team approach invariably maximizes the overall development of a student with disabilities. In addition, sharing expertise and resources among many professionals provides greater problem-solving abilities and enables all individuals involved in the student's educational program to utilize best teaching practices (Rainforth, York, & Macdonald, 1992). And, unlike traditional IEP teams, collaborative teams meet on a regular basis to interact, plan, and modify a student's educational program continually. For example, a collaborative team that meets twice a month is stumped on how to help a student who has autistic behaviors communicate with parents, friends, and teachers. The speech therapist can share with team members the relatively new technique of "facilitated communication," a form of augmentative communication, and all team members can be trained to implement facilitated communication in an effort to help this student communicate. At a future collaborative team meeting, the team will discuss the initial results of the new facilitated communication program and if it should be continued, changed in some way, or dropped.

It should be noted that the formation of collaborative teams usually is not required by administrators. Thus, a team approach will only work if team members have a strong commitment to work together and to share information and ideas with the goal of helping the student achieve maximum development. However, most professionals will be interested in working collaboratively on the student's IEP. This should be particularly true for regular physical educators who can often benefit from the expertise of others to develop and implement individualized physical education programs for their students with disabilities.

Rainforth et al. (1992) coined the term *collaborative teamwork* to refer to the interaction and sharing of information and responsibilities among team members. Rainforth and her colleagues noted that the term was developed as a hybrid of the "transdisciplinary model" and the "integrated therapy model." In the transdisciplinary model, parents and professionals share information and techniques that previously had been the exclusive domain of individual disciplines. For example, physical therapists could share information on positioning that could help a student in the classroom. Unfortunately, the transdisciplinary model often resulted in teachers or paraprofessionals conducting therapy in isolated, nonfunctional ways. For example, a paraprofessional may have learned how to perform range-of-motion activities on a student with cerebral palsy, but she conducts the program away from his peers while his peers work on another activity. In the integrated therapy model, therapy is conducted within functional contexts. For example, speaking in sentences could be practiced and encouraged during lunch, recess, physical education, and other natural contexts. The collaborative model focuses on team members sharing information and working together to provide students with disabilities necessary educational and therapeutic services within functional activities. Thus, this same paraprofessional who has learned how to perform range-of-motion activities might perform these activities during warm-ups in regular physical education. In addition, the student remains with the group while range of motion is performed. Characteristics of collaborative teamwork as outlined by Rainforth et al. (1992, p. 16) can be found in Table 3.1. Note how equal participation, shared responsibility, and the utilization of functional settings are critical aspects of collaborative teamwork.

The collaborative model allows team members to integrate their programs into a student's daily life routines. In addition, team members are encouraged to work together to help students in various settings. For example, a speech teacher, along with a student's parents, may accompany a student to a local YMCA to work on that student's ability to communicate with YMCA staff. Parents and family members are particularly important as they can practice physical education skills at home or take their child to local recreation facilities to follow up on community-based recreation training. As noted above in the story of Juan, team members also can be of tremendous assistance to the regular physical educator. For example, the student's occupational therapist can accompany a student with disabilities into regular physical education to help position a student for a particular activity as well as to help determine appropriate rule and equipment modifications, or an adapted physical educator can team teach with the regular physical educator to ensure that all students, including students with disabilities, receive as individualized a program as possible.

PHYSICAL EDUCATION INCLUSION TEAM (PEIT)

One can consider the physical education inclusion team (PEIT) a subset of the collaborative team. Generally speaking, the PEIT is comprised of all collaborative team members who can contribute to the successful development and implementation of the physical education portion of the stu-

Table 3.1.   Characteristics of collaborative teamwork

1. Equal participation in the collaborative teamwork process by family members and the educational service providers on the educational team
2. Equal participation by all disciplines determined to be necessary for students to achieve their individualized educational goals
3. Consensus decision making about priority educational goals and objectives related to all areas of student functioning at school, at home, and in the community
4. Consensus decision making about the type and amount of support required from related service personnel.
5. Attention to motor, communication, and other embedded skills and needs throughout the educational program and in direct relevance to accomplishing priority educational goals
6. Infusion of knowledge and skills from different disciplines into the design of educational methods and interventions
7. Role release to enable team members who are involved most directly and frequently with students to develop the confidence and competence necessary to facilitate active learning and effective participation in the educational program
8. Collaborative problem solving and shared responsibility for students learning across all aspects of the educational program

dent's IEP. During regular collaborative team meetings, physical education concerns should be discussed by the PEIT. In addition, ongoing discussion between PEIT members should continue outside the IEP meeting. For example, during a particular collaborative team meeting, the regular physical educator notes that Juan's class will be working on a gymnastics unit, and she is not sure if it is appropriate to include Juan in gymnastics activities. The team reviews Juan's IEP and notes that gymnastic activities are not a prioritized goal for Juan. Through discussion among team members, it is decided that Juan can participate with his peers during warm-ups. After warm-ups, Juan will work on pushing his wheelchair (one of Juan's goals) around and across the mats when it is his turn as an alternative to tumbling. In addition, while Juan is waiting for his turn, he will work on holding a striking implement and hitting a ball off a tee (another one of Juan's goals) with a peer who is also waiting his turn.

COLLABORATIVE TEAM MEMBERS

A variety of professionals can be involved in the collaborative team. While each team member has specific responsibilities, the collaborative model suggests that each member can assist other professionals in carrying out their responsibilities. The following describes the specific responsibilities of the collaborative team members as well as how they can assist regular and adapted physical educators in successfully including students with disabilities in regular physical education.

Adapted physical education (APE) specialists are trained specialists (usually with a master's degree in physical education with an emphasis on physical education for students with disabilities) whose major role is to assist in the identification and remediation of physical education-related problems of individuals who have disabilities (Sherrill, 1993). Services include assessment, program planning, writing individual physical education programs, direct implementation of habilitative programs for students with disabililties, consulting with regular physical educators and parents, and fitness and leisure counseling, including sports, for persons with disabilities (Sherrill, 1993). When available (i.e., if a school system has an APE specialist), the APE specialist should be the physical education integration team coordinator. The APE specialist can assist the regular physical educator in including students with disabilities in regular physical education in a variety of ways. First, the APE specialist can take all the information provided by the other team members, including specific information about the student's physical and motor skills, and present it to the regular physical educator in a way that is meaningful and practical. Second, the APE specialist can provide specific information to the regular physical educator regarding ways to modify physical education activities so as to safely and successfully include the student with disabilities. This can be accomplished through counseling sessions, team teaching, or providing written modifications to lesson plans. The APE specialist knows more about how specific types of disabilities impact on physical education; thus, he or she is the most important member of the team.

Regular physical education (RPE) teachers are specifically trained to teach physical education to students without disabilities. The RPE will know more about what happens in regular physical education than any other team member. He or she also will have a great deal of knowledge about all the components of physical education (physical fitness, fundamental motor skills, individual and team sports, and games). Perhaps of greatest importance, the regular physical educator will know what units will be taught at what point in the year, what teaching approach is used, what equipment is available, how many students are in each class, and what the class is like. Most RPEs will have had at least one course in adapted physical education during their formal training. Others will have had more courses as well as practical experiences, and still others will have had inservice training in adapted physical education. Realistically, most RPEs will have had very little training or experience in working with students who have disabilities, and thus may be a little apprehensive about including a student with disabilities in the regular program. It is the responsibility of all team members to make RPEs feel as comfortable as possible with the notion of inclusion. On the other hand, it is the responsibility of the RPE to have an open mind about inclusion, provide opportunities for interaction between students with and without disabilities, and be a role model for students who do not have disabilities by accepting each student and respecting the students' individual differences.

The special education teacher is the primary advocate and program planner for the student with disabilities (Stainback & Stainback, 1985). His or her role is to develop and assist in the implementation of the student's IEP including initiation and organization of inclusive activities. In addition, his or her job is to coordinate all support and related services a student may need to benefit from special education (Stainback & Stainback, 1985). The special education teacher will know more about the student with disabilities than any other team member, with the possible exception of the student's parents. Information the special education teacher has that could facilitate inclusion in regular physical education includes a student's developmental history, health and medical background, behaviors and behavior plans, communication and cognitive skills, self-help skills, and likes and dislikes. In addition, as coordinator of all the student's services, the special education teacher can quickly communicate information to other team members. The special education teacher can also assist in training of peer tutors and paraprofessionals who may work in regular physical education.

The building principal is responsible for everything that takes place in his or her school, including physical education programs and programs for students with disabilities. Thus, while not directly involved in program planning or implementation, the building principal has a vested interest in the success of the inclusive physical education program. Principals who support inclusive physical education can have a direct impact on the attitudes of regular physical education staff who may be reluctant to implement the program. In addition, principals can help team members gain important resources such as extra support, special equipment, and gym time. Finally, the principal can also act as a go-between with other administrators such as directors of physical education or special education at the school-system level.

The school nurse will be an invaluable resource to the team regarding a student's health and medical state. School nurses are mainly responsible for: 1) diagnosing and treating minor injuries and illnesses, 2) handling medical emergencies and contacting other emergency personnel, and 3) monitoring and administering prescription medications. In some schools, nurses are also responsible for specific health care procedures such as suctioning a student's tracheotomy (hole in throat used for breathing), postural drainage for students whose lungs fill with fluid (e.g., students with cystic fibrosis), clean intermittent catheterization to help students who do not have bladder control (e.g., some students with spina bifida), and tube feeding students who cannot receive adequate nutrition through oral feeding (some students with severe gastrointestinal problems). Since the school nurse has direct access to the student's parents and physicians, the school nurse can act as a link between a student's parents and physicians and the school. For example, if a question arises as to the effects of vigorous exercise on a student with a seizure disorder, the school nurse can quickly contact the student's parents and physicians to get an immediate answer. The school nurse should act as a consultant to the team, and team members should feel free to contact the nurse if they have any questions regarding a particular student's health or medical state. For example, the nurse should be consulted when a student with a seizure disorder is involved in activities such as swimming or gymnastics or when a student with allergy-induced asthma is required to go outside for physical education.

Physical therapists (PT) utilize various techniques to relieve pain and discomfort, prevent deformity and further disability, restore or maintain functioning, and improve strength and motor skill performance (Sherrill, 1993). Direction in gait training and use of a wheelchair, walker, braces, or other assistive devices is one of the more important roles of the physical therapist. The physical therapist will know more about the student's physical condition than any other team member. As such, he or she should be included in decisions regarding contraindicated activities or positions, selection of motor skills for training, positioning and limb use for optimum functioning, and modifications to equipment and rules of the game. For example, if a student who is learning to walk with a walker is placed in a regular third grade physical education class, the physical therapist can provide information regarding what warm-up activities are appropriate or inappropriate, how to modify appropriate warm-up activities and what alternative warm-ups could be used at other times, how far and how fast the student should be expected to walk, the student's aerobic capacity, strength, and flexibility, and suggestions for modifications to activities in regular physical education.

Occupational therapists (OT) utilize various techniques to: 1) improve, develop, or restore functions impaired or lost through illness, injury, or deprivation; 2) improve ability to perform tasks for independent functioning when functions are impaired or lost; and 3) prevent, through early intervention, initial or further impairment or loss of function (*Federal Register*, August 23, 1977, p. 42479). One of the major focuses of occupational therapists is assisting persons to perform activities of daily living (ADL) as independently as possible through training or adapted equipment. Another major focus, particularly with children, is the presentation of sensorimotor integration activities designed to assist children with disabilities to fully utilize and integrate vestibular information (information from the inner ear that tells the person where his or her head is in relation to gravity), tactile information (sense of touch and feedback from touch sensors on the skin), and visual information. The OT can be an important resource on the team regarding a student's abilities (and possible adaptations) in: 1) self-help and personal hygiene skills needed in the locker room prior to and after a physical education class; 2) fine motor skills, fundamental manipulative skills, and sport-specific manipulative skills; and 3) skills related to sensory integration such as static and dynamic balance, tactile awareness, and proprioception.

Therapeutic recreation (TR) therapists are responsible for: 1) assessment of leisure function, 2) therapeutic recreation services, 3) recreation programs in schools and community agencies, and 4) leisure education (*Federal Register*, August 23, 1977, p. 42479). Recreation covers an array of programs including music, art, dance, drama, horticulture, camping, and sports and fitness. Therapeutic recreation was recently reemphasized in PL 101-476 (IDEA). Recreation therapists can provide the team with information regarding recreation/leisure assessment, availability of community recreation facilities, and suggestions for adaptations in performing recreation/leisure programs. This information can be particularly important to the physical educator who is assisting the student with disabilities to transition from a school-based physical education program to a postschool recreation program.

Speech therapists' responsibilities include "identification of children with speech or language disorders, diagnosis and appraisal of specific speech or language disorders, referral for medical or other professional attention necessary for the habilitation of speech or language disorders, provision of speech and language services for the habilitation or prevention of communicative disorders, counseling and guidance of parents, children, and teachers regarding speech or language disorders" (*Federal Register*, August 23, 1977, p. 42480). Speech therapists can assist team members in understanding a particular student's receptive and expressive language abilities. For example, speech therapists can explain to members and peers how best to communicate with certain students. Some students might understand verbal cues and simple demonstrations while other students might need sign language or physical assistance. Similarly, speech therapists can explain to team members as well as peers how particular students communicate. Expressive language can include speech, sign language, communication boards, electronic devices such as

Canon communicators or speech synthesizers, or facilitated communication. Knowing how best to present information to students as well as understanding how a student might express his or her desires is extremely important for successful inclusion.

Audiologists are trained professionals who work with students with hearing impairments. The major role of the audiologist is to determine a student's hearing loss and hearing abilities and recommend special augmentative hearing devices such as hearing aids. In addition, audiologists often consult with speech therapists to determine a particular student's potential for speech and language development. An audiologist can assist the regular physical educator by explaining a student's hearing loss and specifying his or her residual hearing abilities. In collaboration with the speech therapist, the audiologist can then recommend ways to communicate with a student who has a hearing impairment. For example, an audiologist might suggest that a student who is in regular physical education and who has a severe hearing loss (wears hearing aids) may need to have verbal directions repeated by a peer or have demonstrations to supplement verbal commands. In addition, the audiologist can explain safety precautions for this student such as avoiding contact to the ear while wearing hearing aids or taking the aids out when swimming.

Vision therapists (VT) are trained professionals who work with students who are visually impaired. The vision therapist's major goal is to help a student with a visual impairment become as functional and independent as possible given limited visual abilities. For students with low vision, goals include learning orientation and mobility skills necessary to move about in various school and community environments and learning adapted techniques for classwork such as reading large print, using felt tip markers, using a magnifying glass, and using computers. For students who have very limited vision or who are blind, goals include orientation and mobility skills such as using a cane and a sighted guide and learning adaptive techniques for classwork such as braille and computers. Vision therapists work very closely with other professionals, and their expertise on particular children as well as general adaptations for students with visual impairments can be invaluable for adapted physical education specialists and regular physical educators. For example the vision therapist can instruct the regular physical educator and peers who do not have disabilities in how to make the student with a visual impairment feel more comfortable in the gym environment, how to interact appropriately with the student, and how to assist the student. Vision therapists can also provide ideas for adapted equipment, safety precautions, and rule modifications such as guide ropes for running, beeper balls for softball, and tandem bike riding. Many vision therapists have easy access to adapted equipment such as beeper balls and balls with bells, while others are knowledgeable about special sports programs designed for persons with visual impairments, such as the United States Association for Blind Athletes (USABA).

Paraprofessionals are hired to assist teachers in implementing a student's individual education program. In inclusive programs, the paraprofessional is often the person who has the most one-on-one contact with the student with disabilities. Paraprofessionals vary greatly in their backgrounds and training—from certified special education teachers to persons with high school degrees who have virtually no prior experience with students who have disabilities. Additionally, paraprofessionals are utilized differently by different teachers. Some paraprofessionals are responsible only for assisting students in activities of daily living such as dressing, feeding, and bathrooming, while others are given much more responsibility in terms of assisting the teacher in educational assessment, program design, and program implementation. Regardless of the exact role of the paraprofessionals, their close contact with the student with disabilities enables them to provide unique insight into the needs and interests of the student. Thus, paraprofessionals can provide valuable information to the team regarding a student's: 1) behaviors at certain times during the day, 2) communication skills, 3) likes and dislikes, and 4) preferred positions, adaptations, and activities. In many programs the paraprofessional accompanies the student with disabilities in physical education, so she or he will not only know about the student but also how the student reacts to physical education activities. (More information about the role of the paraprofessional and techniques for training and evaluating the paraprofessional will be provided in later chapters.)

Parents are often overlooked resources in the education of their children with disabilities even though by law they should be an integral part in the development of a student's individualized education program. Parents probably know more practical information about their child than any professional. In addition, parents often have developed successful management and training techniques at home that can be useful in the classroom and in physical education. For example, parents may have techniques for positioning a student so that he or she can get dressed quickly, something that could be important in the locker room. Parents can also share their goals and expectations for their child as well as their personal recreation interests so that the physical educator can gear the program to meet the unique needs of the family. It is much easier to get support from home when parents are included in the decision process.

Students with disabilities should be included on the team whenever possible. Who else knows more about his or her own abilities, interests, and needs than the student? Also, a student with disabilities who is included in the process of developing his or her educational program is more likely to be more committed to and motivated to work on specific program goals. For example, an elementary-age student with spina bifida might be encouraged to find alternative ways to move when the class is doing locomotor patterns. Similarly, a high school–age student who is blind can choose a cardiovascular training program (e.g., aerobic dance, stair climber, stationary bike, walking the track) that meets his or her interests. Students who are given choices tend to be more motivated learners.

MEETING WITH THE PHYSICAL EDUCATION INTEGRATION TEAM (PEIT)

The PEIT should be viewed as a subset of the collaborative team. Logistically, PEIT meetings are easiest to conduct during part of regular collaborative team meetings. (Other PEIT meetings can be set up as needed and depending on the schedules of team members.) The PEIT portion of the collaborative team meeting should be organized with one team member (usually the adapted physical education specialist) serving as the team leader. This team leader can take on the responsibility of leading this portion of the meeting, soliciting information from key members, documenting decisions that were made during the meeting, and keeping all team members informed (via phone calls or memos). While it may be difficult to get all team members together for ongoing team meetings, it is imperative that all key team members, particularly the regular physical educator, attend at least one preplanning meeting prior to the inclusion of the student with disabilities in regular physical education. In fact, the regular physical educator need only attend the PEIT portion of the collaborative team meeting if time constraints are a problem.

One important part of the PEIT meeting is for team members to introduce themselves and offer their assistance to the regular physical educator. Often regular physical educators are not part of the "special education loop," and thus might not be familiar with the roles of various specialists or who various specialists are. One way of introducing team members to the regular physical educator (as well as to each other) is to utilize the concept of *role release* (Woodruff & McGonigel, 1988). Role release is a systematic way for team members to share ideas about their discipline and begin to work collaboratively to develop and implement the best possible program for a student with disabilities. Role release in introductory meetings should include the following: 1) *role extension* in which all team members begin to acquire knowledge about each other's disciplines (e.g., each team member describes his or her role in the educational program of the student); 2) *role enrichment* in which team members begin to share information about basic practices (team members share their best teaching practices related to a particular student); and 3) *role expansion* in which team members exchange best teaching practices across disciplines (team members explain how other team members can utilize these best teaching practices in their settings). Role release in future meetings should include: 1) *role exchange* in which team members begin to implement teaching techniques from other disciplines, and 2) *role support* in which team members back each other up as they assume the roles of each other's disciplines. By the end of the first meeting, the regular physical educator should feel that he or she has real resources to whom to go in order to answer specific questions about the student's physical education program. In addition, the regular physical educator should have a greater understanding of the student's overall educational program (not just physical education) and how he or she can assist other team members in meeting other educational goals.

A great deal of information should be presented at the initial meeting so that team members can make informed decisions regarding the development of the student's individualized physical education program and strategies for inclusion. Various team members will be able to provide different aspects of the information. Vision teachers can provide information about a student's visual abilities, physical therapists can provide information about a student's motor abilities and physical fitness, the regular physical educator can provide information about the regular physical education curriculum and class format, and the student and his or her parents can provide information about the student's likes and dislikes. Key information and the team member most likely to provide this information are presented in Table 3.2.

While future team meetings are important and should be planned, some members may not be able to attend on a regular basis. In such cases, the team leader should request information from team members to share with the team. For example, if the regular physical educator cannot attend a meeting, he or she can provide information to the team leader regarding how well the student is doing, what modifications and teaching approaches have been effective or ineffective, and what the next physical education unit will include. Similarly, the student's physical therapist can communicate to the group via a memo regarding any physical changes in the student that may affect his or her physical education program. Team members also should feel comfortable contacting each other if they have specific questions about the student's physical education program. For example, a student's vision therapist may contact the regular physical educator to detail changes in the student's vision, or the physical educator may want to contact the student's social worker to determine if changes in the home have any impact on the student's recent behavior problems in physical education. While formal team meetings provide the best means for discussing issues affecting the student's program, the most important point is that team members feel comfortable communicating with each other whenever the need arises.

AN EXAMPLE OF A PEIT MEETING

Sarah is a 13-year-old student who will be a first-year student (sixth grade) at a local middle school. Sarah enjoys holding and throwing various-sized balls, pushing her wheelchair in various directions and being pushed really fast by her peers, bowling, listening to music, and being around her peers without disabilities. Sarah has severe, spastic hemiplegic cerebral palsy (she is learning how to push her wheelchair with direction), mental retardation, a significant vision and speech impairment, and she receives medication to control a seizure disorder. The PEIT for Sarah includes the following team members: Sarah's parents, special education teacher, physical therapist, occupational therapist, speech therapist, vision therapist, nurse, adapted physical education specialist, and regular physical educator. The adapted physical education specialist serves as the team leader. (See Figures 3.1a and 3.1b for examples of a team meeting agenda and minutes form.)

In previous PEIT meetings the team developed a long-term plan for Sarah which included the following goals: 1) push wheelchair with direction, 2) acquire skills needed to participate partially in bowling using a ramp, 3) swim using a flotation device, 4) play miniature golf using a ramp,

5) independently participate in aerobic dance, and 6) partially participate in modified games of basketball and softball. The APE specialist and regular physical educators review the progress Sarah has made toward these goals. For example, Sarah has just completed a unit on softball with her peers. She learned how to hold the bat using one hand and hit a ball off a tee so that it traveled 5' in the air. In addition, she can push her wheelchair down the first base line (with verbal cuing), a distance of 10' in 30 seconds, a tremendous improvement from the previous month.

Other team members ask the regular and adapted physical educators specific questions regarding their areas of interest. For example, the speech therapist notes that Sarah is improving on her ability to communicate with her picture board that is taped to her lap tray, and she wants to know if Sarah is using the board in physical education. The regular physical educator notes that he has seen Sarah use her pictures several times to communicate with him and with peers. Similarly, the vision and physical therapists discuss changes they have seen in Sarah over the past month and query the regular physical educators and APE specialist as to similar changes they might have seen. On Fridays, Sarah goes with the APE specialist and several peers who do not have disabilities to the local YMCA to swim and then to the local bowling alley to bowl. The APE specialist reviews the progress she has made in these IEP goals. He notes that Sarah can now push the ball down the ramp without any extra verbal cues. In addition, he notes that she will take her wallet out of her purse and give the checkout person $1 for shoes after a verbal cue. She also points to the picture of a shoe on her picture board after a verbal cue. (The speech therapist was thrilled to hear this!) The occupational therapist, who assists Sarah at the bowling alley, notes that Sarah is gaining much more control of her "good" hand, and she is able to take things out of her purse and wallet independently within 30 seconds of a verbal command. (This was one of the occupational therapist's goals.) Sarah has not made any notable gains in swimming in the past month, but she really enjoys swimming using a flotation device. In addition, she is continuing to work on her dressing and undressing skills. The team comments that Sarah should continue her bowling and swimming program on Fridays.

The regular physical educator then reviews the next unit, which is track and field. He briefly explains the activities that will take place in this unit, and then asks team members for suggestions for Sarah. The physical therapist notes that Sarah should continue to work on her wheelchair mobility skills. In addition, she gives the regular physical educator some new stretches for Sarah's upper body that she can do during warm-ups with her assistant. The APE specialist suggests that Sarah train for specific Special Olympics wheelchair events so that she can culminate her training with an actual track event. The team meeting concludes with the team leader reviewing Sarah's program and noting in the minutes any actions that should take place by the next meeting. The next meeting is set for the first county-wide inservice day (approximately 6 weeks away) in which the team will discuss how well Sarah's program is going. At that time, team members are expected to provide brief written evaluations of Sarah's progress in her physical education goals (responsibility of regular physical educators and APE specialists) as well as related goals. For example, the speech therapist will come into regular physical education to evaluate Sarah's functional use of the picture board. The APE specialist reminds team members that they should feel free to contact each other by memo or phone if they need more information in the interim.

SUMMARY

There are many individuals who are involved in the education of students with disabilities. While each may have unique goals and objectives for the student, they all want to see the student reach his or her full potential. The best way to provide services to students with disabilities is for all of these individuals to cooperate by sharing information and working together. Such a team approach allows a variety of professionals to provide input and assist in making important decisions

Table 3.2. Information and the team members who can provide it

Information regarding the student:	P/S	SE	MD	PT	OT	VT	ST	PY	RPE	APE
• Specific disability of the student with emphasis on how this disability will affect his or her abilities in regular physical education	x	x	x	x	x	x	x		x	
• Medical and health information regarding the student particularly as it relates to contraindicated activities	x	x	x	x						
• Behaviors of student including what behaviors to expect, what generally causes behavior outbursts, and what behavior program is in place for the student	x	x						x		
• Communication abilities of students including how the student communicates, how well the student understands verbal directions, how best to communicate with the student	x	x					x			
• What special equipment (if any) the student uses, and whether this equipment will be brought into regular physical education	x				x	x				x
• Personal hygiene skills of student including locker room skills, ability to dress and undress, and ability to take a shower and perform personal grooming skills	x	x		x	x					
• Motor skills including general information regarding physical fitness, fundamental motor skills, and perceptual motor abilities	x			x	x					x
• Specific information regarding recreation activities that are available in the student's community or neighborhood	x								x	x
• Interests of student and student's parents, particularly as the student reaches high school and begins to develop interests in particular lifetime leisure skills and possibly sports (including sports for persons with disabilities)	x									

(continued)

Table 3.2. *continued*

	P/S	SE	MD	PT	OT	VT	ST	PY	RPE	APE
• Special sports opportunities such as Special Olympics, wheelchair sports, and so forth	x									x
• Specific goals developed for student that are not directly related to physical education but that can be worked on in the physical education setting	x	x	x	x	x	x	x	x	x	x
2. Activities that take place in regular physical education:										
• How long a typical physical education class is, and how the period is broken down (e.g., 10 minutes for locker room, 25 minutes for activity)									x	
• The daily routine in regular physical education (e.g., warm-up activities, skill stations)									x	
• The typical teaching style (movement education, direct teaching, highly structured, and so forth)									x	
• Minimal skills needed in the locker room									x	

P/S = parent and/or student, SE = special education teacher, MD = physician, PT = physical therapist, OT = occupational therapist, VT = vision therapist, ST = speech therapist, PY = psychologist, RPE = regular physical education specialist, APE = adapted physical education specialist.

Team Meeting Agenda

Team meeting for:_____   Date:_____ Time:_____

Location of meeting: _____

Facilitator:_____   Recorder: _____

Agenda Items and Description	Outcomes Desired	Time

a.

Figure 3.1.   a. Form to Record PEIT Meeting Agenda.   b. Form to Record PEIT Meeting Minutes. From Rain-forth, B., York, J., & Macdonald, C. (1992). *Collaborative teams for students with severe disabilities: Integrating therapy and educational services* (pp. 272–273). Baltimore: Paul H. Brookes Publishing Co. Copyright © 1992 by Paul H. Brookes Publishing Co.; reprinted by permission.

Team Meeting Minutes

Team meeting for:_____   Date:_____

                                                  Start time:_____ Finish time:_____

Participants: _____

_____

Facilitator:_____   Recorder:_____

Priority Sequence	Agenda Items and Key Points	Follow-up Needed: Who? What? When?
1. 2.	Anecdote: Follow-up:	

Next meeting:

Date/time: _____   Location:_____

Facilitator:_____   Recorder:_____

Agenda items:_____

b.

regarding the student's program. In addition, each professional has information that can help other professionals do their jobs better. For example, knowing how to communicate with a student (information provided by the speech therapist) will help the physical therapist provide her services more effectively.

Regular physical educators who are asked to include students with disabilities in their regular physical education programs may feel isolated and uninformed about the student's abilities and disabilities. In many cases, students with disabilities are still being "dumped" into regular physical education programs on the first day of school! A team approach provides the regular physical educator with a wealth of resources to help him or her develop and implement an individualized program as well as answer specific questions as they arise. In some situations, team members might accompany the student into regular physical education. For example, the vision therapist may accompany a student who is blind into regular physical education while a physical therapist might accompany a student with cerebral palsy into regular physical education. In any event, specialists can provide the regular physical educator with important information that will help him or her provide the best physical education program to students with disabilities.

DEVELOPING AN INCLUSIVE PHYSICAL EDUCATION PROGRAM

Chapter 4

Planning
for Inclusion in
Regular Physical Education

*The best thing that has happened with inclusion is that we have all become better physical education teachers. With inclusion, our regular physical education staff was forced to use a larger array of teaching strategies and materials to accommodate students with disabilities. These teachers quickly found out that individualizing instruction and creating a variety of accommodations helped **all** the students in their physical education classes. These teachers have become aware of the fact that* all *students learn differently and that adaptations create a positive atmosphere and facilitate development in* all *their students.*

—Ginny Popiolek

Lee is a 15-year-old student with mental retardation and cerebral palsy who will be attending Jefferson High School in the fall. The physical education staff at Jefferson have attended several in-services regarding inclusion and have been given specific information about Lee. In the spring they had an opportunity to observe Lee in the classroom and during physical education at Washington Middle School. In addition, Lee's adapted physical education (APE) specialist and his parents have met with the physical education staff to outline what they would like to see for Lee during his high school years.

This is the first time that the physical education staff at Jefferson have had to include a student with such significant disabilities into their regular physical education program. They have successfully included students with learning disabilities, mental retardation, and even a student who was deaf, but Lee's disabilities present a completely different problem. What could Lee do? What part of the high school curriculum was appropriate for Lee, and what parts were inappropriate? What adaptations and supports would Lee need to be safely, successfully, and meaningfully included in regular physical education?

There are many questions the physical education staff at Jefferson have regarding including Lee in regular physical education. How can these staff members make an informed decision regarding Lee's program? The physical education staff need a systematic way to develop a program for Lee so that he can work on his individualized education program within regular physical education.

Students with disabilities can receive an individualized, appropriate physical education program within the regular physical education setting. However, the Physical Education Inclusion

Ginny Popiolek is an itinerant APE specialist for the Harford County Public Schools, Bel Air, Maryland.

Team (PEIT) must address several issues before placing a student with disabilities in regular physical education. For example: What goals will be prioritized for each student? Which goals can be incorporated into the regular program? What modifications will be necessary? What in-service training should be provided to the regular physical educator, the paraprofessionals, and peer tutors? Successful placement of students with disabilities in regular physical education involves much more that just placing the student in the regular setting. The purpose of this chapter is to outline a systematic approach to including students with disabilities in regular physical education. The focus of this approach is making critical decisions utilizing an *ecological approach* to programming and preparing personnel *prior to* inclusion. Information in this chapter is derived in part from the model developed by the author. (See also Table 4.1.)

AN ECOLOGICAL APPROACH TO PLANNING

The model outlined in this chapter follows a *functional* (Block, 1992; Brown et al., 1979; Kelly et al., 1991) or an *ecological approach* (Rainforth et al., 1992) to planning and programming. The

Table 4.1. Model for including students with disabilities in regular physical education

1. **DETERMINE WHAT TO TEACH**
    - Determine student's present level of performance.
    - Prioritize long-term goals and short-term instructional objectives.
2. **ANALYZE THE REGULAR PHYSICAL EDUCATION CURRICULUM**
    - What RPE activities match the student's IEP?
    - What RPE activities do not match the student's IEP but still seem important for the student?
    - What RPE activities are inappropriate for a particular student?
    - What is the teaching style of the regular physical educator?
3. **DETERMINE MODIFICATIONS NEEDED IN REGULAR PHYSICAL EDUCATION**
    - How often will student receive instruction?
    - Where will student receive instruction?
    - How will student be prepared for instruction?
    - What instruction modifications are needed to elicit desired performance?
    - What curricular adaptations will be used to enhance performance?
    - How will performance be assessed?
4. **DETERMINE HOW MUCH SUPPORT THE STUDENT WITH DISABILITIES WILL NEED IN RPE**
    - Base on type of activities and abilities (cognitive, affective, and psychomotor) of student.
    - Utilize the "continuum of support" model (Block & Krebs, 1992).
5. **PREPARE REGULAR PHYSICAL EDUCATOR**
    - Discuss the amount of support that will be provided.
    - Discuss the availability of consultation with APE and special education teacher.
    - Explain that he or she is responsible for the entire class, not just the student with disabilities.
    - Explain that his or her work load should not be increased.
6. **PREPARE REGULAR EDUCATION STUDENTS**
    - Talk about students with disabilities in general.
    - Role-play various types of disabilities.
    - Invite guest speakers with disabilities to your class.
    - If the student attends special education class, allow other students to visit the special education classroom and meet student.
    - Talk specifically about the student who will be coming to RPE (focus on abilities).
    - Discuss ways regular students can help student with disabilities and RPE teacher.
7. **PREPARE SUPPORT PERSONNEL**
    - Discuss specific student with whom they will be working.
    - Discuss the student's physical education IEP.
    - Discuss their responsibilities in RPE.
    - Discuss to whom they can go if they have questions.

ecological approach reflects the interaction of the individual student and the environment in which he or she will function. In the case of physical education, an ecologically referenced program focuses on the student's abilities and interests in relation to the skills the student will need to be successful in his or her present setting (i.e., physical education, playground skills, activities seen in the student's neighborhood) as well as skills the student will need to be successful in future settings (i.e., community-based recreation). Team members develop an individualized plan that includes all the skills, activities, and environments that are most important to that student (Rainforth et al., 1992).

The ecological approach is considered a "top-down" model in which planning begins by envisioning where the student will be upon graduation from the program and what skills the student will need to be successful in this future setting (Auxter & Pyfer, 1989; Kelly et al., 1991; Rainforth et al., 1992). Contrast this approach to a developmental model or "bottom-up" approach in which activities are based upon the scope and sequence of normal development of young children without regard to the relevance of these skills to success in current and future physical education/recreation environments.

For example, in the developmental approach, a student would be evaluated using a developmental test such as the Peabody Developmental Scales or Bayley Developmental Scales, or norm-referenced tests such as the President's Council on Physical Fitness Test or the Bruininks-Oseretsky Test of Motor Impairment. Results from these tests reveal the student's approximate developmental age level, then teachers typically develop programs for the student that move him or her up the developmental scales. A student who can only jump 24″ would be encouraged to jump 30″; a student who cannot yet balance on one foot would practice one-foot balance activities; and a student who scored below the 20th percentile on sit-up performance would practice sit-ups. Note how these activities, while related to the student's present level of performance, are not referenced to the skills the student will need to be successful in his or her current or future life circumstances. Does it matter that the student is at the 20th percentile in sit-ups or can only jump forward 24″? Will these discrepancies in performance affect the student's success in regular physical education, playground skills, neighborhood skills, or skills the student will need to be successful in community recreation?

In the ecological approach, assessment is referenced directly to activities that take place in the student's present and future environments. For example, a sixth-grade student with Down syndrome would be evaluated on the skills needed in regular sixth-grade physical education, skills needed to participate with peers in intramurals and neighborhood sports and recreation programs, and skills needed to participate independently in community-based recreation programs when the student graduates from school. Information from such an assessment would lead to programming that is directly related to skills the student will need to be successful now and in the future. The model that follows utilizes the ecological approach to program planning. Note how this approach actually facilitates the inclusion of students with disabilities in regular physical education.

A SYSTEMATIC APPROACH TO INCLUDING STUDENTS WITH DISABILITIES IN REGULAR PHYSICAL EDUCATION

1. *Determine what to teach.* The first step in the planning process is to determine what to teach. That is, what are the most critical skills a student will need to be successful in his or her present and future physical education/recreation environments? There are several factors that will determine what skills to teach. These include factors such as the student's strengths and weaknesses, the student's age, the student's interests as well as his or her parents' interests, what recreation facilities and programs are available in school and in the community, the time allotted to teach the skills, and the support available. (See Table 4.2.)

Table 4.2.   Factors to consider when prioritizing goals and objectives

General factor	Specific reference to physical education
Student's strengths and weaknesses referenced to current and future needs (severity of disability)	What are the student's abilities referenced to regular physical education activities and community play/recreation activities?
How much time is available to teach skills, and what is the chance the student will acquire these skills?	Younger students can be "exposed" to a variety of skills, while older students should begin to focus on skills needed to participate in specific lifetime leisure activities.
Student's interests	What recreational/sport activities does the student prefer?
Parents' interests	What recreational/sport activities do the student's parents prefer?
Peer interests	What activities do peers participate in on the playground, in the neighborhood, and in community recreation?
What recreation facilities are available in the community?	Prioritize activities that will be available to the student in community (e.g., are there bowling alleys or recreation centers? Are they accessible?)
What equipment/transportation is available?	Does the student need special equipment (e.g., bowling ramp, flotation devices?) Is transportation to community recreation facilities available?
What support services (in terms of personnel) are available?	Who will be available to assist the student in physical education and recreation? Are specially trained persons to work with student needed (e.g., vision therapist for student who is blind)?

Evaluation of a student's strengths and weaknesses should be referenced to the skills the student will need to be successful in his or her current and future physical education/recreation environments. For young children, assessment is referenced to skills the student will need in regular elementary school physical education, skills needed to be successful during recess, and skills needed to be successful in neighborhood games. For older students, assessment should be referenced to the skills that the students will need in regular middle school and high school physical education and the skills that the students will need to be successful in community recreation programs. In addition, the students' interests in particular physical education/recreation activities as well as the interests of the their parents and peers should be considered. For example, a ninth-grade student with spina bifida who is interested in learning how to play wheelchair tennis will be more motivated to practice and accept instruction in tennis versus another physical education activity that has been "forced" upon him. In addition, this student will be even more motivated if his parents play tennis and if tennis is popular with the student's friends. Figure 4.1 provides a simple form that is designed to facilitate curricular decisions.

Table 4.3 provides a more detailed description of present level of performance referenced to school and community settings for a 15-year-old student with mental retardation. Note how traditional assessment information about the acquisition of motor skills, fundamental motor pattern performance, and physical fitness are embedded in the ecologically referenced assessment. Ideally, this evaluation should follow a team approach utilizing the expertise of key members of the collaborative team. The vision therapist can assist the regular educator or the adapted physical education specialist in assessing ball skills that require eye–hand coordination skills (e.g., striking, catching, dribbling, volleying), while the physical therapist can assist physical educators in assessing

Form for Curricular Decision Making

Directions: List all of the activities preferred or typically engaged in under the following headings. Scan across the list and place activities that are in more than one column under "Targeted Activities."

Student preferences	Parents' preferences	Activities in RPE	Activities played by peers	Community leisure activities
_____	_____	_____	_____	_____
_____	_____	_____	_____	_____
_____	_____	_____	_____	_____
_____	_____	_____	_____	_____
_____	_____	_____	_____	_____
_____	_____	_____	_____	_____

Targeted Activities: 1. _____ 2. _____

3. _____ 4. _____

Figure 4.1.   Sample form for making initial curricular decisions.

locomotor patterns and physical fitness. (See chap. 5, this volume, for more detailed information on ecologically referenced assessment procedures.)

In some cases, results from this evaluation will reveal that a student has skills similar to his or her age peers and thus does not need any special physical education program. In other cases, a clear discrepancy will appear between a student's abilities and the skills he or she needs to be successful in regular physical education and community activities. If a deficit does exist, then information from the evaluation can be used to develop an individual education program that includes a long-term plan, long-term goals, and short-term instructional objectives.

Table 4.4 provides an example of a student's long-term plan including long-term goals and short-term instructional objectives. The *long-term plan* is the overall purpose of your program and what skills you would like to see a particular student acquire upon graduation from the program. This might include acquiring the ability to participate independently in two or three defined lifetime leisure skills in the community, maintain a certain level of physical fitness, or participate in organized community sports programs including special sports programs for persons with disabilities. The long-term plan guides the entire educational program and helps keep the team focused as to what specific skills you want the student to have upon completion of your program (Kelly et al., 1991). The long-term plan will be based on what is available in the student's community and the student's unique skills. For example, it does not make sense to have a long-term plan that includes swimming if there are no pools in the student's community. Similarly, it would be inappropriate to target volleyball for a particular student if: 1) the student has a significant disability and can only play volleyball with assistance and with modifications to the game, and 2) the only volleyball league in the community is a high-level competitive league in which players and coaches want to play regulation games without modifications. However, softball might be appropriate for this same student if the community softball league has different divisions including a recreation level division in which modifications needed for this student would be tolerated by other players. Thus, the student's abilities and what is available in the community will dictate what activities make up each student's long-term plan.

Table 4.3.   Present level of performance statement from IEP for Sue, a 15-year-old student with mental retardation

---

Present level of performance statement with reference to activities in RPE

Tennis: Sue walks slowly to retrieve the ball, but can only reach balls hit within 5' of her. She is able to get into a side position for a forehand and swing forcefully (no step or body rotation). She is able to get into a backhand position after verbal cues and demonstrate a backhand (no step or body rotation). She hits balls tossed directly to her three out of five times with a forehand and two out of five times with a backhand. She has the strength to hit the ball over the net from 15' away.

Golf: Sue can hold a golf club and swing with a stiff pattern (no leg or arm bend, very little body rotation) with verbal cues. She can hit the ball off a tee with a 5 iron three out of five trials, and the ball travels approximately 25 yards.

Soccer: Sue walks slowly and occasionally jogs to get the ball. She can kick with her toe so that ball travels 10'–15'. She can trap slow moving balls that are kicked directly to her. She does not understand team concepts, and often sits down in the middle of the field when tired or bored.

Volleyball: Sue can set and bump a ball that is tossed directly to her with verbal cues. She can serve a ball over the net from 10' away. She cannot hit the ball in the course of a game; she seems afraid of getting hit by the ball.

Basketball: Sue can dribble a ball several times while standing in place, but not while moving forward. She can make a regulation basket from 5' away (one out of five trials). She is able to demonstrate a chest and bounce pass with verbal cues from 10' away, and she can catch bounce passes (not chest passes) when ball is passed gently from 10' away. She does not understand team concepts and prefers to wander around the court.

Softball: Sue can hit a softball off a tee (not pitched) so that ball travels 15'–20'. She will jog to first base with verbal cues as well as to the other bases (she often needs someone to point her in the right direction). Sue can throw overhand (no stepping or body rotation) approximately 10'. Sue tries to bend over and pick up grounders and catch balls tossed directly to her from 10' away. She tends to sit down in the outfield, but will stay more focused with verbal cues when playing catcher.

Aerobics: Sue tries to follow the routine but tends to be out of sync compared to her peers. She does exert more effort in aerobics than any other activity, but she tires easily. (After 3–4 minutes, she stands and rests.) She has adequate flexibility and strength.

Weight   Sue can do six exercises on the Universal machine with verbal cues and occasional assistance
Training: for positioning. She needs assistance to set correct weight. Her strength is similar to that of her peers.

Present level of performance statement from IEP with reference to community-based recreation (Sue's parents took Sue to various recreation sites and reported results to her teacher.)

Tennis: (See previous assessment.) Sue reiterated her interest in tennis.

Aerobics: (See previous assessment.) Sue reiterated her interest in aerobics.

Mini-golf: Sue had some difficulty maneuvering her wheelchair through the miniature golf course, but was able independently to play all but three of the holes. Sue was not interested in miniature golf.

Bowling: Sue was able to hold a regulation ball and roll it using a regular pattern and grip. She was not very accurate and uninterested in learning how to bowl.

Karate: Sue was able to do all the upper body movements, and she was able to replace lower body movements with arm movements. Sue was not interested in karate.

Yoga: Sue was not interested in yoga, so she was not assessed in this area.

Once a long-term plan is in place, the next step is to write long-term goals that eventually lead to the student achieving the end of the long-term plan. Long-term goals are part of the IEP process and describe what specific skills a teacher expects a student to acquire in the course of a year. For example, a long-term plan for a particular student might be to play tennis upon graduation. A long-term goal for the student might be demonstrating the ability to hit a tennis ball using a

Table 4.4. Long-term plan, long-term goals, and short-term instructional objectives for Sue, a 15-year-old student with mental retardation

LONG-TERM PLAN: Sue will demonstrate the ability to participate independently (with occasional cues from peers as needed) in recreational softball and tennis as well as fitness activities at a local health club.

Long-Term Goal 1: Sue will improve her cardiovascular endurance.

Short-Term Instructional Objectives:

1. Sue will pedal a stationary Lifecycle at the University Health Club at level 2 maintaining an RPM level of 70 continuously for 20 minutes with verbal reinforcement every 5 minutes three out of four days.
2. Sue will participate in an aerobics class during regular physical education performing movements as best as she can so that her heart rate (as measured by a peer) will be 120–150 bpm for 25 minutes three out of four days.

Long-Term Goal 2: Sue will develop the skills needed to participate in modified and regulation individual and team sports.

Short-Term Instructional Objectives: (specific to softball)

1. Using a regulation softball bat and encouraged to "choke up" 2" (tape cue markers), Sue will hit a regulation softball off a tee so that ball rolls at least 60' (distance to first and third base) three out of four trials.
2. After hitting ball off tee, Sue will run to first base independently so that she arrives at first base in 7 seconds or less three out of four trials.
3. Sue will play catcher during a softball game demonstrating the following behaviors independently three out of four trials:
   a. put on face mask
   b. find correct position behind plate
   c. squat in correct position and maintain position for duration of each pitch
   d. move glove in direction of ball when ball is pitched

Long-Term Goal 3: Sue will demonstrate the ability to play doubles tennis with peers at a beginner's level.

Short-Term Instructional Objectives:

1. Sue will hit a backhand demonstrating the components listed below when ball is hit within 10' of her so that ball travels over net and into opposing players' court five out of ten trials 2 days in a row.
   Components of the backhand:
   —stand facing opposing player
   —move to ball
   —set up in sideways position
   —bring arm back horizontally across body so that head of racquet is behind body
   —shift weight and step forward with front foot
   —bring arm forward horizontally and contact ball slightly ahead of body
   —follow through with arm and racquet moving toward opposing player
2. Sue will hit a forehand demonstrating the components listed below when ball is hit within 10' of her so that ball travels over net and into opposing player's court five out of ten trials 2 days in a row.
   Components of the forehand:
   —stand facing opposing player
   —move to ball
   —set up in sideways position
   —bring arm back horizontally away from body so that head of racquet is behind body
   —shift weight and step forward with front foot
   —bring arm forward horizontally and contact ball slightly ahead of body
   —follow through with arm and racquet moving toward opposing player

Long-Term Goal 4[a]: Sue will develop the skills needed to participate in community-based leisure activities in inclusive environments.

Short-Term Instructional Objectives:

1. Sue will enter the University Health Club, show her ID card, locate locker room, put her gym bag in a locker, lock the locker, then locate the weight room using natural cues only (including asking health club staff for assistance) with 100% accuracy 4 out of 5 days.
2. Sue will follow picture cards and complete a 6-machine Nautilus weight training circuit performing the exercise for each machine correctly and completing one set of 10–12 repetitions per machine independently (or asking YMCA staff for assistance) with 100% accuracy 4 out of 5 days.

(continued)

Table 4.4.   (*continued*)

3. Sue will demonstrate appropriate behavior in the locker room and in the weight room as noted by: (a) changing clothes quickly without acting inappropriately, (b) only saying "hi" to strangers or responding appropriately when a stranger initiates a conversation in the locker room, and (c) not acting inappropriately or talking to others while others are working out unless others initiate conversation in the weight room 100% of the time 4 out of 5 days.

ᵃSue participates in community-based recreation twice per week instead of regular physical education.

backhand strike when the ball is hit to the student at a moderate speed. A student with a more significant disability might have participating in a community aerobic/conditioning class with minimal assistance as part of the long-term plan, and the long-term goal for this student might be to demonstrate the ability to sustain movements and to engage in appropriate behavior for the first 10 minutes of a 45-minute aerobics class. Long-term goals should be based on assessment results and in particular a student's present level of ability in a particular activity. (See Table 4.4 for an example.)

Once long-term goals are in place, the next step is to write short-term instructional objectives that lead to acquisition of the long-term goals. Short-term instructional objectives also are part of the IEP process and usually are written in anticipation of the student achieving a particular objective in 2–3 months. In addition, these objectives are written in behavioral (measurable) terms so that any observer could immediately tell if the student has acquired a particular objective. (See Table 4.4 for an example.) It should be noted that at this point in the process we are not concerned with where the student will work on the goals and objectives or how much support or special equipment the student will need. Rather, we are only concerned that the overall plan and specific goals and objectives have been prioritized for this student and reflect his or her present level of performance, age, skills needed now, and what skills will be needed in the future.

2.   *Analyze the regular physical education curriculum.* Each student has been evaluated and a long-term plan including long-term goals and short-term instructional objectives has been established. The next step is to determine if the student's individual program matches the regular curriculum. This step requires a careful analysis of the regular physical education curriculum, including an analysis of the yearly plans for various grade levels, unit plans and daily lesson plans for specific activities, and the general teaching style of the regular physical educator. This information can then be used to determine when a particular student can work on his or her individual goals and when alternative activities might be needed (i.e., which activities in regular physical education directly match the student's IEP objectives, which activities somewhat match the student's IEP, and which activities do not match the student's IEP and require alternative activities) (see Figure 4.2). Note that no effort is made at this point to detail specific ways to accommodate a student in the regular program or how to work on specific IEP goals and objectives. Such information will be determined later in the process. At this point, we just want to get a general idea of how well the student's IEP fits into the regular physical education curriculum.

Table 4.5 contains a yearly plan for a typical second-grade physical education program with initial considerations for including John, a student who is blind, and Table 4.6 contains a yearly plan for a typical 10th-grade physical education program with initial considerations for including Sue, a student with severe mental retardation. Note that the activities in regular physical education at the lower elementary level (kindergarten through third grade) are generally going to match the goals and objectives for most students with disabilities. That is, most elementary-age students need some foundational skills before they can apply these skills to popular sports and recreational activities. In the case of John, who is blind, he needs to work on understanding movement concepts and developing skillful locomotor and manipulative patterns. These goals match very nicely with the regular program (even though he may need special accommodations to par-

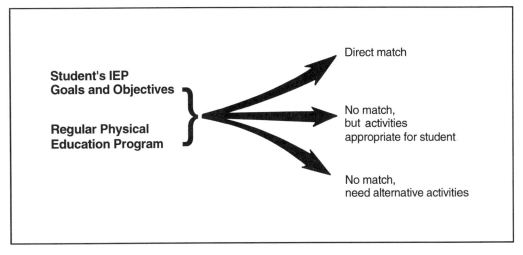

Figure 4.2. Possible outcomes of analysis of regular physical education curriculum.

ticipate and receive instruction). Even when his IEP does not directly match what the other students are doing (e.g., gymnastics and rhythms), these activities are deemed important enough and beneficial enough to John that it is recommended that he participate in these activities with his peers.

The story is a little different for middle school and high school students. A quick glance at Sue's IEP in relation to the regular 10th-grade curriculum reveals that she can work on her IEP goals while her peers participate in the tennis unit in September, aerobics unit in December, weight training unit in February, and softball unit in May. The other units do not match Sue's IEP goals, so Sue may need to participate in alternative activities (i.e., her IEP goals and objectives) while her peers participate in these other activities. For example, when the class is playing soccer in October, Sue could go to the tennis court to work on her tennis goals with peers rotating in to assist and play with her. Similarly, Sue could work in the weight room with various peers in March when the class is working on field hockey and lacrosse. However, Sue certainly could benefit from the endurance and stretching activities in track and field (perhaps walking around the track with peers at a vigorous pace and participating in warm-ups), so she could be included in this unit.

Table 4.5. Yearly plan for second-grade physical education

September	■ Rules; introduction of general movement concepts
October	■ Movement concepts and locomotor patterns
November	■ Throwing and catching
December	■ Striking and kicking
January	■ Movement concepts and locomotor patterns
February	□ Rhythm
March	□ Tumbling
April	□ Throwing and catching
May	■ Striking and kicking
June	■ Review all skills

Note: Movement concepts and locomotor patterns will be incorporated via warm-up activities in all units.

■ = Activity directly matches John's IEP goals.
□ = Activity does not directly match, but is appropriate for John to participate.

Table 4.6.   Yearly plan for 10th-grade physical education

September	■ Tennis
October	−Soccer
November	−Volleyball
December	■ Aerobics (females)/Wrestling (males)
January	−Basketball
February	■ Weight Training
March	−Field Hockey/Lacrosse
April	□ Track and Field
May	■ Softball
June	□ Golf

■ = Activity directly matches Sue's IEP goals.
□ = Activity does not directly match, but is appropriate for Sue to participate.
− = Activity does not match Sue's IEP goals and is inappropriate for Sue.

Similarly, Sue could participate in golf with her peers to see if she enjoys this activity. (Golf may replace tennis as a lifetime sport.)

The important point is that inclusion does not necessarily mean that students with disabilities have to do the same thing that their peers without disabilities do. While students without disabilities might be able to afford being "exposed" to a variety of activities in regular physical education and still leave the program with the ability to participate successfully in two or more lifetime leisure activities, students with disabilities will only acquire critical lifetime leisure skills if training focuses intensely on these skills (Wessel & Kelly, 1986). Thus, decisions need to be made as to what activities will be most beneficial for the student and which ones really will not help the student achieve IEP goals. This does not mean that a student will require programming away from regular physical education. Sue certainly can participate in warm-up activities with her peers during regular physical education. Additionally, while Sue's peers are working on their activities such as basketball in the gym, Sue could be practicing hitting a tennis ball back and forth with a peer or hitting a softball off a tee with a peer in the corner of the gym or in the hall. Peers without disabilities can be rotated into the station to assist and participate with Sue so that Sue still receives the social benefits of integration while working on her specific IEP goals.

Once there is a general idea of what is going to be taught throughout the year and when it will be taught, the next step is to analyze each physical education unit that matches the student's program. Unit plans usually can be obtained from regular physical educators a week or so prior to the introduction of that unit. (More seasoned teachers may have their unit plans from previous years in a file for your use.) Table 4.7 contains an example of a 10th-grade softball unit plan. An analysis of the softball unit suggests that Sue can work on many of the softball skills highlighted in her IEP during this unit (with modifications as needed). In addition, Sue could easily be accommodated in the modified game that includes peers without disabilities. However, some physical education programs at the high school level only work on the actual game rather than skills. It would be much more difficult to integrate Sue into such a program since her softball skills are still very weak. By analyzing the unit ahead of time (even 1 week before the unit begins), you can begin to make decisions about how Sue will work on her goals during the unit, including what modifications might be needed to make Sue more successful. Again, more detailed accommodations and modifications will be developed later in the process.

Finally, an analysis of a general daily lesson plan should be conducted so that you can further determine where the student's IEP goals and objectives can be implemented and where the student may have difficulty with specific activities. Again, most regular physical educators can quickly outline their typical daily lesson plan. Most physical education lesson plans begin with some type

Table 4.7. Sample 4-week softball unit plan

WEEK 1

Introduction to game
- equipment
- field dimensions
- basic rules
- basic concepts and positions

Warm-up activities
- stretching major muscles of upper and lower body
- strengthening abdominals, arms, and legs
- cardiovascular endurance activities (e.g., jogging around the base path)

Introduction to basic softball skills (emphasis on learning correct movements)
- striking
- fielding
- throwing
- base running

Lead-up games to work on skills
- base running relays, hot-box, 500
- pepper, 500
- home run derby, spot hitting

WEEK 2

Continue warm-up activities (have students lead warm-ups)

Team concepts and team strategies
- base running strategies; hitting ball to various places in field; hitting cut-off person
- view video of softball game that shows these techniques

Continue refinement of skills
- throwing from greater distances; throwing with varying force
- fielding balls hit to the side; fielding high flies in the outfield
- hitting faster-pitched balls; hitting balls in different parts of strike zone

WEEK 3

Continue warm-up activities (have students lead warm-ups)

Review of all softball skills

Introduce games:
- 10 v. 10 with outfield players practicing throwing balls back and forth during down time and batting team practicing hitting balls off a tee behind backstop while waiting
- modified game of softball for students who have less skill (including students without disabilities who have limited softball skills)

WEEK 4

Continue warm-up activities (have students lead warm-ups)

Continue to review softball skills

Continue games with less instruction (both regulation and modified)

Some anticipated accommodations for Sue:
1. have peer assist her during warm-ups (demonstration and occasional physical prompt)
2. have peer assist Sue as she moves from station to station and at station as needed
3. have adapted physical education specialist write activities for Sue to do at each station
4. use smaller ball (tennis ball) for throwing and catching with mitt
5. use lighter bat (whiffle ball bat) and have ball on tee for striking
6. have Sue play in outfield with a peer during games
7. allow Sue to run to a closer base when running to first and allow a peer to run with her around other bases until she understands where to go
8. have Sue play in recreational, noncompetitive game

of warm-up activity followed by some type of skill activity, which is then followed by some type of game activity. In addition, physical education at the middle school and high school levels will include locker room activities (e.g., dressing, showering, grooming) immediately prior to and after each physical education class. Table 4.8 outlines a typical daily lesson plan for a 10th-grade class with considerations for Sue.

Table 4.8.   General daily lesson plan for 10th-grade physical education with comments regarding Sue[a]

1. *Locker room* (change into physical education uniform) (approximately 5 minutes)
2. *Squads/Attendance* (students sit in squads while attendance is taken) (2 minutes)
3. *Warm-ups* (students are led by teacher in several stretching, strength, and aerobic activities) (7–10 minutes)
4. *Skill focus* (work on specific skills related to team or individual sports—as little as 5 minutes to as many as 30 minutes depending on where we are in unit. The beginning of the unit focuses more on skill development whereas the end of the unit focuses more on games)
5. *Games* (play lead-up and regulation games related to team or individual sports (5–30 minutes)
6. *Locker room* (shower, grooming, put on street clothes) (approximately 10 minutes)

[a]Sue will need assistance in locker room both prior to and after class. (Teacher assistant can assist initially, but peers whose lockers are near Sue's will eventually learn how to assist Sue.) Sue should be able to participate in warm-ups with minimal cues from peers. Sue will need modified ways to practice skills and to participate in group activities. (Have APE specialist or team provide suggestions.)

An alternative way to determine what activities take place in regular physical education is called an *ecological inventory* (Brown et al., 1979). An ecological inventory provides a detailed analysis of all the activities students without disabilities typically do during a particular activity (in this case, physical education). The analysis begins with identifying subenvironments and activities that take place within each subenvironment. This is followed by a "discrepancy analysis" that determines how the student with disabilities currently performs each activity and provides suggestions for modifications so that the student could be more successful. Figure 4.3 provides an example of an ecological inventory with discrepancy analysis. While the ecological inventory is more difficult to develop compared to a simple daily lesson plan, the information from the inventory provides much more detailed information regarding daily routines and potential problems students with disabilities will have with regular activities. Special education teachers often have experience developing ecological inventories and, with the assistance of the regular physical educator, can quickly develop such an inventory for the team.

One final analysis of the regular curriculum is how the particular *teaching style* a particular teacher uses affects the program. (See Mosston, 1981, for a more thorough review of teaching styles.) There are many different teaching styles, but most revolve around two basic types: a *direct approach* and an *indirect approach*.

In the direct approach, each student performs the same basic movement under the direct guidance of the physical educator. Each student knows exactly what is expected of him or her, how particular skills are to be performed, when to perform these skills, and where to perform these skills. Obviously such an approach provides the teacher tremendous control over a class yet still allows for some individualization. However, creativity and the process of "learning how to learn" or discovering the best way to perform a particular skill are not provided in this approach. For example, a teacher might be working on the overhand throw with a second-grade class. She might have all students stand a certain distance from the wall and, on her verbal cue, shift weight to the back foot, reach back with the throwing arm, shift weight forward, rotate the body, and throw the ball to the wall. Some teachers who use this approach are quite inflexible, expecting all children to perform a particular movement the same way, at the same time, and with the same requirements for success. Obviously, such an approach would not be very accommodating for a student who has a disability. In contrast, teachers can use the direct approach and still accomodate varying abilities. For example, in the throwing example above, a teacher might allow some students to stand closer to or farther away from the wall, give some students larger balls and other students smaller balls, or even allow a student with cerebral palsy to throw using a different pattern.

In the indirect approach, students are encouraged to discover the best way to perform certain skills by actively exploring and experimenting with equipment, rules, distances, and patterns. Such an approach allows for more creative learning and encourages students to problem-solve.

Ecological Inventory with Discrepancy Analysis

Student's name: John Schwartz   Student's birthdate: 8–10–82   Teacher: M. Block (APE specialist)

Environment: RPE—Soccer   Initiation of program: 6–21–92   Suggested assistant: Steve Smith
                                                                                    (peer tutor)

	What are the steps that a person without disabilities uses?	What assistance does the student with disabilities currently need?	What adaptations or levels of assistance might help this student?
Subenvironment: Locker room			
Activity 1:	Locate locker room.	V	Teach student to use natural cues on wall; add arrows on walls.
Activity 2:	Enter locker room.	I	None needed
Activity 3:	Locate empty locker.	V	Teach student to ID lockers without locks; color-code one locker.
Activity 4:	Take off clothes.	PP	Wear pull-on clothes; practice dressing at home; use Velcro instead of buttons.
Activity 5:	Place clothes in locker.	I	None needed
Activity 6:	Put on exercise clothes.	P	Use pull-on clothes; equip shoes with special ties; use Velcro instead of buttons.
Activity 7:	Lock locker.	P	Repeated practice; perhaps longer lock or key lock might be easier than combination lock.

(continued)

Figure 4.3. Sample ecological inventory with discrepancy analysis for 10th-grade physical education. (For more information on this chart, see Block, M.E. [1994]. All kids can have physical education the regular way. In M.S. Moon [Ed.], *Making school and community recreation fun for everyone: Places and ways to integrate.* Baltimore: Paul H. Brookes Publishing Co.) (Key: see page 66.)

Figure 4.3. *(continued)*

	What are the steps that a person without disabilities uses?	What assistance does the student with disabilities currently need?	What adaptations or levels of assistance might help this student?
Subenvironment: Gym—Attendance			
Activity 1:	Locate gym.	V	Natural cues on walls; put extra cues on walls.
Activity 2:	Find squad and sit down.	V	Teach student to ID members of squad; have squad members cue student if he appears lost.
Activity 3:	Sit quietly with squad.	I	None needed
Subenvironment: Gym—Warm-up			
Activity 1:	Stand up with squad.	V	Have peers provide cues.
Activity 2:	Perform 10 jumping jacks.	VP	Have peers provide cues; do jumping jacks with arms only.
Activity 3:	Perform sitting-leg stretch.	VP	Have peers provide cues; have peer tutor provide physical assistance as needed.
Activity 4:	Perform 10 sit-ups.	VP	Pair up with peer tutor; perform 5 rather than 10.
Activity 5:	Perform 10 push-ups.	VP	Have peers provide cues; perform modified, knee push-ups.
Activity 6:	Run continuously for 3 minutes.	V	Have peers provide cues; alternate run/walk for 10 minutes.

(continued)

Figure 4.3. *(continued)*

	What are the steps that a person without disabilities uses?	What assistance does the student with disabilities currently need?	What adaptations or levels of assistance might help this student?
Subenvironment: **Gym—Soccer stations**			
Activity 1:	Locate squad and station.	V	Have peers provide cues.
Activity 2:	Practice shooting.	VP	Shoot from closer distance; shoot at wider goal; use lighter ball.
Activity 3:	Wait turn.	I	None needed
Activity 4:	Move to next station.	V	Have peers provide cues.
Activity 5:	Passing/trapping	VP	Stand closer to peer; use partially deflated ball; use tape markings on foot to cue correct contact point; pass to stationary partner.
Activity 6:	Wait turn.	I	None needed
Activity 7:	Move to next station.	V	Have peers provide cues.
Activity 8:	Dribbling	VP	Dribble with partially deflated ball or Nerf ball; work on dribbling straight ahead without obstacles; work on walking, then jogging, while dribbling.
Activity 9:	Wait turn.	I	None needed
Activity 10:	Go back to original squads.	V	Have peers provide cues.

(continued)

Figure 4.3. *(continued)*

	What are the steps that a person without disabilities uses?	What assistance does the student with disabilities currently need?	What adaptations or levels of assistance might help this student?
Subenvironment: Soccer game			
Activity 1:	Listen to instructions by teacher.	V	Have peer tutor reexplain rules in simpler terms.
Activity 2:	Put on assigned pinny.	PP	Have peer provide assistance.
Activity 3:	Go to assigned position.	V	Have peers provide cues.
Activity 4:	Play game.	VP	John will play a wing fullback, and a non-skilled peer will play opposite him.
Activity 5:	Watch flow of game.	V	Have peer tutor provide cues.
Activity 6:	Interact with teammates.	V	Have peer provide cues.
Activity 7:	Shake hands with other team.	V	Have peers provide cues.
Activity 8:	Take off pinny.	PP	Have peer assist student.
Activity 9:	Put pinny away.	V	Have peers provide cues.
Activity 10:	Walk to locker room.	V	Have peers provide cues.
Subenvironment: Locker room			
Activity 1:	Locate locker room.	V	Use natural cues on wall; use additional wall cues.
Activity 2:	Enter locker room.	I	None needed
Activity 3:	Locate locker.	V	Tape colored sign on locker; have peer provide cues as needed.

(continued)

Figure 4.3. *(continued)*

	What are the steps that a person without disabilities uses?	What assistance does the student with disabilities currently need?	What adaptations or levels of assistance might help this student?
Activity 4:	Take off gym clothes.	PP	Have peer provide assistance as needed.
Activity 5:	Place exercise clothes in gym bag.	I	None needed
Activity 6:	Get towel, soap, and shampoo.	V	Have peer tutor provide cues as needed.
Activity 7:	Locate shower.	V	Place extra sign on wall, have peer provide cues.
Activity 8:	Turn on water and modulate water temperature.	PP	Practice starting with cold and gradually add hot; have peer tutor assist.
Activity 9:	Shampoo hair and wash self.	PP	Start from top and work down; practice at home; have peer provide assistance.
Activity 10:	Turn off shower and collect personal items.	PP	Step away from water, turn off hot, then cold; have peer assist as needed.
Activity 11:	Dry self.	V	Start from top and work down; practice; peer can give verbal cues as needed.
Activity 12:	Locate and use deodorant.	V	Have peer provide cues as needed.

(continued)

Figure 4.3. *(continued)*

	What are the steps that a person without disabilities uses?	What assistance does the student with disabilities currently need?	What adaptations or levels of assistance might help this student?
Activity 13:	Put on street clothes.	P	Use pull-on clothes; use special ties for shoes; have peer assist as needed.
Activity 14:	Go to mirror and comb hair/check appearance.	V	Start from top and work down; cue in on hair combed and shirt tucked in; shoes on correct feet; peer gives cues as needed.
Activity 15:	Place all personal belongings in gym bag.	V	Teach student to check area and locker; use picture cue card; peer gives cues.
Activity 16:	Leave locker room and go to class.	V	Use natural cues on wall; use additional wall cues; have peer tutor assist as needed.

Key: I   = independent
      V   = verbal cues or reminder
      PP   = partial physical assistance
      P+ = physical assistance (student tries to help)
      P   = physical assistance (student is passive)
      P− = physical assistance (student fights assistance)

However, it may be more difficult controlling a class using an indirect approach, learning specific skills often takes longer compared to a direct approach, and some students may never problem-solve the movement problem in the way you prefer (e.g., some may never throw overhand even though you had hoped that they would discover that is the best way to throw a small ball for distance). Indirect instruction tends to be very accommodating to students with disabilities, particularly students with physical disabilities who are encouraged to discover their best way to perform particular movements. On the other hand, such an approach can be confusing to students with mental retardation, and the freedom allowed in such programs can promote behavior problems in students with emotional disturbances.

At this point in the process it is best to get a feeling for the teaching approach used in physical education and how this approach matches the unique abilities of a student with disabilities whom you plan to include. Ideally, a student will be placed in a class in which the teacher uses an approach that matches the student's learning style. Realistically, this may not happen. Still, regular physical educators can be encouraged to teach the group of students one way and a particular student with disabilities another way. For example, a teacher might use a command approach when teaching throwing, but at the same time she can encourage a student who has cerebral palsy to explore different ways to throw to see which method is most effective given the student's unique movement abilities. (See chap. 6, this volume, for more detail on various teaching approaches.)

3. *Determine modifications needed for regular physical education.* At this point you should know each student's present level of performance, long-term plan including long-term goals and short-term instructional objectives, and generally where the student will be able to work on these goals and objectives within the regular physical education program. The next step is to determine specific modifications that will be needed to implement each student's individual program within the regular physical education setting. Rainforth et al. (1992) outlined several questions that should guide the decision process when determining specific instructional modifications for students with disabilities. (See Table 4.9.)

3a. *How often will instruction occur?* Students with disabilities may need more instruction than their peers without disabilities to learn even simple skills. Therefore, one of the first decisions to be made in terms of modifications is how often the student with disabilities will receive instruction. For example, if elementary-age students without disabilities receive physical education twice per week, you may want to request that a student with significant disabilities receive regular physical education with peers without disabilities twice per week plus twice per week working in a small group of students (composed of both children with and without disabilities) who need extra help on specific skills. Another possibility is working with the student one-on-one on Mondays to review the activities that will take place during the week. You can give the student extra practice on skills and explain and practice some of the activities that will take place. (See Wessel & Kelly, 1986, for a detailed description of how to determine how often a student should receive physical education.)

The question of "how often" also can include how often an adapted physical education specialist team-teaches with the regular physical educator or how often particular support personnel come in and assist the student with disabilities. For example, a speech teacher may come to regular physical education once a week to assist a student with autism in physical education activities as well as in communication. Having this professional assist the student (with guidance from the regular educator and/or APE specialist) may optimize the student's time in regular physical education, thus giving him or her even more instruction and practice in critical skills. Similarly, the adapted physical education specialist may come into regular physical education once a week to work with the student along with other students without disabilities who need extra help. Such a team approach allows the regular physical educator time to work with a smaller, more skilled group of students without disabilities while the adapted physical educator works with a smaller group of less skilled students (including the student with disabilities).

Table 4.9.   Considerations when determining a student's individual instructional program

1. How often will the student receive instruction?
2. Where will the student receive instruction?
3. How will the student be prepared for instruction?
4. What instructional modifications are needed to elicit desired performance?
5. What curricular adaptations are needed to enhance desired performance?

Adapted from Rainforth, York, & Macdonald (1992).

3b. *Where will the student receive instruction*? The second related question is where instruction will occur. Since our focus is on inclusion, in most cases instruction will occur in regular physical education. Activities that are directly related to the student's IEP can be modified so that the student can work on these goals in a safe and successful setting. Even when regular physical education activities do not match the student's IEP, alternative activities can be presented within the regular setting. For example, an elementary-age student who is working on independent walking can practice this skill (with assistance as needed) while his or her peers without disabilities work on kicking skills. In either case above, you should note where specific IEP objectives (including objectives from other team members) can be embedded into the typical daily physical education routine. (See Figures 4.4 and 4.5 for examples.)

In other cases, regular physical education may not be the most appropriate for particular students, and alternative settings should be identified that include interaction with peers without disabilities. The example above suggests one solution in which a student with disabilities needs extra physical education and receives these services in a small group that includes students without disabilities. Similarly, students with autistic-like behaviors who cannot deal with the stimulating environment of a large gymnasium and 20 or more peers running around may need to begin their programs in a quieter, less-threatening setting. Such a setting may be in the cafeteria or in a work room with one or two peers without disabilities. Gradually, the student can be weaned into the more stimulating regular physical education setting. Finally, older students should receive part of their physical education instruction (i.e., instruction in community-based recreation) at local recreation facilities such as health clubs, bowling alleys, and recreation centers. Again, students without disabilities can be included in these outings to make the experience more normalizing and to promote appropriate social skills. Decisions regarding how often and where to teach particular skills, like all decisions, should be student-based (i.e., what is best for the student). Factors such as age and severity of disability, availability of support personnel, and availability of transportation and recreation facilities in the community will no doubt influence the team's decision as to how often and where the student will receive community-based physical education.

One cautionary note here. Other team members may wish to target physical education as a good place to work on their goals. For example, a physical therapist might ask physical education staff to do particular stretching activities during physical education for a student with cerebral palsy, a speech teacher may ask physical education staff to encourage a particular student to practice answering "wh" questions (*who, what, where, why*), or an occupational therapist might ask you to assign a peer to help a student with spina bifida in the locker room so that the student can work on independent dressing and undressing skills. While these requests are often appropriate and easily implemented by physical education staff, others' particular goals should not take precedence over specific physical education goals. For example, some special education teachers integrate their students with disabilities into regular physical education to improve social and communication skills without regard to whether the students improve in physical education/recreation. Such teachers may push to have their students participate with their peers without disabilities in all regular physical education activities including activities that you as a physical educator do not feel are safe or appropriate (e.g., an 18-year-old student who is blind participating in field hockey when your goal is to have this student acquire skills needed to participate independently in beep baseball, weight training, aerobics, swimming, and hitting golf balls at a driving range). In such cases you must make it perfectly clear that participating in regular physical education activities just so the students can talk with their peers is not good use of their physical education period. Furthermore, by participating in field hockey this student is missing out on necessary practice time in his targeted activities. Again, most requests are reasonable and can be easily accommodated, but make sure all team members understand that the purpose of physical education is to teach students specific motor, fitness, sport, and recreation skills and should not be considered a "dumping ground" for everyone else's goals and objectives.

Activity in physical education	Physical education IEP objectives (written generally)				
	Improve endurance	Improve strength	Develop tennis skills	Develop softball skills	Access local YMCA
1. Walks to locker room.	X				
2. Changes clothes, puts clothes in locker.					
3. Goes to squad.					
4. Sits in squad (does sit-ups with peer).		X			
5. Participates in warm-ups.		X			X
6. Participates in skill activities (choosing stations).		X	X	X	
7. Participates in game.		X	X	X	
8. Walks to locker.	X				
9. Showers, changes clothes.					
10. Walks to class.	X	X			

Figure 4.4. Selected objectives for physical education IEP and where they will be embedded within the regular program.

	IEP objectives					
Activity in physical education	Walking faster	Appropriate behavior with peers	Dressing/undressing	Say "hi"/"bye"	Making choices	Follow one-cue directions
1. Walks to locker room.	X	X				
2. Changes clothes, puts clothes in locker.		X	X			X
3. Goes to squad.	X	X				X
4. Sits in squad (does sit-ups with peer).		X		X		X
5. Participates in warm-ups.	X				X	
6. Participates in skill activities (choosing stations).	X	X			X	X
7. Participates in game.		X				X
8. Walks to locker.	X	X				X
9. Showers, changes clothes.	X	X	X			X
10. Walks to class.	X	X		X		X

Figure 4.5. Selected objectives from IEP (including IEP goals from other team members) and where they will be embedded within the regular program.

3c. *How will the student be prepared for instruction?* Preparation for instruction can involve several factors. For students with physical disabilities such as cerebral palsy, preparation might include relaxation techniques, techniques to normalize muscle tone, range-of-motion activities, and positioning to facilitate active, independent movement (Rainforth et al., 1992). Physical educators can incorporate specific range-of-motion and relaxation activities in their warm-ups. (Either the entire class can do them or the student can do these activities while his or her peers do other forms of warm-ups.) Such exercises can help the student demonstrate more functional arm or leg use during physical education. In other situations, preparation may take place back in the classroom. For example, a student with a significant physical disability normally sits in a wheelchair during academic classes. While sitting in the chair might be the best position for this student in terms of academic work such as using eye-gaze when working on the computer, sitting in a chair may not be the best position for functional arm and hand use. For physical education this student might be better positioned in a prone stander or side-lyer so that he or she will have more range of motion in the arms for pushing balls down a ramp. (See Table 4.10 for an example of a positioning decision.) The student's physical therapist would be the best resource to determine how to help the student warm up and what the best position is for students during certain activities. Therapists also can develop easy-to-follow picture cards that show you how to warm up and

Table 4.10. Considerations in selecting positions for two sample activities for students with significant physical disabilities

	Activity	
Questions to ask	Warm-up exercises	Basketball play
1. What positions do peers without disabilities use when they engage in the activity?	Lying down, standing, moving	Standing, moving
2. Which of these positions allow easy access to activity materials and equipment?	Sitting better than standing	Standing better than sitting
3. Do the positions allow for proximity to peers?	Yes, sitting on mat with peers	Yes, stander is easy to move near peers
4. Do the positions promote efficient movement as needed to perform the task?	Sitting on mat allows participation in many warm-up activities	Standing allows free movement of hands for holding/pushing
5. What positions provide alternatives to over-used postures and equipment?	Usually sits in chair, stretching on mat is good alternative	Usually sits in chair, stander is good alternative
6. If positioning equipment is required, is it unobtrusive, cosmetically acceptable, and not physically isolating?	No equipment needed	Prone stander, while fairly obtrusive, is nicely decorated; peers are used to it.
7. Is the positioning equipment safe and easy to handle?	None needed	Should be placed in stander by therapist or teacher, easy to move
8. Is the equipment individually selected and modified to individual learner needs?	None needed	Fit to student by physical therapist
9. Is the equipment available and easily transported to natural environments?	None needed	Easily wheeled into gym
Final position	*On mat*	*Prone stander*

Adapted from Rainforth, York, & Macdonald (1992).

position students. In some cases, the teacher or teacher assistant can warm up the student and place him or her in particular pieces of equipment prior to physical education.

Another consideration for preparing students for instruction is working with students who have behavior problems. Some students may have difficulty transitioning from quiet, classroom activities to the stimulation of the gymnasium. These students may need to be reminded several times that physical education is their next class. In addition, some students such as those with autism may need strategies to help them cope with transition, such as being the first or last person in the gym, sitting in a smaller squad, and sitting at the end of a squad in order to watch the first few warm-up activities. Students who have behavior problems might need to be reminded of the rules of the gymnasium and any specific consequences/reinforcers that may be presented during physical education. Such simple reminders prior to entering the gymnasium often help the student refocus on appropriate behaviors. A concerted effort by the classroom teacher and physical educator to make transitions smoother for students with disabilities can prevent many behavior problems.

3d. *What instructional modifications are needed?* There are many factors related to instruction that can be modified to accommodate students with disabilities in regular physical education. Such factors as teaching style, length of instruction, types of cues given, and type of structure are just a few instructional factors under the control of the teacher. (See Table 4.11 for a more complete list.) Making simple adjustments in how you present various aspects of your lesson can help students with disabilities be more motivated, more successful, to follow directions, and to improve the quality of their practice and rate of skill development. The team should work together to determine how instruction will be modified to meet the unique needs of students with disabilities.

For example, one of the easiest and best ways to individualize instruction for students with disabilities is to vary how you prompt and communicate with students. Some students will respond quite well to verbal cues given to the whole class while other students may need extra verbal cues, demonstrations, or even physical assistance to understand directions and perform skills correctly. One consideration when instructing students is level of cues presented or "prompt hierarchy" (Snell & Zirpoli, 1987). Prompts are cues given to students that help them make responses they do not or cannot do without these cues. Instructional prompts range from nonintrusive prompts such as a student following natural cues in the environment (student sees peers stand up and run around the gym, and the student quickly stands up and runs with peers) to intrusive prompts such as physical assistance (physically helping the student hold a bat and then strike a ball off a tee). (See Table 4.12 for a list of prompts ranked from least to most intrusive.) Each type of prompt can be further broken down into levels. For example, physical assistance can vary from

Table 4.11. Factors to consider in making instructional modifications to accommodate students with disabilities[a]

Teaching style (direct, indirect)

Class format and size of group (small/large group; stations/whole class instruction)

Level of methodology (verbal cues, demonstrations, physical assistance)

Starting/stopping signals

Time of day when student is included (some do better in morning v. afternoon)

Duration (of instruction, expected participation, length of activities)

Order of learning (in what order will you present material and instruction?)

Instructional setting (indoors/outdoors; part of gym/whole gym)

Eliminate distractors (extra lighting, temperature, etc.)

Provide structure (set organization of instruction each day)

Level of difficulty (control complexity of instruction, presentation of information, organization)

Level of motivation (make setting and activities more motivating)

[a]See Chapter 6, this volume, for an in-depth discussion of these modifications.

Table 4.12.   Least- to most-intrusive level of prompts

Natural cues in environment
⇓
Verbal cues
⇓
Pointing/gestures
⇓
Picture cards
⇓
Demonstration
⇓
Physical prompting
⇓
Physical assistance

physical assistance in which the student passively allows the teacher to help him, physical assistance in which the student resists assistance, and physical assistance in which the student actively tries to perform movement. Ideally, students will follow natural prompts in the environment, but many students with disabilities will need extra prompts to understand directions and instruction.

Physical educators should find out from the speech therapist or the special education teacher which level of prompt is needed for a student to understand directions and instruction. However, most physical educators and peers will quickly discover on their own how best to prompt students. For example, while the class receives verbal instructions on the activities of the day, a student with mental retardation may need to have directions repeated in a simplified way by a peer, or the peer may demonstrate what the teacher conveyed verbally. At a skill station, some students can read directions on how to perform various skills while a student with mental retardation can use picture cards. Students should be given the level of prompt that will ensure their success in the activity. In addition, if a student will not be able to respond to a verbal cue or demonstration, then start with physical prompts or assistance so that the student will not fail the task or be confused. For example, if a student with cerebral palsy needs physical assistance to toss a ball, it makes no sense to give him a verbal cue first, then point, then gesture, then demonstrate, then touch, and finally physically assist the student. Time will be wasted, and the student will probably experience failure for at least five out of six cues. However, since the ultimate goal is to have students follow natural cues whenever possible, an attempt should be made to fade extra prompts systematically during the course of the program. For example, students with mental retardation can learn to focus on natural cues in the locker room at the YMCA for locating an empty locker and eventually walk to the weight room independently.

Another consideration when instructing students with disabilities is to determine how they will communicate with you. Again, many students with disabilities will be able to respond like their peers without disabilities with clear, concise speech. However, some students will speak in one- or two-word sentences; other students may communicate with gestures or signs; still others may communicate by pointing to pictures or via facilitated communication; and still others may use sophisticated computer-assisted speech synthesizers or keyboards. Regardless of how a student communicates, it is important that you understand each student's mode of communication. This does not mean that you necessarily have to learn sign language or how to facilitate a student. Still, you should discuss each student's communication skills with the speech therapist or the special education teacher so that you can effectively communicate with each student who participates in your program. (See chap. 6, this volume, for more specific suggestions for modifying instruction.)

3e. *What curricular adaptations will be used to enhance performance*? Perhaps the greatest challenge to the physical education team is finding ways to accommodate students with disabilities who cannot perform the skill the same way or at the same level as their peers. The goal at this level is to create adaptations that allow the student to participate and acquire skills in a safe, successful, and challenging environment.

There are many ways to adapt specific situations, skills, or activities to enhance a person's performance. For some, adaptations might be as simple as giving a student with limited strength a lighter bat. For other students, such as students with visual impairments, a simple adaptation might involve assigning a peer to assist in retrieving balls. Still other students, such as those with more significant disabilities, may need special equipment such as ramps, special switches, and major changes to the rules of games as well as physical assistance to participate successfully in regular physical education. Chapters 6 and 7 in this text provide an extensive review of specific strategies for modifying the curriculum to accommodate students with disabilities in regular physical education. (See Tables 4.13 and 4.14 for a list of some of these strategies.) Suggestions include: 1) accommodating students who have problems with fitness, 2) accommodating students

Table 4.13. Curricular adaptations to accommodate individuals with specific limitations[a]

A. *Does the student have limited strength, power, or endurance?*
   1. Lower targets.
   2. Reduce distance/playing field.
   3. Reduce weight/size of striking implements, balls, or projectiles.
   4. Allow student to sit or lie down while playing.
   5. Use partially deflated balls or suspended balls.
   6. Decrease activity time/increase rest time.
   7. Reduce speed of game/increase distance for students without disabilities.

B. *Does the student have limited balance?*
   1. Lower center of gravity.
   2. Keep as much of body in contact with the surface as possible.
   3. Widen base of support.
   4. Increase width of beams to be walked (in gymnastics unit).
   5. Extend arms for balance.
   6. Use carpeted rather than slick surfaces.
   7. Teach students how to fall.
   8. Provide a bar to assist with stability.
   9. Teach student to use eyes optimally.
   10. Determine whether balance problems are related to health problems.

C. *Does the student have limited coordination and accuracy?*
   1. For catching and striking activities, use larger, lighter, softer balls.
   2. Decrease distance ball must travel and reduce speed at which it is thrown.
   3. For throwing activities, use smaller balls.
   4. In striking and kicking, use stationary ball before trying one that is moving.
   5. Increase the surface area of the striking implement.
   6. Use a backstop.
   7. Increase size of target.
   8. In bowling-type games, use lighter, less stable pins.
   9. Concentrate on safety.

Adapted from Sherrill (1993).

[a]See Chapter 7, this volume, for a detailed explanation and examples of each of these modifications as well as Chapter 6, this volume, for two models (i.e., Developmental and Ecological Task Analysis) for making specific curricular modifications.

Table 4.14. Curricular adaptations when modifying group games and sports[a]

1. *Can you vary the purpose/goal of the game?* (For example, some students play to learn complex strategies, others play to work on simple motor skills.)
2. *Can you vary number of players?* (Play small games such as 2 v. 2 basketball.)
3. *Can you vary movement requirements?* (Some students can walk while others can run; some can hit a ball off a tee while others hit a pitched ball; more-skilled students may be forced to use more complex movements while less-skilled students use simpler movements.)
4. *Can you vary the field of play?* (Set up special zones for students with less mobility; make the field narrower or wider as needed; shorten the distance for students with movement problems.)
5. *Can you vary objects used?* (Some students use lighter bats or larger balls; some use a lower net or basket.)
6. *Can you vary the level of organization?* (Vary typical organizational patterns; vary where certain students stand; vary the level of structure for certain students.)
7. *Can you vary the limits/expectations?* (Vary the number of turns each student receives; vary the rules regarding how far a student can run, hit, etc.; vary how much you will enforce certain rules for certain players.)

From Morris, G.S.D., & Stiehl, J. (1989). *Changing kids' games.* Champaign, IL: Human Kinetics Publishers. Copyright © 1989 by Gordon S. Morris and Jim Stiehl. Reprinted by permission.

[a]See Chapter 6, this volume, for a more detailed explanation of the Games Design Model.

who have problems with balance, 3) accommodating students who have problems with coordination, and 4) specific modifications to traditional games and team sports. The physical education inclusion team should work together to examine the student's abilities referenced to the requirements of specific skills and rules of games to determine which adaptations to implement. In addition, deciding which modifications to employ should be weighed against the student's age, what equipment is closest to that which peers who do not have disabilities use, and what equipment will likely be available in the community. (See Table 4.15 for a sample checklist with application to physical education.) For example, a seventh-grade student with mental retardation is integrated into an introductory tennis unit. Due to limited strength and coordination, this student is given a shorter, lighter racquet (racquetball racquet versus tennis racquet) and is allowed to hit a ball off a tee or a ball that is gently tossed to the student by a peer. These adaptations allow the student to practice the skill and improve performance. While this student may someday have the strength and control to use a regulation tennis racquet and hit a moving ball, the student needs these adaptations to participate successfully at this time. In addition, these adaptations will not affect the student's ability to participate in tennis in the community later in life (e.g., hitting a ball against the wall using a tee or trying to hit balls that bounce off the wall).

Even students with very significant disabilities can be accommodated via adaptations to equipment and rules. (See Tables 4.16 and 4.17 for examples.) As with considerations regarding prompts and cues given to students, each student should be provided the necessary adaptations that will promote meaningful participation and success. Still, special equipment and changes to rules should be systematically faded away whenever possible so that students can participate in activities using the same rules and equipment as their peers. In addition, caution should be taken when making adaptations that stigmatize the student or dramatically change the game for nondisabled students. For example, allowing a high school student to use a Mickey Mouse balloon as a substitute for a volleyball only accentuates the differences rather than the similarities between this student and his or her peers. A better adaptation might be having a peer catch a regulation volleyball for this student and then hold it while he or she hits it. Similarly, forcing all children to walk rather than run in a soccer game to accommodate a student who uses a walker would ruin the game for the students without disabilities. A better solution could be setting up a small zone for this student in which he or she is the only player allowed to kick the ball. (See chaps. 6 and 7, this volume, for more detail on modifications.)

Table 4.15.   Considerations in determining the appropriateness of adaptations (with suggested applications for the physical education curriculum)

Questions to ask	Sample applications
Will the adaptation increase the student's participation in the activity?	Lower basket or shorter distance to first base allow student to play team sports with peers.
Will it allow the student to participate in an activity that is preferred or valued by the student, his or her friends and family members?	Modifications allow student to participate in team sports, popular group games, playground activities, community sports, and so forth.
Will it continue to be useful and appropriate as the student grows older and enters other environments?	Bowling ramp can be used in regular bowling facilities, flotation devices can be used in community pools, adapted golf club can be used at local driving range.
Will it take less time to teach the student to use the adaptation than to teach the skill directly?	Use flotation device rather than teaching swimming, have student hit ball off tee rather than hit pitched ball.
Will the team have access to the technical expertise needed to design, construct, adjust, and repair the adaptation? (Will physical educator be taught how to use equipment and do simple maintenance?)	Special switches are provided to hit or toss balls. APE specialist and physical therapist will show regular PE teacher how to use switches.
Will use of the adaptation maintain or enhance related motor and communication skills?	Adapted switches promote independent arm and hand movements and participating with peers promotes socialization and communication.

Adapted from York & Rainforth (1991).

4.   *Determine the support that the student will need in regular physical education.* One of the final steps in developing the program for a student with disabilities is to determine who (if anyone) will provide assistance to the student with disabilities. Some students, such as those with spina bifida, may not need any special assistance, while students with learning disabilities or mental retardation may need peers to give them extra cues to follow directions. Students with significant disabilities or complex health care needs may need a trained teacher assistant or a professional to provide assistance. How much and what type of personal support a student will need will depend on the age of the student, the type of activities being presented, the physical, cognitive, and social skills of the particular student, and the medical condition of the student.

For example, a student with mental retardation and no behavior or medical problems could be assisted by a peer during physical education. In fact, such a student could be the responsibility of the entire class rather than assigning one student helper. The physical educator might tell the class, "If you are near John and he looks confused or looks like he needs help, please assist him." Similarly, a student with muscular dystrophy may only need someone to retrieve balls, while a student who is blind could have a peer help him or her move from one station to another.

Even students with more significant disabilities often can be assisted by a peer in their class. For example, a student with significant athetoid cerebral palsy is in a ball skill unit in first grade. The class is broken down into stations, and this student relies on assistance from his peers to help him at each station. At a throwing station, this student is assisted by students who are either resting or waiting their turns. These peers have been taught by the APE specialist how to place the ball in this student's hand and how to position his chair so that he can throw. These peers also push the student's wheelchair from station to station during transitions.

However, a student who needs more specific instruction to perform a skill correctly or who needs more attention (perhaps a student with autism) should have a trained peer tutor, volunteer,

Table 4.16. Chronological age–appropriate activities and sample modifications for elementary-age students with significant disabilities

Age-appropriate activities	Modifications
Manipulative patterns	
Throwing	Pushing a ball down a ramp, grasp and release
Catching	Tracking suspended balls, reaching for balloons
Kicking	Touching balloon taped to floor, pushing ball down ramp with foot
Striking	Hitting ball off tee, hitting suspended ball
Locomotor patterns	
Running	Being pushed quickly in wheelchair while keeping head up
Jumping/hopping	Lifting head up and down while being pushed in wheelchair
Galloping/skipping	Moving arms up and down while being pushed in wheelchair; also, student can use adapted mobility aids such as scooterboards and walkers
Perceptual-motor skills	
Balance skills	Propping up on elbows, prone balance over wedge
Body awareness	Accept tactile input, imitate simple movements
Spatial awareness	Moving arms in when going in between, ducking head under objects
Visual-motor coordination	Track suspended objects, touch switches
Physical fitness skills	
Endurance	Tolerate continuous activity, move body parts repeatedly
Strength	Use stretch bands, use isometric exercises
Flexibility	Perform ROM activities as suggested by PT

From Block, M.E. (1992). What is appropriate physical education for students with profound disabilities? *Adapted Physical Activity Quarterly, 9,* 201–202. Copyright © 1992 by Human Kinetics Publishers. Reprinted by permission.

or teacher assistant who provides support. For example, a student with autism who is easily distracted and who is frightened by the gymnasium comes to physical education with a teacher assistant whom the student has learned to trust. The student feels comfortable with the assistant, and the assistant has been trained in how to help this student work on his physical education goals. As the semester progresses and the student begins to feel more comfortable with the environment and his peers, the teacher assistant encourages peers to play with and assist the student. Similarly, a peer tutor can be trained to assist a student with significant mental retardation in learning to perform various skills prescribed by the APE specialist or PEIT (e.g., throwing using a skillful pattern, striking a certain way). Ideally, peers who assist students for the majority of the class will be older students who are involved in some type of peer mentoring or community service program. Whenever possible, avoid having peers miss their physical education period in order to help a student with a disability.

One final situation may occur when a student has a medical or health condition or a behavior problem that poses a risk to the student and/or his or her peers. In such a situation, a trained staff member should be responsible for providing support. For example, a high school student with significant mental retardation and aggressive behaviors should be supported by a trained teacher assistant, special education teacher, or APE specialist. These professionals, while trained in how to deal with the student's behaviors, also should be trained in how to help the student acquire IEP objectives while in regular physical education. Similarly, a nurse or therapist might support a student with a medical condition in regular physical education so that medical emergencies can be handled quickly and appropriately. Again, these support staff, while trained in dealing with the student's medical condition, should be given specific direction on how to help the student work on his or her IEP goals.

Table 4.17. Chronological age–appropriate activities and sample modifications for middle school, high school, and young adulthood[a]

Age-appropriate activities	Modifications
Team sports	
Soccer skills	Passing/kicking/shooting—push ball down ramp using foot
Soccer game	Set up special zones, use ramps for kicking
Volleyball skills	Track suspended balls, reach and touch balls
Volleyball game	"Buddy" catches ball, student has 3 seconds to touch the ball
Basketball skills	Using switch that shoots ball into small basket, keeping head up and arms out on defense; pushing ball off tray for passing
Basketball game	Buddy pushes student into offensive or defensive zone, ball passed to buddy, student has 5 seconds to activate switch that shoots his ball into small basket
Individual sports	
Bowling	Use a ramp (play at community facility when possible)
Bocce (lawn bowling)	Same as above
Miniature golf	Push ball down ramp using mini-putter
Golf (driving range)	Activate switch that causes ball to be hit
Physical fitness skills	
Endurance	Move body parts during aerobic dance program
Strength	Use stretch bands, isometrics, free weights
Flexibility	Perform ROM activities as suggested by PT during aerobics or during warm-up activities prior to team sports

From Block, M.E. (1992). What is appropriate physical education for students with profound disabilities? *Adapted Physical Activity Quarterly, 9,* 201–202. Copyright © 1992 by Human Kinetics Publishers. Reprinted by permission.

[a]In all activities, utilize the principle of partial participation to ensure that the student is successful.

Block and Krebs (1992) described a "continuum of support to regular physical education" in which they tell how to make decisions regarding personnel who can support students with disabilities in regular physical education. (See Table 4.18.) Readers are referred to this article for more information on how to select and train support personnel.

The important point in selecting support personnel is that the decision regarding *who* assists particular students should be a thoughtful process rather than simply assigning a peer, volunteer, or assistant to work with a student. In addition, it is extremely important that support personnel go through some type of formal training program prior to working with specific students, as well as ongoing training, so that these individuals can provide appropriate, safe support to students with disabilities. Finally, the regular educator and/or APE specialist should take responsibility for informing support personnel about changes to the daily or weekly routine, when new units will start, and what modifications are appropriate for particular activities.

PREPARING TEAM MEMBERS FOR INCLUSION

Steps 1–4 in this model allow one to determine what goals a particular child has and how these goals can be met in regular physical education. At this point, you are just about ready to include the student in regular physical education, but first the regular physical education teacher and the students without disabilities must be made to feel comfortable having a student with disabilities in their regular physical education class (Morreau & Eichstaedt, 1983). Care should also be taken to make sure the support staff (teacher assistants, volunteers, peer tutors) know the student with

Table 4.18. A continuum of support to regular physical education

LEVEL 1: NO SUPPORT NEEDED
 1.1 Student makes necessary modifications on his or her own.
 1.2 RPE teacher makes necessary modifications for student.

LEVEL 2: APE CONSULTATION
 2.1 No extra assistance is needed.
 2.2 Peer tutor "watches out" for student.
 2.3 Peer tutor assists student.
 2.4 Paraprofessional assists student.

LEVEL 3: APE DIRECT SERVICE IN RPE 1x/WEEK
 3.1 Peer tutor "watches out" for student.
 3.2 Peer tutor assists student.
 3.3 Paraprofessional assists student.

LEVEL 4: PART-TIME APE AND PART-TIME RPE
 4.1 Flexible schedule with reverse mainstreaming.
 4.2 Fixed schedule with reverse mainstreaming.

LEVEL 5: REVERSE MAINSTREAM IN SPECIAL SCHOOL
 5.1 Students from special school go to regular physical education at regular school 1–2x per week.
 5.2 Nondisabled students come to special school 2–3x per week for reverse mainstreaming.
 5.3 Students with and without disabilities meet at community-based recreation facility and work out together.

whom they are working as well as their responsibilities to the team. One of the primary reasons why inclusion fails is that those directly involved with the program are not adequately prepared (Grosse, 1991; Lavay & DePaepe, 1987). The next three steps discuss ways to prepare key personnel for inclusion.

   5. *Prepare the regular physical educator.* The first and probably most important person to prepare is the regular physical educator. The PEIT often assumes that regular physical educators are receptive to inclusion and will have the skills necessary to accommodate successfully the unique needs of the student with disabilities. While some regular physical educators feel comfortable having a student with disabilities in their program, many others may feel very threatened (Minner & Knutson, 1982; Santomier, 1985). For example, many feel that they do not have the training, students with disabilities will take too much of their time, it will be dangerous, and the students without disabilities will not accept the special student. While these may sound like excuses, most regular physical educators rarely have the in-depth training needed to include students with disabilities successfully. For example, a typical undergraduate physical education teacher preparation program includes only one course on adapted physical education, and most of these courses focus on identifying various types of disabilities rather than on practical suggestions for developing and implementing individual programs within the regular setting.

   One of the most important steps in preparing the regular physical educator is to define his or her specific role. Vandercook and York (1990) described the roles of regular education teachers in facilitating the inclusion of students with disabilities in their regular education classes. The role they outlined can be applied to regular physical educators as follows: 1) the regular physical education teacher should view the student with disabilities as a member of the class rather than as a visitor; 2) the regular physical educator should contribute information about the regular physical education curriculum, instructional strategies, teaching style, management techniques, routines, and rules; 3) the regular physical educator should work collaboratively with support personnel, family members, and peers in developing physical education programs and in including the student with disabilities in typical physical education activities; 4) the regular physical educator should provide a model of appropriate interaction and communication with the student with disabilities (set expectations for acceptance and inclusion that would transfer to peers without disabilities); and 5) the regular physical educator should be willing to give it a try. This last rule should not be taken lightly. Many physical educators refuse to allow the student to participate in regular physical education, or if they allow the student into the gym, they make only a minimal effort to include the student in physical activities appropriately.

For inclusion to be truly successful, the regular physical education teacher must learn to feel comfortable with the notion of having students with disabilities come to regular physical education. This can be accomplished in several ways. First and foremost, those physical educators who feel most threatened should be assured that they will receive both direct and consultative support from an adapted physical education specialist and a special education teacher. The adapted physical education specialist and the special education teachers can assist in the development of the individual program for the student with disabilities, obtaining and setting up adapted equipment, and developing appropriate modifications to the regular program. The special educator can also provide specific information about students' specific skills and weaknesses, any medical/health concerns, communication skills, behaviors, and likes and dislikes. In addition, regular physical educators should be assured that students with disabilities, especially students with significant disabilities, will receive support through peer tutors, paraprofessionals, the special education teacher, or the APE specialist. The regular physical educator should never be left alone with the student until he or she feels comfortable with the situation. Finally, assurance should be given that including a student with disabilities should not cause the regular physical educator any more work. In fact, others helping the regular physical educator plan and implement the program for the student with disabilities might actually make his or her job easier. For example, if a teacher assistant comes into the gym with a particular student, the regular physical educator could send several students who need extra practice (along with instructions for the teacher assistant) to work with the teacher assistant and the special student. This way the regular physical educator could work with a smaller group of students on specific skills and strategies.

Another method of helping the regular physical educator is to provide desensitizing workshops. These workshops can change preconceived notions about persons with disabilities, foster more positive attitudes, and provide suggestions for modifications. Clark, French, and Henderson (1985) outlined several activities which could be used to desensitize the regular physical education teacher including: 1) invite guest lecturers who have disabilities, 2) visit special education classes and get to know the students better, 3) show videotapes on athletes with disabilities, 4) do role-playing activities in which the regular physical educator has to move about in a wheelchair or is blindfolded while doing typical physical education activities, 5) brainstorm with the collaborative team about modifications for specific physical education units, 6) visit other schools that are successfully including students with disabilities in regular physical education, and 7) have an APE specialist team-teach with the regular physical educator early in the semester to show some concrete ways of accommodating the student with disabilities. When provided prior to inclusion, these and similar activities can facilitate acceptance and confidence in regular physical educators.

Finally, it is extremely important that the regular physical educator understand that his or her responsibilities are still with the entire class, not just one or two students. The regular physical educator should not spend any more time with the student who has disabilities than with his or her students without disabilities. However, the regular physical educator should feel comfortable talking with, correcting, and reinforcing the special student just as he or she would students without disabilities. In addition, activities should continue to be challenging to all students, and the regular program should not be compromised. (See chap. 6, this volume, for more detail.) For example, skill hierarchies could be extended to accommodate students with disabilities yet provide challenging activities at the other end of the hierarchy for more skilled students. (See Figure 4.6.) Similarly, modifications to group activities and team sports should be made so that students with disabilities can be included. However, these modifications should not detract from the program for the students without disabilities. It is important that regular physical educators understand the impact of certain modifications to games on the entire class, and they should strive to implement only those modifications which allow a student with disabilities to participate without drastically affecting students without disabilities. (See chaps. 6 and 7, this volume, for more detail.)

6. *Prepare the regular education students.* A second consideration for successful inclusion is the attitude of students without disabilities toward having a student with disabilities in their regular physical education program. Peer acceptance can be the critical difference between successful and unsuccessful inclusion. Unfortunately, the initial response of many students without disabilities is negative. Some will be scared of students with disabilities, particularly students with physical disabilities. Others will immediately reject students with disabilities because they feel that these students will detract from their physical education program. Still others may be sympathetic toward students with disabilities and try to "mother" these students. While none of these responses will facilitate successful inclusion, these responses are understandable given that most students without disabilities know very little about students with disabilities. Thus, an important part of the process of including students with disabilities is to prepare students without disabilities.

Clark et al. (1985) and Stainback and Stainback (1985) suggested several ways in which teachers can help students without disabilities develop a more positive attitude toward students with disabilities. First, students without disabilities should learn about persons with disabilities in a positive manner. One method to change attitudes is to bring in guest speakers who have disabilities who participate in sports such as wheelchair racing or basketball, sit-skiing or skiing for the blind, or Special Olympics. These persons can dispel stereotypes that persons with disabilities cannot play sports. Local sports organizations affiliated with national sports associations (e.g., United States Association for Blind Athletes, National Wheelchair Sports Association, Special Olympics) are excellent resources for recruiting speakers.

A second method for changing attitudes is role-playing in which students without disabilities are given a disability. This technique has been used for years in Red Cross adapted aquatics classes as well as in physical education programs in which students with disabilities are to be included (Mizen & Linton, 1983). In physical education, students can be blindfolded and asked to move through an obstacle course, sit in chairs and play volleyball or basketball, or have one arm tied up while trying to hit a softball. The teacher should facilitate discussions regarding how a peer with a disability might feel when he or she is trying to participate in these activities. Discussions should also include the fact that in some situations a person with a disability is actually at an advantage. For example, a person who is blind can move around his or her house when the lights go out much better than a sighted person.

A final method for changing attitudes is to discuss the purpose of sports rules and how these rules can be modified to include all students successfully. Discussion should include the concept of "handicapping" (e.g., in sports such as golfing and horse-racing) in order to equalize competition. Encourage students to discuss ways of "handicapping" (i.e., making rule modifications) to equalize competition in physical education. For example, a student who is blind might have difficulty hitting a pitched ball and running to first base. A fair modification for this student might include allowing him to hit a ball off a tee when he is batting. When he must run to first base, a

_____ will:

1. _____ touch ball with hand/head stick when ball is placed on lap tray.
2. _____ hold ball on lap tray.
3. _____ hold ball on lap tray while he or she is pushed in wheelchair around gym.
4. _____ push ball off lap tray.
5. _____ drop ball to floor.
6. _____ drop ball to floor, then reach down to touch ball before it bounces three times.
7. _____ drop ball to floor, then reach down to touch ball before it bounces two times.
8. _____ drop ball to floor, then reach down to touch ball before it bounces one time.
9. _____ push ball to floor with two hands so that ball bounces up to approximately waist height.
10. _____ push ball to floor with two hands two times in succession.
11. _____ push ball to floor with two hands three times in succession.
12. _____ push ball to floor with one hand two times in succession.
13. _____ push ball to floor with one hand three times in succession.
14. _____ push ball to floor with one hand five times in succession.
15. _____ push ball up and down repeatedly with one hand.
16. _____ dribble ball while standing still for 10 seconds.
17. _____ dribble ball while standing still for 20 seconds.
18. _____ dribble ball while walking forward slowly.
19. _____ dribble ball while walking forward at normal walking speed.
20. _____ dribble ball while walking forward quickly.
21. _____ dribble ball with dominant hand while jogging forward.
22. _____ dribble ball with dominant hand while running forward.
23. _____ dribble ball with nondominant hand while walking forward.
24. _____ dribble ball with nondominant hand while jogging forward.
25. _____ dribble ball with nondominant hand while running forward.
26. _____ dribble ball with either hand while weaving through cones.
27. _____ dribble ball using a cross-over dribble while weaving through cones.
28. _____ dribble ball with either hand while moving in a variety of directions.
29. _____ dribble and protect ball while guarded by opponent going at full speed.

Cue Key (prompts can be given by physical educator, teacher assistant, or peer tutor):

I   = independent
IN   = indirect cue
V   = verbal cue
G   = gestural cue
M   = model
T   = touch prompt
PP   = partial physical assistance
P+   = physical assistance (student tries to help)
P   = physical assistance (student passively participates)
P−   = physical assistance (student fights assistance)

Performance Key:

+   = student performs skill 4/5 trials
+/− = student performs skill, but not 4/5 trials
−   = student does not perform skill

Figure 4.6. Extension of traditional skill station for dribbling a basketball. (From Block, M.E., Provis, S., & Nelson, E. [1994]. Accommodating students with special needs in regular physical education: Extending traditional skill stations. *Palaestra, 10*[1], 32–38.)

peer can guide the student toward first base. Since it takes longer for the student to run to first base, we can also move the base closer to home plate. Moving the base closer to home plate would also make it more challenging for the students without disabilities to get this student out. Ideally, several distances to first base should be developed so that very skilled students run farther than average students, who run farther than students with lower skills. If students are involved in the process of developing modifications to accommodate students with different abilities, then they are more likely to "buy in" to these modifications and be more accepting when they are implemented.

In addition to general methods designed to change attitudes, discuss with students the specific disabilities (and abilities) of the student who will be integrated into regular physical education. Focus on how similar this student is to them. For example, stress how this student is the same age they are, likes to wear similar clothes, enjoys playing and watching sports, hates the food in the cafeteria, and argues with his mom about bedtime. Discuss positive ways in which they can assist the student during physical education such as retrieving balls, locating stations, and moving from one part of the gym to another. Also, students should be allowed to visit this student in his or her special class or in other inclusive classes during the day such as art, history, industrial arts, or music. Similarly, the student with disabilities should be encouraged to visit the regular physical education class, and the students without disabilities should be encouraged to introduce themselves and chat with the student. When the students are prepared ahead of time, many of the fears, misconceptions, and stereotypes can be shattered before they begin.

Preparing peers is an important part of successful inclusion, but encouragement should not stop once the student enters the program. Too often students with disabilities are ignored in physical education because their peers without disabilities do not know how to interact with or assist them. The teacher should provide ongoing encouragement to students without disabilities (both through modeling and direct suggestion) to talk to the student with disabilities, to provide feedback and positive reinforcement, to correct gently or redirect the student when he or she misbehaves, and to ask the student if he or she needs assistance. Rather than having one peer assigned to one student, the entire class should take responsibility for the special student. For example, if a student who has mental retardation does not know to which station to go, one of her peers can assist her. Similarly, if a student who is blind has lost the ball she was dribbling, one of her peers can retrieve it for her. Students without disabilities should be continuously prompted and reinforced for interacting with the student with disabilities. As the year progresses and students without disabilities begin to feel more comfortable with the special student, interactions will become more spontaneous.

7. Prepare support persons. One final, often-neglected step is preparing support persons who will be assisting the student with disabilities in regular physical education. These support persons, whether trained teacher assistants, peer tutors, or community volunteers, are committed to helping the student with disabilities, yet they often have no formal training or experience working with students with disabilities or in physical education. While such support persons are given some direction by the special education teacher in how to work with the student in regular education classrooms, they are rarely given direction when in physical education. This may be due to miscommunication between the regular physical educator and the special educator. That is, the regular physical educator assumes the special educator has provided the support person with a list of physical education activities, while the special educator assumes that the regular physical educator is guiding the support person on how to provide specific physical education activities to the student with disabilities. What results are confused and often frustrated support persons who have no idea what they should be doing with the student with disabilities in regular physical education and often make up their own physical education program. Obviously, such a situation prevents the student from developing necessary motor, fitness, and leisure skills, and can even be dangerous depending on what activities the support person chooses to attempt. For example, a student with

Down syndrome might have positive atlanto-axial instability (a condition of the vertebrae of the neck that can lead to paralysis), and this student should not be allowed to participate in forward rolls during a gymnastic unit. Yet, no one has informed this person's peer tutor of this problem, and he has been given no direction on what to do and what not to do by the regular physical educator. Seeing other children in the class doing forward rolls during a gymnastics unit, the peer tutor assumes that his student should be doing the same activity. Such a scenario is frightening, yet this scenario and similar ones take place all too often because no one has taken responsibility in preparing support persons.

Training of support persons should be an ongoing responsibility of all collaborative team members. This training should focus on both general information about their role as a support person as well as specific information about the student with whom each will be working and how he or she will facilitate the inclusion of the student in regular physical education. The following provide some suggestions regarding information that various collaborative team members should present to support persons: 1) provide general information (perhaps in the form of a brochure or handout) regarding their role as a support person and what is expected of them; 2) provide information regarding the philosophy of the program and the general goals that have been developed for all students (i.e., opportunities to interact with peers without disabilities, improved social behavior, improved communication skills, and improved independence in a variety of functional skills); 3) provide resources and key personnel to whom they can go with questions if they need help (e.g., go to the regular physical educator or adapted physical education specialist if they have questions about modifying specific physical education activities; go to the physical therapist if they have specific questions about positioning or contraindicated activities); 4) provide a detailed description of the student, including IEP objectives, medical/health concerns, unique behaviors, likes and dislikes, and who special friends are; 5) describe specific information regarding safety/ emergency procedures (e.g., what to do if a student has a seizure or an asthma attack, make sure particular students get water every 10 minutes); 6) provide specific information regarding what typically happens in physical education including yearly outline, unit and daily lesson plans, daily routines, rules and regulations, typical teaching procedures, and measurement and record-keeping procedures; 7) provide general suggestions for modifying activities (e.g., use a balloon or suspended ball when speed and weight of ball are a concern; lower goals or targets, make them larger, or bring them closer to the student for more success); 8) provide several alternative activities when regular program activities are deemed inappropriate (e.g., when a forward roll is contraindicated, the student can be working on fitness goals or fundamental motor patterns; when the class is playing field hockey, the student can be working on alternative striking activities that would facilitate the acquisition of lifetime leisure skills such as croquet, golf, or tennis); and 9) provide several suggestions for facilitating interactions with peers without disabilities.

SUMMARY

Once a school system or school adopts a philosophy of inclusion, it is tempting to place students with disabilities immediately into as many regular programs as possible. One of the first places students will be placed is regular physical education since physical education is viewed as a non-academic program. Unfortunately, regular physical educators often have the least training in terms of working with students with disabilities. This may lead to poor attitudes toward the student with disabilities (which quickly transfer over to the students without disabilities), lackluster haphazard programming or no programming at all, and ultimately a waste of valuable learning time for the student with disabilities. It has been suggested in this chapter that preparing all key personnel prior to inclusion can prevent such a downward spiral from occurring. Preparation should include collaborative team members developing individual goals for the student, comparing individual goals to what takes place in regular physical education, anticipating the need for certain modifications and adjustments prior to implementation and developing appropriate accommodations, and finally, preparing regular physical educators, peers without disabilities, and support persons. While carefully preparing for integration might take several weeks or even months, the end result is a smooth and positive transition into regular physical education that is supported by regular physical education staff and peers without disabilities.

Chapter 5

Assessment to Facilitate Successful Inclusion

The best thing about inclusion in physical education is the positive reactions of the peers without disabilities. The students without disabilities become more aware of what our students with very severe disabilities can do if given proper instruction, adapted equipment, and support. For example, we take our 19- to 21-year-old students out to bowl at the University of Minnesota. The regular college students can't believe that our students can bowl and are amazed at the special equipment our students use. One regular student even asked if he could try one of the bowling balls that has a handle.

We also take our students swimming in the community. Even though our students have severe disabilities, they are quite comfortable in the water with their flotation devices. There have been several instances when teens without disabilities watch us literally throw our students into the pool. Many of these students without disabilities are actually less skilled and less comfortable in the water than our students. They are amazed at how well our students do in the water and suddenly look at our students with more respect.

—Kathy King

David is a ninth grader who has a significant visual impairment. He has just moved to Jefferson County, and he will be attending Monroe High School. David did not receive physical education at his previous school because they thought the severity of his visual impairment precluded traditional physical education. Rather, David received orientation and mobility training during physical education. At Monroe, all students receive physical education in the regular setting, even students with disabilities like David. Programs are modified and individualized as needed to ensure that all students receive a program that meets their unique needs. But how does the physical education inclusion team (PEIT) decide what is appropriate to teach David and other students with different abilities? How does the PEIT determine David's present strengths and weaknesses? How does the PEIT decide how to teach and modify particular skills? And once the program is implemented, how does the PEIT determine if David is making adequate progress toward his goals?

The previous chapter outlined an ecological approach to the decision process for developing and implementing a physical education program for students with disabilities in the regular set-

Kathy King is a special education teacher and adapted aquatics instructor at Anwatin Middle School in Minneapolis, Minnesota.

ting. However, all programming decisions should be based on information obtained from assessment data. Without such assessment data, programming decisions would be based on "best guesses" or assumptions that in turn could result in a poor or inappropriate physical education program.

Assessment is a critical yet often misused part of the overall program. According to PL 101-476, IDEA, part of the IEP process must include assessing all students with disabilities to determine their present levels of performance. Assessment data can then be used by the collaborative team to make informed decisions regarding specific diagnoses, types and intensity of services, instructional plans, amount and type of supports, and ultimate least restrictive placement. In addition, assessment should be an ongoing process that begins with the development of the student's IEP and continues during the implementation of the program. Unfortunately, what often happens is that assessment tools are used improperly, assessment data are misinterpreted, or decisions are made based on a specific disability label or school philosophy (Davis, 1984; Grosse, 1991).

The purpose of this chapter is to outline assessment procedures that can facilitate the inclusion of students with disabilities into regular physical education. The chapter begins with a brief review of the legal basis for assessment as outlined in PL 101-476. This will be followed by a review of traditional assessment procedures, then a detailed review of an ecological approach to assessment. Finally, an example of how an ecological assessment is conducted will be presented.

It should be noted here that the term *assessment* will be used synonymously with the term *evaluation* which is used in IDEA. Thus, assessment will be defined rather broadly as the process of collecting and interpreting data in order to plan and implement physical education programs for students with disabilities. The term *test* will be used to describe specific tools used to collect assessment information.

LEGAL BASIS FOR ASSESSMENT IN PHYSICAL EDUCATION

Evaluation procedures are clearly outlined in PL 101-476. Table 5.1 contains excerpts from the *Federal Register* (August 23, 1977, pp. 42496–42497) that present the legal description of evaluation procedures.

All of the procedures outlined in Table 5.1 should be adhered to when conducting a physical education assessment. For example, placement decisions (including the decision whether to place a student in regular versus adapted physical education specialist) cannot be made until a student is given a full and individual evaluation of motor needs. This evaluation should be conducted by "trained personnel" (ideally an adapted physical education specialist), and the evaluation should draw upon information from all team members including preferences of the student and his or her parents. In addition, testing materials must be appropriate for the student's age and abilities. For example, it would be inappropriate to give an 18-year-old the Peabody Developmental Motor Scales that are designed for students birth to 6 years old. Similarly, it would be inappropriate to give a student who uses a wheelchair a standard physical fitness test that is designed for able-bodied students. Decisions regarding placement and scope of the program should be based on assessment that is more relevant to the student's needs, abilities, and future placements. The following section contrasts traditional approaches to assessment in adapted physical education versus an ecological approach to assessment.

TRADITIONAL VERSUS ECOLOGICAL APPROACHES TO ASSESSMENT

Traditional Approach to Assessment

How adapted physical education decisions are made varies from school system to school system. Still, there are traditional ways in which adapted physical education specialists (or other team members

Table 5.1.   Legal description of evaluation procedures outlined in PL 101-476

PROTECTION IN EVALUATION PROCEDURES

121a.530   **General**
 (a) Each state educational agency shall insure that each public agency establishes and implements procedures which meet the requirements of 121a.530–121a.534.
 (b) Testing and evaluation materials and procedures used for the purposes of evaluation and placement of handicapped children must be selected and administered so as not to be racially or culturally discriminatory.

121a.531   **Preplacement Evaluation**
 Before any action is taken with respect to the initial placement of a handicapped child in a special education program, a full and individual evaluation of the child's educational needs must be conducted in accordance with the requirements of 121a.532.

121a.532   **Evaluation Procedures**
State and local educational agencies shall ensure, at a minimum, that:
 (a) Tests and other evaluation materials
  (1) are provided and administered in the child's native language or other mode of communication, unless it is clearly not feasible to do so.
  (2) have been validated for the specific purposes for which they are used; and
  (3) are administered by trained personnel in conformance with the instructions provided by their producer.
 (b) Tests and other evaluation materials include those tailored to assess specific areas of educational need and not merely those which are designed to provide single general intelligent quotients;
 (c) Tests are selected and administered so as best to ensure that when a test is administered to a child with impaired sensory, manual, or speaking skills, the test results accurately reflect the child's aptitude or achievement level or whatever other factors the test purports to measure, rather than reflecting the child's impaired sensory, manual, or speaking skills except where those skills are the factors which the test purports to measure);
 (d) No single procedure is used as the sole criterion for determining an appropriate educational program for a child; and
 (e) The evaluation is made by a multidisciplinary team or group of persons, including at least one teacher or other specialist with knowledge in the area of suspected disability.
 (f) The child is assessed in all areas as related to the suspected disability, including, where appropriate, health, vision, hearing, social and emotional status, general intelligence, academic performance, communicative status, and motor abilities.

121a.533   **Placement Procedures**
 (a) In interpreting evaluation data and in making placement decisions, each public agency shall:
  (1) draw upon information from a variety of sources, including aptitude and achievement tests, teacher recommendations, physical condition, social or cultural background, and adaptive behavior;
  (2) insure that information obtained from all of these sources is documented and carefully considered;
  (3) insure that the placement decision is made by a group of persons, including persons knowledgeable about the child, the meaning of the evaluation data, and the placement options; and
  (4) insure that the placement decision is made in conformity with the least restrictive environment rules in 121a.550–121a.554.
 (b) If a determination is made that a child is handicapped and needs special education and related services, an individualized education program must be developed for the child in accordance with 121a.340–121a.349 of subpart C.

121a.534   **Reevaluation**
Each state and local educational agency shall insure:
 (a) that each handicapped child's individualized education program is reviewed in accordance with 121a.340–121a.349 of subpart C, and
 (b) That an evaluation of the child, based on procedures which meet the requirements under 121a.532, is conducted every three years or more frequently if conditions warrant or if the child's parent or teacher requests an evaluation.

responsible for physical education for students with disabilities) use and conduct assessments. Traditional procedures can be broken down into four major categories: 1) classification, 2) development of IEP, 3) placement, and 4) instruction.

1. *Classification.* Traditionally, the first step in the assessment process is to determine if a student needs specialized physical education services. In some school districts, students qualify for adapted physical education services simply because they have a particular diagnosis. For example, students who use wheelchairs usually qualify for adapted physical education because it is assumed that the goals for these students are completely different from their peers without disabilities. However, students with learning disabilities often do not get adapted physical education services because it is assumed that they do not have any special motor or fitness needs. Such practices are in direct violation of the law that specifically mandates that all students with disabilities be evaluated to determine if they require special physical education services. (See legal description in Table 5.1.) More importantly, no one has taken the time to assess each student's strengths and weaknesses before determining who qualifies for adapted physical education. Many students with learning disabilities in fact have motor and learning problems that justify specialized physical education, while many students who use wheelchairs can do quite well in regular physical education without any special support.

Others who try to determine if a student qualifies for adapted physical education use *norm-referenced* or *standardized tests*. A standardized test is one in which a student's score is compared to the scores of others on the same test (Safrit, 1990). That is, a student's score is compared to a set of norms. Norms are established by testing a representative sample of subjects from a particular population. For example, for a test to be valid for children 2–6 years of age, a large sample of children ages 2–6 should be tested to develop norms. These norms can then be analyzed and organized so as to describe scores that correspond to a certain percentage of the population. For example, a particular score on a test might represent a point below which 75% of the norm sample scored (75th percentile). School systems can then establish minimal cut-off scores that correspond to who does or does not qualify for adapted physical education. Such an approach is by far the most widely used approach (Ulrich, 1985). Many states even have set criteria based on standardized test results for determining who qualifies for adapted physical education services. Sherrill (1993) noted that students in Alabama and Georgia who score below the 30th percentile on standardized tests of motor performance qualify for adapted physical education services. Sherrill herself suggested that, in fact, students who consistently score below the 50th percentile should qualify for special physical education service.

For example, the Bruininks-Oseretsky Test of Motor Proficiency (BOT), the standardized test most often used by adapted physical education specialists (Ulrich, 1985), is frequently used to determine which students qualify for adapted physical education. (See Figure 5.1 for examples of BOT items.) The BOT is a valid, norm-referenced test designed to measure specific motor abilities of children 4½–14½ years of age. Areas evaluated include running speed and agility, balance, bilateral coordination, response speed, strength, upper-limb coordination, visual-motor coordination, and upper-limb speed and dexterity. A school system might decide that a student with a total score below the 30th percentile qualifies for adapted physical education. But what information does data collected from the BOT give the team that would help the team determine if a student needs adapted physical education services? Will a student who performs at the 20th percentile have difficulty in regular physical education activities? Will a student who does poorly on subtest items such as response speed or bilateral coordination do poorly with activities in regular physical education without extensive support? Does the BOT reliably predict how well a second grade student will do in a unit that focuses on locomotor patterns or how well a middle school student will do in a softball unit?

SUBTEST 5 / Item 7

Touching Nose with Index Fingers—Eyes Closed

With eyes closed, the subject touches any part of his or her nose first with one index finger and then with the opposite index finger, as shown in Figure 26. The subject is given 90 seconds to touch the nose four consecutive times. The score is recorded as a pass or a fail.

Trials: 1

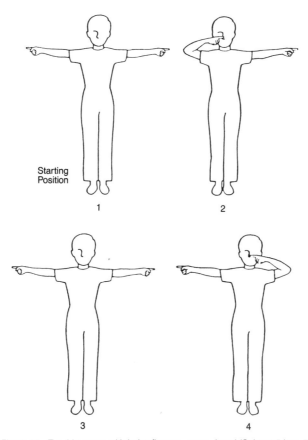

Figure 26   Touching nose with index fingers—eyes closed (Subtest 5 Item 7)

ADMINISTERING AND RECORDING

Have the subject stand facing you. Say: **Hold your arms straight out to the side. Close your hands and point with your first** (index) **fingers** (demonstrate). **Touch your nose with the tip of one of your fingers and then put your arm straight out again** (demonstrate). **Then touch your nose with the other fingertip and put that arm straight out again** (demonstrate). **Now do it with your eyes closed and your head still. Keep touching your nose until I tell you to stop. Ready, begin.**

Begin timing. If necessary, provide additional instruction. For example, remind the subject to touch the nose with the tips of the index fingers and to return one arm to an extended position before moving the other arm. Start counting as soon as the subject is moving the arms and touching the nose correctly in a continuous movement. During the trial correct the subject and start counting over if she or <u>he:</u>

(continued)

Figure 5.1.   Select items from the Bruininks-Oseretsky Test of Motor Proficiency. (From Bruininks, R.H. [1978]. *Bruininks-Oseretsky Test of Motor Proficiency—Manual* [pp. 82–85]. Circle Pines, MN: American Guidance Service. Reprinted with permission.)

Figure 5.1. (*continued*)

    a. fails to maintain continuous movements
    b. fails to touch the nose with the index finger
    c. fails to alternate arms
    d. fails to extend arms fully after touching nose
    e. moves head to meet the finger
    f. opens eyes.

Allow no more than 90 seconds, including time needed for additional instruction, for the subject to touch the nose correctly four consecutive times (twice with each finger). After 90 seconds, tell the subject to stop.

On the Individual Record Form, record pass or fail.

SUBTEST 5 / Item 8

Touching Thumb to Fingertips—Eyes Closed

With eyes closed, the subject touches the thumb of the preferred hand to each of the fingertips on the preferred hand, moving from the little finger to the index finger and then from the index finger to the little finger, as shown in Figure 27. The subject is given 90 seconds to complete the task once. The score is recorded as a pass or a fail.

Trials: 1

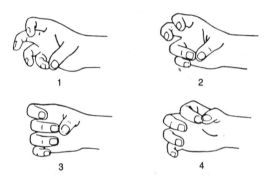

Figure 27 Touching thumb to fingertops—eyes closed (Subtest 5 Item 8)

ADMINISTERING AND RECORDING

Have the subject sit beside you at a table. Have the subject extend the preferred arm. Then say: **You are to touch your thumb to each of the fingertips on this hand. Start with your little finger and touch each fingertip in order. Then start with your first finger and touch each fingertip again as you move your thumb back to your little finger** (demonstrate). **Do this with your eyes closed until I tell you to stop. Ready, begin.**

Begin timing. If necessary provide additional instruction. During the trial correct the subject and have the subject start over if he or she:

    a. fails to maintain continuous movements
    b. touches any finger except the index finger more than once in succession
    c. touches two fingers at the same time
    d. fails to touch fingers above the first finger joint
    e. opens eyes.

Allow no more than 90 seconds, including time needed for additional instruction, for the subject to complete the task once. After 90 seconds, tell the subject to stop.

On the Individual Record Form, record pass or fail.

(*continued*)

Figure 5.1.   *(continued)*

SUBTEST 5 / Item 9

Pivoting Thumb and Index Finger

The subject touches the tip of the right index finger to the tip of the left thumb, then pivots the hands to touch the tip of the left index finger to the tip of the right thumb. The subject continues to pivot the hands touching finger to thumb, in an upward or downward motion. See Figure 28. The subject is given 90 seconds to complete five consecutive pivots correctly. The score is recorded as a pass or a fail.

Trials: 1

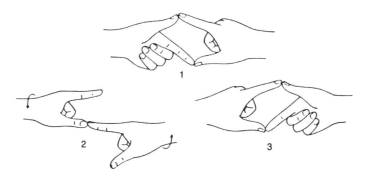

Figure 28   Pivoting thumb and index finger (Subtest 5 Item 9)

ADMINISTERING AND RECORDING

Have the subject sit beside you at a table. Say: **Touch your first** (index) **finger of each hand to the thumb of your other hand** (demonstrate). **Watch how I separate one thumb and finger and move them** (demonstrate). If necessary, place the subject's thumbs and index fingers in the correct starting position. Then say: **Keep moving your thumbs and fingers this way until I tell you to stop. Ready, begin.**

Begin timing. If necessary, provide additional instruction. (For young subjects, it may be helpful to remind them of the "Eency Weency Spider" song, which uses the same action.) Start counting pivots as soon as the subject establishes a continuous motion. During the trial correct the subject and start counting over if she or he:
a. fails to maintain continuous movements
b. places the thumbs or index fingers incorrectly.

Allow no more than 90 seconds, including time needed for additional instruction, for the subject to complete five consecutive pivots correctly. After 90 seconds, tell the subject to stop.

On the Individual Record Form, record pass or fail.

Similarly, why does performance at or below the 20th percentile on the American Alliance of Health, Physical Education, Recreation, and Dance (AAHPERD) Health-Related Fitness Test (HRFT) qualify a student for adapted physical education services? The HRFT measures health-related physical fitness for students ages 5–18 years. Areas evaluated include cardiovascular endurance (1-mile run), percent body fat (skinfold), muscular strength (sit-ups), and flexibility (sit and reach). Does a student's performance on any or all of these items predict how well a student will do in regular physical education? Will limited abdominal strength as measured by sit-ups help determine if a high school–age student will be unsuccessful or need modifications to popular lifetime leisure activities such as softball, tennis, or golf? It should be clear that the BOT, the

AAHPERD Health-Related Fitness Test, and similar tests are not related to what really takes place in regular physical education. Yet these types of tests are often used to make decisions regarding who qualifies for adapted physical education services.

2. *Development of individualized education program.* Once it has been determined that a student requires special services, the next step is to determine on what specific skills the student should work. The development of the student's individualized education program (IEP) is an important process because the IEP will guide the specific activities the student will work on for the next year. In most cases, information taken from the classification assessment is used to develop the student's IEP. This makes the assessment tools used for classification critical. Unfortunately, in the traditional approach, the use of standardized tests forces practitioners to follow a developmental or "bottom-up" approach. In the bottom-up approach, deficiencies at the lower end of the developmental continuum become the focus of a student's physical education program without regard to how these skills affect the acquisition of real-life skills (Kelly et al., 1991). In practice, IEP goals are the items a student fails on developmental tests or tests of motor abilities.

For example, a student who does poorly on upper-limb speed and dexterity (e.g., sorting playing cards quickly) might have as a goal on his IEP improving upper-limb response speed with specific activities such as repeatedly touching nose with index fingers, touching thumb to fingertips, or pivoting thumb and index finger. Similarly, a student who fails items #121 (stand on tiptoes for 5 seconds with eyes open) and #128 (stand on one foot with hands on hip for 5 seconds) on the gross motor scale of the Peabody Developmental Motor Scales (Folio & DuBose, 1974) would have an IEP goal to improve static balance and a short-term instructional objective of standing on tiptoes and balancing on one foot. While upper-limb response speed and static balance may be a problem for this student, is working on these nonfunctional skills in isolation an appropriate objective? How do these goals relate to skills the student will need to be successful in current and future physical education and recreation environments? Again, while the long-term goals may be appropriate, the short-term instructional objectives are nonfunctional, splinter-type skills that bear no relation to the skills a student needs to be successful in regular physical education.

3. *Placement.* Once it has been determined that a student qualifies for adapted physical education services and has an IEP, the next step in the assessment process is to make a decision regarding where the student will receive these services. IDEA mandates that placement decisions be based on the concept of the least restrictive environment (LRE). Remember, LRE mandates that students with disabilities be educated with their peers without disabilities, and that separate programming should occur only when education in the regular setting cannot be satisfactorily achieved with the use of supplementary aids and services. Unfortunately, most school systems interpreted LRE as permission to provide a "cascade of services" or a continuum of placements from least- to most-restrictive rather than as a mandate to provide proper support to students in the regular setting (Snell & Janney, in press). This is no more evident than in adapted physical education in which a variety of LRE models have been described (e.g., Dunn & Fait, 1989; Jansma & Decker, 1990; Sherrill, 1993). An example of Jansma and Decker's (1990) cascade of placement options is listed below:

1. Full-time regular physical education
2. Part-time adapted and part-time regular physical education, flexible schedule
3. Part-time adapted and part-time regular physical education, fixed schedule
4. Full-time adapted physical education, regular school
5. Full-time adapted physical education, special school
6. Full-time adapted physical education, residential
7. Full-time adapted physical education, home
8. Full-time adapted physical education, hospital

In theory, information obtained from assessment data is used to place students along the continuum. In reality, placement decisions tend to be an either/or decision process: regular physical education with no support or separate physical education. Again, there tends to be a domino effect that begins with the use of a standardized assessment tool to determine classification which influences IEP goals and in turn influences placement. That is, the use of standardized tests to develop IEP goals usually results in goals and objectives that bear no resemblance to activities that take place in regular physical education. For example, it is difficult for the regular physical educator to see how working on upper-limb speed and dexterity (IEP goals based on results of standardized assessments) are related to lessons on locomotor patterns and body awareness. Thus, he or she concludes that the student should be placed in a separate adapted physical education class.

4. *Instruction.* The last and perhaps most relevant aspect of assessment is how to help a student acquire the targeted goals on his or her IEP. Unfortunately, decisions at this level still will be based on standardized test results which focus on motor abilities, developmental level, and physical fitness. Again, these tests are usually conducted in such a way that they bear no relation to critical physical education skills. For example, poor performance on sit-ups on the HRFT does not indicate *why* the student is having trouble doing sit-ups nor how to help this student improve his physical fitness as it relates to real-life physical education and recreation skills. Most teachers have the student practice sit-ups. But what if the student did poorly because of lack of motivation? A poorly motivated student may need a different type of instruction versus a student who actually has poor abdominal strength. Similarly, how do you cue a student who might have trouble with upper-limb activities? Do you just give him extra practice on upper-limb skills or do you need to modify instruction? Perhaps the skill needs to be broken down into smaller steps, perhaps the student needs physical assistance, or perhaps the student needs adapted equipment. Unfortunately, information from standardized assessment tools does not provide information regarding instruction. Thus, teachers are forced to make instructional decisions based on what they think is best for a particular student.

AN ECOLOGICAL APPROACH TO ASSESSMENT

If the traditional approach to assessment is not effective, then what is the alternative approach? Many professionals are recommending a functional or ecological approach to assessment in which programming decisions are based on a "top-down" model (Auxter & Pyfer, 1989; Block, 1992; Wessel & Kelly, 1986). As described in the previous chapter, the ecological approach to programming provides a much more real-world approach that emphasizes the end of the developmental continuum rather than the beginning. Thus, the first step in a top-down assessment model is to identify current and future recreation environments (top of the model) that are appropriate for each student. This is followed by assessment to determine: 1) what specific skills are needed for a student to be successful in the identified recreation environments, 2) which of these skills the student currently possesses, and 3) which skills the student still needs to acquire. Kelly et al. (1991) viewed this process in terms of a pyramid in which the top of the pyramid represents the ultimate goal of the program with lower levels representing skills needed to reach the top. (See Figure 5.2.)

The top-down approach forces the teacher to focus on critical skills a student needs to be successful in current and future recreational environments, while eliminating less functional items. For example, while some items on developmental tests are critical for success in later recreational environments, many more are not functional and can be eliminated. Activities such as crawling reciprocally, standing on tiptoes, walking along a circle, and skipping are items on developmental tests that rarely are related to any functional end-goal in a top-down approach. Yet, these and other nonfunctional items often appear on a student's physical education IEP goals

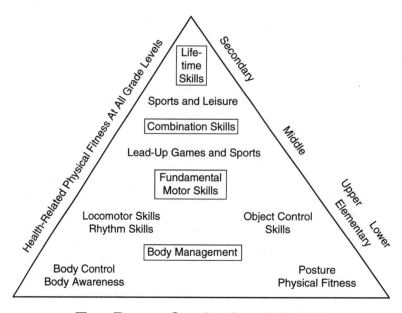

Top-Down Curriculum Model

Figure 5.2. Top-down pyramid. (From Kelly, L.E. et al. [1991]. *Achievement-based curriculum: Teaching manual.* Charlottesville: University of Virginia; reprinted with permission.)

because the student was unable to perform these items on a particular developmental test. These items would not have to be taught in a top-down approach since these skills are not related to functional outcomes.

The ecological assessment model can be broken down into seven interrelated phases that help answer the following four, real-life questions: 1) what do we teach? 2) where do we teach it? 3) how do we teach it? and 4) how effective is our program? (See Table 5.2.)

Phase 1: What skills should we teach? It is impossible to teach all skills to all students. While many students without disabilities will acquire skills quickly enough to learn a variety of lifetime leisure skills, students with disabilities often take much longer to learn just a few skills. Therefore, it is important to target just a few key activities that you will focus on for particular students (Block, 1992; Kelly et al., 1991). The first phase of the assessment process defines what skills are critical in the student's present and future environments (Kelly et al., 1991; Rainforth et al., 1992). Information that assists in defining critical skills the student needs in his or her present or future environments include the student's and parents' interests, peer interests, and an analysis of the activities that are available in the community now and in the future.

One rather simple way of determining which activities are important for a particular student is to ask key persons in the student's life (e.g., student, parents, peers, persons in community) what they perceive to be critical skills (Voeltz, Wuerch, & Bockhaut, 1982). Student and parent preferences can be measured simply by asking them at the IEP meeting what they would like to see in the physical education program. IDEA actually requires that the parents and student be involved in the development of the IEP from the beginning. Seeing what the student's peers do in physical education, during recess, and in their neighborhood also is a simple process which involves examining the regular physical education curriculum and observing students without disabilities during play. Peers also can be questioned either formally or informally as to the recreation activities they typically engage in after school. This information can then be used to determine

Table 5.2. Seven phases of an ecological assessment approach

Phase 1: Delineate what to teach.

Phase 2: Determine student's present level of performance on targeted skills.

Phase 3: Develop student's IEP based on present level of performance.

Phase 4: Determine where to teach skills.

Phase 5: Determine how to teach skills.

Phase 6: Determine level of support needed to teach skills.

Phase 7: Conduct ongoing evaluation.

what activities are popular for the age-matched student without disabilities. Activities that are appropriate and important for students without disabilities are usually appropriate for students with disabilities (with modifications as needed to accommodate individual abilities). This information can then be used to develop a list of critical activities and skills for particular students. Figure 4.1 in the previous chapter provides a simple checklist for noting students', parents', and peers' preferences for making curriculum decisions.

Student and parent preferences as well as what is available in the school and community will help shape the list of activities that might be targeted for a particular student. Note that a student's particular abilities (or disabilities) are not the focus at this point in the assessment process. Only after specific activities and skills are defined do we begin to ask how well the student can perform these skills and what modifications are needed for the student to be successful. For example, at this level of assessment we might decide that locomotor patterns are appropriate for a 7-year-old student who uses a wheelchair because running, jumping, leaping, skipping, and hopping are skills used in regular physical education and they are popular activities enjoyed by peers at home and during recess. In addition, the student's parents want her to improve her wheelchair skills. Locomotor patterns for this student involve learning how to move her wheelchair forward, backward, around obstacles, up and down ramps, and with increasing speed.

Other factors to consider when prioritizing goals for students with disabilities include availability of transportation, availability of assistance, and chance the student will acquire the skills needed to participate in the activity with minimal support and modifications. Helmstetter (1989) described a checklist designed to weigh these criteria when prioritizing goals for students with disabilities. (See Figure 5.3.) Activities in which the majority of the criteria are met should be high priority activities. For example, the team lists 10 activities as possible targeted activities for a 13-year-old student who uses a wheelchair. All of the 10 activities have met the first level of analysis; that is, these are popular activities that are available at some level in the student's school and in the community. The team then examines these 10 activities using the criteria listed in Figure 5.3 to determine which of these activities are most appropriate for this particular student. Weight training, aerobics, swimming at a local health club, wheelchair road-racing, and tennis emerge as the activities that scored the highest on the checklist. Thus, these activities become prioritized activities for this particular student.

Phase 2: Determine student's present level of performance. We now have a reference of how to measure present level of performance. That is, rather than assessing all the possible motor patterns, motor and perceptual-motor abilities, and fitness attributes of a particular student, we need to assess the student only on the critical skills and abilities directly related to the targeted activities. For example, we should measure throwing, catching, striking, and running skills if we have identified softball as a targeted skill, but there is no need to measure kicking or skipping skills. These motor skills will be measured in terms of *how well* the student performs the skill

Criteria	Activity											
	1	2	3	4	5	6	7	8	9	10	11	12
1. Can be used in current environments	—	—	—	—	—	—	—	—	—	—	—	—
2. Can be used in future environments	—	—	—	—	—	—	—	—	—	—	—	—
3. Can be used in four or more different environments	—	—	—	—	—	—	—	—	—	—	—	—
4. Affords daily opportunities for interaction with non-disabled persons	—	—	—	—	—	—	—	—	—	—	—	—
5. Increases student independence	—	—	—	—	—	—	—	—	—	—	—	—
6. Helps maintain student in, or promotes movement to, a least restrictive environment	—	—	—	—	—	—	—	—	—	—	—	—
7. Is chronological age-appropriate	—	—	—	—	—	—	—	—	—	—	—	—
8. Student will acquire in 1 year the necessary skills to participate in the activity	—	—	—	—	—	—	—	—	—	—	—	—
9. Parents rate as a high priority	—	—	—	—	—	—	—	—	—	—	—	—
10. Promotes a positive view of the individual	—	—	—	—	—	—	—	—	—	—	—	—
11. Meets a medical need	—	—	—	—	—	—	—	—	—	—	—	—
12. Improves student's health or fitness	—	—	—	—	—	—	—	—	—	—	—	—
13. If able, student would select	—	—	—	—	—	—	—	—	—	—	—	—
14. Student shows positive response to activity	—	—	—	—	—	—	—	—	—	—	—	—
15. Advocacy, training, and other support can be arranged so that student can participate in the activity in the absence of educational services	—	—	—	—	—	—	—	—	—	—	—	—
16. Related service staff support selection of activity	—	—	—	—	—	—	—	—	—	—	—	—
17. Transportation is no barrier	—	—	—	—	—	—	—	—	—	—	—	—
18. Cost is no barrier	—	—	—	—	—	—	—	—	—	—	—	—
19. Staffing is no barrier	—	—	—	—	—	—	—	—	—	—	—	—
20. Environments are physically accessible	—	—	—	—	—	—	—	—	—	—	—	—
TOTAL	—	—	—	—	—	—	—	—	—	—	—	—

Figure 5.3. Checklist for prioritizing goals. Twenty examples of criteria used for setting priorities (rating of: 3 = strongly agree with statement, 2 = agree somewhat with statement, 1 = disagree somewhat with statement, 0 = disagree strongly with statement) for 12 different activities. (Reprinted with permission from Helmstetter, E. [1989]. Curriculum for school-age students. In F. Brown & D.H. Lehr [Eds.], *Persons with profound disabilities: Issues and practices* [p. 254]. Baltimore: Paul H. Brookes Publishing Co. Adapted by Helmstetter from Dardig, J.C., & Heward, W.L. [1981]. A systematic procedure for prioritizing IEP goals. *The Directive Teacher, 3,* 6–7.)

(qualitative assessment; see Figure 5.4) as well as *how much* of the skill the student can do (quantitative assessment such as how far, how many, and how fast; see Figure 5.5 for an example).

As noted in Chapter 4, skills or characteristics associated with skilled performance such as physical fitness, general motor abilities, and perceptual skills should also be measured, but only as they relate to the skills under each targeted activity. The top-down pyramid pictured in Figure 5.2 shows how fitness and motor abilities are directly related to the skills at the top of the pyramid. This is an important difference between an ecological approach to assessment traditional assessments which measure fitness, motor abilities, and perceptual-motor skills without reference to real skills.

For example, cardiovascular endurance is usually measured by having a student run/walk a certain distance for a certain period of time. While this measure may be useful to determine a student's overall cardiovascular integrity, it does not indicate if the student has adequate cardiovascular endurance to participate in real-life activities such as softball, soccer, basketball, swimming, or other targeted activities. A better measure of cardiovascular endurance for younger children would be an appraisal of their ability to sustain various animal walks and locomotor patterns during the course of a physical education class. If the student needs to stop and rest after just a few locomotor patterns (maybe 2 minutes of exercise) while his peers do not need to rest until they complete several locomotor patterns (up to 10 minutes), then the student is functionally deficient in cardiovascular endurance.

For older students, a better measure of cardiovascular endurance is to determine how long the student can be active in the targeted individual and team sports. Such a measure, while not standardized or norm-referenced, can still be objectively collected during the course of the semester to determine progress. If, for example, a student needs to sit out and rest after 2 minutes of a game of soccer, improvement can be gauged by measuring how long the student can stay actively engaged in the game by the end of the unit. Other fitness measures such as strength and flexibility, as well as measures of motor abilities, perceptual-motor abilities, and functional motor patterns, should be also measured with specific reference to how these factors relate to the skill targeted for the student. (See Table 5.3 for another example of how abilities can be measured as they relate to functional skills.)

Table 5.3. Analysis of underlying abilities and how they affect kicking

Strength	Flexibility	Endurance	Eye–foot coordination	Balance	Coordination
Stand on one foot.	Bend leg in back swing.	Kick several balls during practice.	Accurately contact foot to ball.	Stand on one foot during backswing, contact, and follow-through.	Interaction between upper and lower leg
Lift kicking leg up.	Bring leg forward to contact ball.				Interaction between arms and legs
Forcefully move leg forward to kick ball.	Follow through.				Ability to plant foot next to ball
Keep arms out to side for balance.	Extend arm out to side for balance.				
Kick ball a certain distance.					

CLASS RECORD OF PROGRESS REPORT

CLASS: _____   DATE: _____

AGE/GRADE: _____   TEACHER: _____

SCHOOL: _____

OBJECTIVE: CATCHING A BALL

SCORING: ASSESSMENT: _____ Date X = Achieved O = Not Achieved / = Partially Achieved REASSESSMENT: _____ Date ⊗ = Achieved Ø = Not Achieved	SKILL LEVEL 1		SKILL LEVEL 2				SKILL LEVEL 3	PRIMARY RESPONSES: N = Not Attending NR = No Response UR = Unrelated Response O = Other (Specify in comments)
			Three Consecutive Times					
	Focuses eyes on ball.	Stops ball with hands or hands and arms.	Focuses eyes on ball.	Extends arms in preparation to catch ball, with elbows at sides.	Contacts and controls ball with hands or hands and arms after one bounce.	Bends elbows to absorb force of ball.	Two or more play or game activities at home or school demonstrating skill components over six-week period.	
NAME	1	2	3	4	5	6	7	COMMENTS
1.								
2.								
3.								
4.								
5.								
6.								
7.								
8.								
9.								
10.								

Recommendations: Specific changes or conditions in planning for instructions, performance, or diagnostic testing procedures or standards. Please describe what worked best.

_____

_____

_____

_____

_____

_____

Figure 5.4. Sample qualitative analysis of catching skill for preschool children. (Adapted with permission from Wessel, J.A., & Curtis-Pierce, E. [1990]. *Ball handling activities: Meeting special needs of children.* Belmont, CA: Fearon Teacher Aids.)

QUANTITATIVE ANALYSIS FOR SKILL ASSESSMENT

CLASS: _____   DATE: _____

AGE/GRADE: <u>Preschool</u> _____   TEACHER: _____

SCHOOL: _____

SKILL: <u>Catching</u> _____

NAME	Catch balloon tossed from 2'	Catch balloon tossed from 4'	Catch 8" Nerf ball from 2'	Catch 8" Nerf ball from 4'	Catch 8" Nerf ball from 6'	Catch tennis ball from 3'	Catch tennis ball from 6'	Catch tennis ball tossed to side from 6'		
	1	2	3	4	5	6	7	8	9	10
1.										
2.										
3.										
4.										
5.										
6.										
7.										
8.										
9.										
10.										

Figure 5.5. Sample quantitative analysis of catching skill for preschool children.

Phase 3: Development of the student's IEP. Now that we have targeted specific activities and we know the student's present level of performance on these activities, we can formulate the student's IEP including long-term goals and short-term instructional objectives. This should be a fairly simple process now since we have narrowed down the activities that constitute the student's program. For example, tennis is one key activity for Sarah, and we have evaluated this student on her forehand, backhand, and serve. In addition, we have measured such fitness skills as strength (being able to hit the ball over the net from various distances), flexibility (ability to demonstrate adequate range of motion in strokes and adequate range of motion for running and positioning legs), and perceptual skills such as eye–hand coordination (ability to hit stationary or moving ball at various heights, speeds, and trajectories) and balance (ability to move, stand, and hit ball without losing balance or falling). (Results of Sarah's assessment are in Table 5.4.) Based on the results of this assessment, long-term goals and short-term instructional obectives have been established for Sarah. (See Table 5.5.) Note how these goals and objectives are directly related to the student's overall program goal (i.e., to play a functional game of tennis). In addition, note how the goals and objectives are directly related to the student's present level of performance on tennis

Table 5.4. Functional assessment of tennis skills for Sarah, a high school–age student with Down syndrome (written in paragraph form)

Forehand—Demonstrates full range of motion in stroke. Has adequate strength to hold regulation racquet. Has strength to hit ball over net into server box from 20' away (near baseline). Can hit ball off tee consistently, but can only hit moving ball when ball is tossed from 5' away 1 out of 5 trials. Qualitatively, student shows side orientation, brings arm back horizontally, and swings forward horizontally. Problems appear to be keeping eye on ball and timing.

Backhand—Demonstrates full range of motion in stroke. Has adequate strength to hold regulation racquet. Has strength to hit ball over net into server box from 10' away (not from baseline). Can hit ball off tee consistently, but can only hit moving ball when ball is tossed from 5' away 1 out of 10 trials. Qualitatively, student shows side orientation, brings arm back horizontally using two-hand pattern, and swings forward horizontally. Problems appear to be keeping eye on ball and timing.

Serving—Demonstrates full range of motion in stroke. Has adequate strength to hold regulation racquet. Has strength to hit ball over net into server box from 10' away (not from baseline). Hit self-tossed ball 1 out of 10 trials. Qualitatively, student stands facing net, tosses ball by bending legs and tossing underhand with arm, brings racquet up over head, and strikes into ball with good follow-through toward ground, combination arm and leg, brings arm back horizontally using two-hand pattern. Problems appear to be accuracy in toss, keeping eye on ball, and timing.

skills. It should be clear that the type of assessment that is used is critical in determining what types of IEP goals and objectives will be established. Remember in the traditional approach how standardized tests resulted in nonfunctional goals and objectives such as standing on one foot for increasing periods of time or doing more sit-ups. In contrast, balance and fitness skills are incorporated into functional goals and objectives (in Sarah's case, functional tennis goals) in the ecological approach.

Phase 4: Where should we teach these skills? Once a list of activities and skills has been delineated, the student's present level of performance determined, and the IEP written, the next decision to be made is where best to teach these skills. As noted in Chapter 4, data collection at this level involves comparing the student's targeted goals to the activities that take place in regular physical education or community recreation. (See Figure 5.6 for example.) Again, most likely, there will be plenty of overlap, in which case the student should be placed in regular physical education with support as needed. Even if some regular physical activities appear to be different from those targeted for the student, the student's targeted activities can be presented in regular physical education. For example, softball, bowling, swimming, and fitness have been targeted for a particular student, but the regular physical education program is beginning a basketball unit. Fitness activities can be worked on while other students are working on warm-up activities at the

Table 5.5. Sarah's IEP goals and objectives based on functional assessment of tennis skills

Long-term plan:	To have Sarah develop the skills needed to play a beginner's level game of tennis with peers
Long-term goal:	Sarah will demonstrate the ability to perform a functional forehand and backhand so that she can hit a ball back and forth with instructor.
Short-term instructional objective:	1. Sarah will demonstrate the ability to hit a tennis ball that is tossed to her from 5' away using the components of a skillful forehand so that she contacts tennis ball 4 out of 5 trials and so that ball travels over net 3 out of 5 trials.
	2. Sarah will demonstrate the ability to hit a tennis ball that is tossed to her from 5' away using the components of a skillful, two-handed backhand so that she contacts tennis ball 4 out of 5 trials and so that ball travels over net 3 out of 5 trials.

Directions: List the activities/goals targeted for the student in the left-hand column, activities that take place in regular physical education or community recreation in the middle column, and how well these activities match in the next column. (Use the key listed below.) Then provide suggestions for how the student can participate in regular physical education/community recreation.

Student's Goals	Activities in RPE/Recreation	Match	Suggestion for Placement

Key:
+   Activities directly match; regular physical education.
+/−   Activities can reasonably be modified; regular physical education.
−   Activities have no relation to student's goals; alternative activities needed in RPE.
O   Activities have no relation to student's goals; alternative activities needed outside RPE.

Figure 5.6.   Comparison of student's goals to activities in RPE.

beginning of the class. While other students work on shooting skills, the student can work on hitting a softball placed on a tee into a modified basket. While other students are working on dribbling, the student can work on pushing his wheelchair toward first base, and while other students work on passing, the student can work on throwing a ball to a peer. While it may be more difficult to incorporate alternative activities into some regular physical education units, most activities like the example above can be easily adapted.

Note that placement decisions are made on skills that are needed in present and future environments, and students should receive training in the environments where these skills will be used. For elementary-age children, most critical skills will take place in the regular classrooms of the school the student attends. This is true for physical education where the activities conducted in regular physical education are often the same ones that are important for students with disabilities. As students reach middle school and high school, a greater number of skills may be more appropriately taught in the community (Brown et al., 1991; Sailor, Gee, & Karasoff, 1983). This is particularly true for upper-level high school students who may spend 75% or more of their school day in the community learning job and community skills (Brown et al., 1991). In terms of physical education, lifetime leisure skills should be taught in the community environment where they will be used eventually. Thus, if a student's program is vastly different from the program that takes place in regular physical education and if this alternative program involves lifetime leisure activities, instructional training should take place in the community. Again, to promote integration, students without disabilities should be invited on these community trips to participate alongside students with disabilities.

Another aspect of where to teach the student is how well the student performs the routines in regular physical education. These routines can be evaluated to determine what skills the student can do independently, what skills with which the student might need assistance, and what activities might need to be modified. As noted in Chapter 4, one way of analyzing the regular routine and how well a particular student performs these routines is an *environmental inventory with a discrepancy analysis*. Such information can assist the regular physical educator and the adapted physical education specialist to determine what tasks the student can do independently or with support, what tasks need training, and what tasks need to be modified to meet the student's unique needs. (See Figure 4.3.)

   Phase 5: Determine how to teach the skill. The next decision is how to help the student achieve the goals outlined in his or her program. Again, Chapter 4 outlined several factors that should be considered when making instructional decisions. Figure 5.7 presents a checklist to guide the decision process regarding implementing instructional modifications. Such factors include the following: 1) will I need to modify instruction? 2) will I need to modify the curriculum? 3) how should I communicate with the student? 4) do I need to break the skill down into smaller components? 5) do I need to teach the skill differently? and 6) will I need to use adapted equipment? Each of these questions should be answered through assessment.

   As noted in Chapter 4, one of the most important questions regarding instruction is how to communicate with the student. One simple way to determine how to communicate with the student is to set up a meeting with the student's speech therapist. He or she can describe the best ways to communicate with the student (e.g., verbal versus demonstration versus assistance) as well as how the student will communicate with you. A more ecologically valid approach (i.e., directly related to physical education) is to evaluate how the student responds to different types of cues in

---

Student's name: _____   P.E. class/teacher: _____

Who will implement modifications?

RPE teacher   Classmates   Peer tutor   Teacher assistant   Specialist

Instructional component	Things to consider	Selected modifications/Comments
Teaching style	Command, problem-solving, discovery	_____
Class format and size of group	Small/large group; stations/whole class instruction	_____
Level of methodology	Verbal cues, demonstrations, physical assistance	_____
Starting/stopping signals	Whistle, hand signals, physical assistance	_____
Time of day	Early A.M., late A.M., early P.M., late P.M.	_____
Duration of instruction	How long will student listen to instruction?	_____
Duration of expected participation	How long will student stay on task?	_____
Order of learning	In what order will you present instruction?	_____
Instructional setting	Indoors/outdoors; part of gym/whole gym	_____
Eliminate distractors	Lighting, temperature, extra equipment	_____
Provide structure	Set organization of instruction each day	_____
Level of difficulty	Complexity of instructions/organization	_____
Levels of motivation	Make setting and activities more motivating	_____

Figure 5.7.   Checklist to determine instructional modifications to accommodate students with disabilities.

different physical education situations (e.g., large versus small group). (See Figure 5.8 for a sample checklist.) Initially, such an assessment could be used to determine how you will generally communicate with a particular student. For example, if you have a student who has a visual impairment, you might find that a combination of verbal cues and physical assistance seems to work best. For another student who has a specific learning disability, environmental cues such as pictures or symbols on the wall or on the floor might work best. Again, the speech therapist or adapted physical education specialist can assist with this process in regular physical education. Once you have a general idea of how to communicate with particular students, you will want to repeat the same process (informally as you internalize the various types of communication techniques) over and over again in various teaching-learning situations to make sure the student understands the cues you are giving.

The next question to ask, assuming the student is delayed in motor skill development and is not performing the targeted skill correctly, is how to instruct the student. At this level, you are trying to find out if the student: 1) does not know the correct components of the skill and just needs instruction and feedback, or 2) knows the correct components of the skill but cannot perform the skill because of specific motor or sensory impairments. If the student does not know the components, instruction could be as simple as showing the student how to perform the skill using verbal cues, physical assistance, demonstration, and environmental cues. For example, a 7-year-old student with mental retardation has had little instruction on how to perform a skillful, two-handed catch. In this case, instruction might only require giving her information about the correct pattern, specific instruction with corrective feedback, and time to practice the skill. On the other hand, another 7-year-old student with a learning disability might not be able to perform a two-handed catch because of problems with visual-motor perception and body awareness. This student might need more than instruction on how to catch. This student might need supplemental practice and instruction to improve visual-motor perception and body awareness in addition to specific instruction in the components of the catch. Figure 5.9 provides a simple checklist to aid in deciding which students need general instruction and which students need supplemental instruction.

Directions: Instruct student in various situations. (See below.) Note how student responds to each type of cue or combination of cues. You may need to repeat in various instructional situations (e.g., outside versus inside; simple skills versus more complex skills).

	Responds correctly	Delayed response (5–10 seconds)	Does not respond
Verbal cues			
Gestures			
Demonstration			
Environmental cues			
Physical assistance			

Situations in which this assessment was conducted (whether formally or informally):
_____ Inclusive physical education setting with peers without disabilities (large group)
_____ Inclusive physical education setting with small groups (5–7 students)
_____ Inclusive physical education setting: one-on-one instruction

---

Figure 5.8. Sample checklist to determine communication skills of student.

	Yes	No	Comments
Does the student appear to have normal sensory awareness?			
Does the student appear to have normal body awareness?			
Does the student appear to respond to specific instructional cues related to targeted skill?			

Note: If the answer to some or all of the above questions is no, then the student may need to be checked for perceptual problems such as visual-motor problems or problems with body awareness. (Consult with other team members such as the occupational therapist.) If the student does have perceptual problems, he or she may need either supplemental instruction to improve these deficits or compensations to overcome these deficits.

Figure 5.9.   What type of instruction does the student need?

For some students, even breaking a skill down into smaller components may not be enough. For example, students with physical disabilities such as spinal cord injuries or cerebral palsy may not be able to peform skills the way students without disabilities do. Forcing them to perform the skill the way other students do can lead to frustration and potential noncompliance. In addition, the students might not be able to work on other, more functional skills if they are continually asked to learn how to perform a more fundamental skill using a particular pattern. In these cases, the students should be given an alternative way to perform the skill that meets their unique abilities. Again, this decision should be driven by assessment data. Figure 5.10 provides a simple checklist that can help guide this decision.

Caution should be taken when deciding if an alternative pattern should be introduced to particular students. If the alternative pattern does not give the student any advantage over the regular pattern, then it may not be appropriate. For example, if a student is having difficulty kicking a soccer ball due to spasticity in his legs, he may be allowed to pick up the ball and throw it as an alternative pattern. However, this student would not be allowed to use this alternative pattern in league soccer games, so this type of adaptation may not be very functional if the goal is for the student to be integrated into a regular soccer league. In contrast, a student with spastic cerebral palsy might be allowed to throw backwards over the head rather than throwing forward.

	Yes	No	Comments
Does the student have a physical disability that appears to preclude typical performance?			
Is the student having extreme difficulty performing the skill?			
Is the student making little to no progress over several months or years despite instruction?			
Does the student seem more comfortable and motivated using a different pattern?			
Will an alternative pattern still be useful (i.e., functional) in the targeted environments?			
Will the alternative pattern increase the student's ability to perform the skill?			

Note: If the answer to some or all of the above questions is yes, the student may need an adapted pattern.

Figure 5.10.   Does the student need an alternative way to perform the skill?

This student could then use this skill when playing horseshoes, lawn darts, or when competing in the Indian club throw.

The next step is to determine if the student needs some type of curricular adaptation or adapted equipment. Curricular adaptations and adapted equipment such as flotation devices or a shorter racquet allow students to perform functional, lifetime leisure skills more independently. Still, most students should be given every opportunity to learn skills without modifications or special equipment since such adaptations can be costly, difficult to transport, and heighten the difference between students with and without disabilities. If a student is having difficulty with a particular skill and you are considering curricular adaptations or adapted equipment, the questions in Figure 5.11 may be helpful in making the decision. Once the decision has been made to utilize some curricular adaptations or adapted equipment, checklists in Figures 5.12 and 5.13 can be used. Note that some curricular adaptations and pieces of adapted equipment can be used temporarily to motivate or assist a student in learning a particular skill. If modifications or equipment are to be used temporarily, a plan should be developed to wean the student away quickly and easily from these adaptations. For example, arm flotation devices are often used to give young swimmers confidence in the water, but these young swimmers often become dependent on these "floaties." It then becomes extremely difficult to wean the student away from the floaties to swim more independently. A systematic plan should be set up to help the student gradually swim without the aid of such devices.

Phase 6: Determine level of support needed to teach skill. The final step before actually implementing the program is to determine how much support a particular student will need and who will provide this support. Some students can do quite well in regular physical education with no extra support, while other students will need support in the form of peers, volunteers, teacher assistants, or specialists. Again, assessment data should guide this decision process. As noted by York, Giangreco, Vandercook, and Macdonald (1992), collaboration is needed to determine the amount and type of support needed by particular students.

Important factors that should be considered when determining level of support are the student's characteristics, the physical educator's and peers' characteristics, and the setting. These factors taken together will help the team determine the best type of support to provide. For example, York et al. (1992) noted that student characteristics such as particular abilities, previous experiences, and/or other aspects of their intellectual, communication, social, physical, sensory, or

	Yes	No	Comments
Will adaptation increase the student's participation in the activity?			
Will it allow the student to participate in an activity that is preferred or valued by the student, friends, and family members?			
Will it take less time to teach the student to use the adaptation than to teach the skill directly?			
Will the team have access to the technical expertise to design, construct, adjust, and repair the adaptation?			
Will the adaptation maintain or enhance related motor/communication skills?			

Note: If the answer to most of the above questions is yes, then the student may need adapted equipment.

Figure 5.11. Does the student need adapted equipment?

Does the student have limited strength?

Things to consider   Selected modifications (if any) and Comments

     Shorten distance to move or project object.   _____

     Use lighter equipment (e.g., balls, bats).   _____

     Use shorter striking implements.   _____

     Allow student to sit or lie down while playing.   _____

     Use deflated balls or suspended balls.   _____

     Change requirements (a few jumps, then run).   _____

Does the student have limited speed?

Things to consider   Selected modifications (if any) and Comments

     Shorten distance (or make it longer for others).   _____

     Change locomotor pattern (allow running v. walking).   _____

     Make safe areas in tag games.   _____

Does the student have limited endurance?

Things to consider   Selected modifications (if any) and Comments

     Shorten distance.   _____

     Shorten playing field.   _____

     Allow "safe" areas in tag games.   _____

     Decrease activity time for student.   _____

     Allow more rest periods for student.   _____

     Allow student to sit while playing.   _____

Does the student have limited balance?

Things to consider   Selected modifications (if any) and Comments

     Provide chair/bar for support.   _____

     Teach balance techniques (widen base, extend arms).   _____

     Increase width of beams to be walked.   _____

     Use carpeted rather than slick surfaces.   _____

     Teach student how to fall.   _____

     Allow student to sit during activity.   _____

     Place student near wall for support.   _____

     Allow student to hold peer's hand.   _____

Does student have limited coordination and accuracy?

Things to consider   Selected modifications (if any) and Comments

     Use stationary balls for kicking/striking.   _____

     Decrease distance for throwing, kicking, and shooting.   _____

     Make targets and goals larger.   _____

     Use larger balls for kicking and striking.   _____

     Increase surface of the striking implements.   _____

     Use backstop.   _____

(continued)

Figure 5.12. Checklist to determine curricular adaptations to accommodate individuals with specific limitations. (Adapted from Sherrill [1993].)

Figure 5.12. (*continued*)

Use softer, slower balls for striking and catching.   _____

In bowling-type games, use lighter, less stable
  pins.   _____

What can you do to maximize safety?   _____

Note: Some or all of these modifications can be implemented. Also, these modifications can be implemented
for one student, for several students, or for the entire class to make the activity more challenging and success-
oriented.

health functioning are important factors to consider when determining levels of support. In addition, the student's behaviors in terms of his or her ability to follow directions, stay on task, and
maintain control in a crowded, noisy environment are important.

Related to the student's characteristics are the characteristics of the physical educator and the
peers without disabilities. Physical educators and peers who have knowledge about the student
being included, knowledge about successful ways to include students with disabilities, and previous experience with inclusion may need less support, while a physical educator who has limited
knowledge of inclusion or is experiencing inclusion for the first time may need more support.

Things to consider	Selected modifications (if any) and Comments
Can you vary the purpose/goal of the game (e.g., some students play to learn complex strategies, others play to work on simple motor skills)?	_____
Can you vary number of players (e.g., play small games such as 2 v. 2 basketball)?	_____
Can you vary movement requirements (e.g., some students walk, others run; some hit a ball off a tee, others hit pitched ball; skilled students use more complex movements, less skilled use simpler movements)?	_____
Can you vary the field of play (e.g., special zones for students with less mobility; make the field narrower or wider as needed; shorten the distance for students with movement problems)?	_____
Can you vary objects used (e.g., some students use lighter bats/larger balls; some use a lower net/basket)?	_____
Can you vary the level of organization? (Vary typical organizational patterns; vary where certain students stand; vary the level of structure for certain students.)	_____
Can you vary the limits/expectations? (Vary the number of turns each student receives; vary the rules regarding how far a student can run, hit, etc.; vary how much you will enforce certain rules for certain players.)	_____

Note: Use these suggestions to modify rules for both students with and without disabilities to make the game
challenging, safe, and success-oriented.

Figure 5.13.   Checklist to determine curricular modifications for group games and sports. (Adapted from Morris
& Stiehl [1989].)

Finally, the expectations of the setting, in this case physical education, will affect how much support a particular student will need. Figure 5.14 presents a checklist to help facilitate decisions regarding supports. Note how this form reads like a flow chart in which the regular physical educator, in collaboration with other team members, tries to determine how much support he or she would need to provide safely and successfully an appropriate, quality physical education program to the student with disabilities as well as to the students without disabilities. In making this impor-

	Locker room	Warm-ups	Skills	Games
Can you handle having _____ in these situations without extra support?				
If NO, could you handle situation with consultation from specialists? If yes, from which specialists would you like consultative support? (See below.)				
Can you handle situation on your own with consultative support?				
If NO, could peers in class provide enough extra support (without drastically affecting their program)?				
If NO, could an older peer tutor or volunteer provide enough support?				
If NO, could a trained teacher assistant provide enough support?				
If NO, could a regular visit from a specialist provide enough support? If yes, which specialists would you like for direct support? (See below.)				

Comments:

_____

_____

_____

_____

_____

Key:

APE specialist, Adapted Physical Education Specialist (modifications to physical education).
SE, Special Educator (behavior management, personality, interests).
P, Parent (interests, personality, behaviors, homework).
PT, Physical therapist (gross motor needs, adapted equipment, positioning, contraindicated activities).
OT, Occupational therapist (fine motor skills, adapted equipment).
ST, Speech therapist (communication skills).
VT, Vision therapist (visual skills, adaptations, mobility skills).

Figure 5.14. Checklist for determining general supports in regular physical education.

tant decision, the team should weigh such factors as personal needs of the student (e.g., ability to dress out, sit and wait turn, interact with peers), physical needs of the student (performing all of the physical education activities), sensory needs of the student (receiving information, following directions, locating certain places in the gymnasium), comfort level of regular physical educator, teaching style of regular physical educator, level of structure in class, and general make-up and behaviors of regular physical education students.

Again, types of supports that can be provided vary from trained therapists to peers. In many cases, peer tutors and volunteers can provide support to students with milder disabilities, while specialists may be needed to provide more support for students with significant disabilities. (See Table 5.6.) Support provided by specialists often can be faded away so that the student is responding to more natural cues in the environment with occasional support from peers. For example, a student with severe, spastic diplegic cerebral palsy (needs assistance to move his wheelchair) might need a physical therapist or adapted physical education specialist to provide assistance in regular physical education. However, as the peers become more comfortable with the student, the specialist can begin to train peers how to assist the student in throwing balls, pushing his wheelchair, and performing other physical education activities.

Again, there is no clear-cut way to determine how much support a particular student will need. The team should work together to make an informed decision based on as much information as they can collect regarding the student, the teacher and peers, and the environment.

Phase 7: Ongoing evaluation. The final phase of the assessment process is ongoing evaluation. Ongoing evaluation is critical to determine if the student is making progress toward his or her targeted goals. If he or she is not making adequate progress, then ongoing evaluation can quickly discover what the problem might be. If we do not conduct ongoing evaluation or wait until the end of a unit or end of a semester to evaluate the program, a student might miss valuable practice time (Kelly et al., 1991). For example, it was decided that a high school student with Down syndrome would use a racquetball racquet rather than a tennis racquet based on initial assessment of the student's strength and ability to hold a regulation tennis racquet. However, evaluation of the student at the end of the first day revealed that he does very well with the racquetball racquet, but cannot reach most balls hit toward him. A lighter regulation racquet was tried the next day, and the student was able to hold the racquet and reach many more balls. If we had waited until the end of the unit to evaluate the student, he would have had to use an inappropriate piece of equipment the entire time and would probably have had to relearn how to strike a tennis ball using a regulation tennis racquet.

Ongoing evaluation should include all four previous phases of the assessment model. Ongoing Phase 1 evaluation (*what do we teach?*) can be as simple as talking with the student, parents, and peers to find out how they perceive the program to date. If they all perceive that the program is going well and the student is involved in appropriate activities, then your program has social validity. Ongoing Phase 2 evaluation (*where do we teach it?*) could be conducted by measuring the student's progress toward his targeted goals in his current placement; how his special education teacher, teacher assistant, regular physical education teacher, and peers perceive he is doing in regular physical education; and how modifications to various activities are working. Ongoing Phase 3 evaluation (*present level of performance in targeted skills?*) might be the most critical aspect of ongoing evaluation. As the student progresses and acquires new skills, changes should be made to his present level of performance and expectations for future progress. For example, a new goal (hopping) might be targeted for a student who has achieved the goal of demonstrating a consistent, skillful gallop much sooner than expected. However, the goal for a student who is not making anticipated progress in his ability to demonstrate a skillful gallop might be changed to revisit the skill of stepping and sliding. Checklists similar to the ones described in Figures 5.4 and 5.5 can be used to measure progress the student is making both qualitatively and quantitatively.

Table 5.6. Support personnel who can assist students with specific needs

Student challenge	Potential support personnel
Cognitive/learning processes	
Curricular/instructional adaptations or alternatives	Educator, speech-language pathologist, occupational therapist, psychologist, vision or hearing specialist, classmate, support facilitator
Organizing assignments, schedules	Educator, occupational therapist, speech-language pathologist, support facilitator
Communication/interactions	
Nonverbal communication	Speech-language pathologist, teacher, family members
Socialization with classmates	Speech-language pathologist, teacher, psychologist, classmates
Behaving in adaptive ways	Educator, psychologist, speech-language pathologist, classmates
Physical/motor	
Functional use of hands	Occupational therapist, physical therapist, family member, classmate
Mobility and transitions	Physical therapist, occupational therapist, orientation and mobility specialist, educator, family member, classmates
Posture (body alignment)	Physical therapist, occupational therapist
Fitness and physical activity	Physical therapist, physical educator, nurse
Sensory	
Vision	Vision specialist, occupational therapist, orientation and mobility specialist
Hearing	Audiologist, hearing specialist, speech-language pathologist
Health	
Eating difficulty	Occupational therapist, speech-language pathologist, physical therapist, nurse, educator
Medications	Nurse
Other health needs	Nurse
Current and future living	
Career and vocational pursuits	Vocational educator, counselor, educator
Leisure pursuits	Educator, occupational therapist, community recreation personnel
Support from home and community	Social worker, counselor, educator

From York, J., Giangreco, M.F., Vandercook, T., & Macdonald, C. (1992). Integrating support personnel in the inclusive classroom. In S. Stainback & W. Stainback (Eds.), *Curriculum considerations in inclusive classrooms: Facilitating learning for all students* (p. 108). Baltimore: Paul H. Brookes Publishing Co.; reprinted by permission.

Finally, ongoing Phase 4 evaluation (*how well does the student follow the regular routine?*) again can be measured by talking with the student, his peers, and the regular physical educator. If the student is having difficulty in any area on the ecological inventory or is not making anticipated progress on tasks that have been targeted for training, accommodations might need to be implemented. For example, the ecological inventory and discrepancy analysis suggested that a student needed a peer to help him change into his clothes for physical education. However, the student is taking much longer than expected in the locker room, and he and the peer are missing warm-up activities. It is decided to change the support person from a peer to a teacher assistant. In addition, the student comes down to physical education 5 minutes earlier than his peers to make sure he has enough time to change into his uniform. Again, the use of the ecological inventory described in Figure 4.3 can be used to conduct ongoing evaluations.

EXAMPLE OF ASSESSMENT TO FACILITATE INCLUSION

The following is an example of how the ecological approach to assessment might look for one student. John is a 10-year-old student who has recently moved into the Washington school district. John has been diagnosed as having mental retardation and diplegic, spastic cerebral palsy such that he has very limited movement in his legs and some control over his arms, and a seizure disorder which is controlled with medication. John uses a manual wheelchair for mobility, and he can push it forward and maneuver it around obstacles slowly, but independently. John communicates verbally with one- to two-word statements, and he seems to understand most simple directions. John can go to the bathroom and take care of his personal needs with minimal assistance (needs help pulling up pants, buttoning shirt, and transferring out of chair). John enjoys being with his peers and doing the same things they do. He is a big baseball fan, and his favorite team is the Chicago Cubs. John received special education services in his previous placement, but he did not have a specific IEP for physical education. The collaborative team has scheduled a meeting to determine how they should proceed with John's IEP. The adapted physical education specialist, in conjunction with the regular physical educator and the special education teacher, has been asked to assess John in order to make recommendations to the team regarding physical education services.

Phase 1: What do I teach? The first phase of the assessment process is to determine what physical education skills to target for John. Information is collected in order to find out what John likes to do, what his parents like to do, what his peers like to do, and what young adults in the community like to do. (See Figure 5.15.) First, the adapted physical education specialist asks John what he would like to learn in physical education. Since he is a big baseball fan, John wants to learn how to play baseball. He also mentions tennis, and John's father notes that the family often plays tennis, but John watches from the sidelines because of his disability. Both John and his parents would like to see John somehow play tennis with the family on these weekly outings. Finally, John's mother says that she would like to see John move his wheelchair faster, for longer periods of time, and with more precision around obstacles when he goes to the mall or to a grocery store.

Next, the adapted physical education specialist conducts a simple survey in John's school to determine what activities students without disabilities John's age like to do during recess and in their neighborhood after school. This information provides social validity as to the potential activities that might be targeted for John. For example, if John's friends like to play softball and we target football skills, there is very little chance John will acquire the skills needed to play with his peers. The results of the survey revealed that the most popular recreational activities (other than Nintendo and watching television!) are riding bikes, playing soccer in the fall, basketball in the winter, and softball in the summer, and going down to the creek to fish and play in the water.

Form for Curricular Decision Making

Directions: List all of the activities preferred or typically engaged in under the following headings. Scan across the list and place activities that are in more than one column under "Targeted Activities."

Student preferences	Parents' preferences	Activities in RPE	Activities played by peers	Community leisure activities
Baseball	Tennis	Lead-up	Bike riding	Softball
Tennis	Wheelchair	games &	Soccer	Swimming
	mobility	skills to	Basketball	Weight training
		a variety	Softball	Aerobics
		of team	Fishing	wheelchair
		sports		mobility

Targeted Activities: 1. Softball   2. Tennis
                                3. Wheelchair mobility   4. General Fitness

Figure 5.15.   Curriculum decisions for John.

Some of these activities can be targeted for John's physical education IEP while others can be recommended to other team members, including John's parents, in terms of activities they might want to focus on with John.

Next, the adapted physical education specialist conducts a survey in the community in which John lives to determine what recreation activities are popular for young adults. While John will not be graduating from school for some time, the severity of his physical and mental disabilities indicates that he will learn skills very slowly. Therefore, some critical skills that John will need upon graduation should be targeted immediately in John's IEP. The survey reveals that the most popular active recreational activities in John's community are bowling, golf, tennis, aerobic dance, weight lifting, softball, soccer, hiking, biking, and swimming. The team can then make a determination regarding which of these community-based recreation activities are realistic possibilities for John. For example, even though adult coed soccer is a popular sport in John's community, the program is very competitive. There is only one division, and only skilled players participate in the league. This activity would not be appropriate for John given its current parameters. However, adult coed softball is another popular sport in John's community, and this program is large enough to have several divisions. As it turns out, Division C is specifically designed for persons just learning how to play softball or for those who just want to have fun. It would seem plausible that such a division would accept John into the league, especially if John can learn some of the key softball skills such as batting, pushing his chair toward first base, tossing a ball to a peer, and understanding the general rules and etiquette of the game. Swimming, weight training, and aerobics also are activities that might be targeted for John since these activities can easily be adapted to accommodate John's unique needs.

Based on this preliminary assessment, it appears that softball, tennis, wheelchair mobility, and fitness (strength and endurance in pushing his wheelchair) are activities that should be the main focus of John's program. (See Figure 5.15.) Tennis is something in which John and his parents are interested, and it is an activity that John can play now and when he leaves school.

Softball appears to be a popular sport that his peers play during recess and after school. Softball also is a lifetime recreation sport that should be available to John when he leaves school. With John's interest in baseball, softball should be a motivating activity for him. Finally, wheelchair mobility including improved strength, endurance, and control are skills that his parents have targeted. Mobility skills can be worked on in a variety of physical education activities, and improved wheelchair skills will help John both in the targeted physical education skills (tennis, softball) and in community skills (shopping).

Phase 2: Determine the student's present level of performance. The second phase of the assessment is to determine John's present level of performance in motor skills, physical fitness, motor abilities, perceptual motor abilities, and cognitive abilities. However, now the APE specialist has a reference on how to measure these areas. That is, measurement of John's present level of performance will be referenced to skills needed in tennis, softball, and mobility. For example, tennis skills John will need include forehand strike, backhand strike, and wheelchair mobility. These skills will be measured both qualitatively and quantitatively. Qualitative measurement involves analyzing how John performs these skills. (See Figure 5.16 for an example from working with John on softball skills.)

Other areas will be measured in reference to the skills needed in the targeted activities. For example, physical fitness will be referenced to what minimum amounts of strength, flexibility, and stamina are needed to participate in softball, tennis, and mobility. Table 5.7 provides an example of the specific fitness, perceptual, motor, and cognitive requirements as they relate to the skills needed for softball. The adapted physical education specialist can now evaluate John's present level of performance in reference to the requirements of the activities. For example, assessment regarding John's strength revealed that he did not have the grip strength to hold a regulation tennis racquet. However, he was able to hold a racquetball racquet, especially when it was strapped to his hand with an Ace bandage. John also was able to hold a badminton racquet, but the length of the racquet made it difficult for him to control. In addition, it was determined through assessment of the tennis stroke that John did not have the flexibility in his shoulder, arm, and trunk to perform a functional forehand, but he was able to do a fair backhand (move arm into preparatory back position, swing arm horizontally, follow through, and hit the ball with racquetball racquet so that ball traveled forward 5′ on 2 out of 3 trials).

John's wheelchair mobility skills on the softball field were limited. He could push his wheelchair forward slowly toward first base, but not fast enough to be safe in most situations. John was able to hit the ball off a tee on 3 out of 4 tries so that the ball traveled approximately 10′. Cognitively, John understood the general concept and rules of softball. He was able to stay on task during the entire assessment process (15 minutes), and he seemed motivated and receptive to instruction. Notice how the information obtained from this type of assessment is directly applicable to what John needs work on in relation to his targeted skills and how the teacher might go about teaching the skills (e.g., shortening the distance to first base, allowing him to hit a ball off a tee, having assistance when playing the field to compensate for his limited skills).

Phase 3: Develop the student's IEP. The next step is to develop John's IEP. Again, the development of the IEP should be a team approach that is based on assessment information. The bulk of the information regarding the physical education section of John's IEP is based on the assessment of his present level of performance on the targeted skills. Table 5.8 shows the softball portion of John's IEP.

Phase 4: Determine where to teach these skills. The fourth phase of the assessment process is to determine where John will work on these skills. This can be accomplished by examining the curriculum for the fourth, fifth, and sixth grade at John's school. The philosophy of the physical education program at John's school is to expose students to and provide some foundational skills in a variety of individual and team sports including lifetime leisure skills. A basic foundation in a

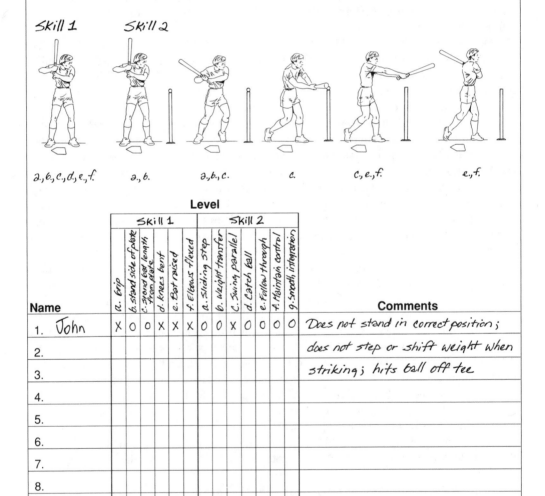

Figure 5.16. Qualitative analysis of John's softball skills. (Adapted from ICAN Lifetime Leisure Skills Program.)

Table 5.7. Fitness, perceptual, motor, and cognitive requirements to play softball

	Strength	Flexibility	Stamina	Perceptual-motor	Fundamental-motor	Cognitive
Batting	Hold bat.	Twist trunk. Bend and extend arms.	Stand at place for up to 5 minutes.	See ball. Timing	Striking	Differentiating balls and strikes
Base running	Leg strength (arm strength if pushing w/c)	Bend legs and arms.	Run to first base and possibly around all bases.	Locate first base. Stay in base path.	Running	Know when to run.
Fielding	Hold mitt.	Bend and move to ball.	Stand in field for entire inning.	Locate ball when hit. Move to ball. Timing. Locate person to whom to throw.	Catch. Throw.	Know where to throw the ball. Know where to stand.

117

Table 5.8. Softball portion of John's IEP

Long-term plan:	John will demonstrate the skills needed to play in a modified game of softball with peers in school and in the community.
Long-term goal:	John will demonstrate functional competency in striking a pitched ball, pushing wheelchair to first base, and throwing ball to peer in practice situations.
Short-term instructional objectives:	1. John will demonstrate the ability to push his wheelchair from home to first base that is 30′ away (1/2 the distance of regulation softball) in 30 seconds or less three out of four trials.
	2. John will hit a pitched Nerf ball holding two hands on bat and using a horizontal striking pattern that includes follow-through across body when ball is tossed slowly from 10′ away three out of four trials.
	3. John will throw a ball overhand so that ball travels a distance of 10′ and within 1′ to either side of peer three out of four trials.

variety of activities will help these students make informed choices on what activities they want to focus when they go to high school. (High school physical education follows an elective format.) The following are the specific activities and when they are targeted during the year:

	5th grade	6th grade	7th grade
1st quarter	soccer	tennis	roller skating/blading
2nd quarter	volleyball	aerobics	badminton
3rd quarter	basketball	weight training	bowling
4th quarter	softball	golf	archery

A general inspection of the middle school physical education curriculum suggests that John's peers will be working on softball in the spring of the fifth grade and tennis in the fall of the sixth grade. John should be integrated into these units (with modifications as needed) so that he can work on his targeted goals. But what happens to John when his class works on other activities? When can John be integrated and when might it be appropriate to remove John so that he can focus on his specific goals and objectives? Badminton in the seventh grade is a sport similar to tennis, and in fact the lighter racquet and birdie might prove to be a useful adaptation for John. Thus, John should probably stay in regular physical education for this activity. Similarly, aerobics, weight training, and roller skating/blading are activities that can help John improve his strength, flexibility, and endurance. Weight training (improving strength and flexibility) can concentrate on the muscle groups that John uses to propel his wheelchair, and aerobics can improve John's endurance. For roller skating/blading, John can practice pushing his wheelchair following the same course his peers follow on their skates/blades. When the class goes to a local roller rink as the end of the unit, John can go along and push his wheelchair. Golf, bowling, and archery are lifetime leisure activities that are available in John's community. John might find these lifetime leisure sports enjoyable, and some or all of these activities might be so interesting to John that they might become targeted goals for him when he enters high school. Therefore, he will stay in regular physical education part of the time for these activities (2 days per week) so that he can learn what they are about. He will receive specialized adapted physical education the other 3 days in the week to work on his targeted goals.

That leaves soccer, volleyball, and basketball. While these activities can be accommodated so that John can have a safe and successful experience, they do not appear to be high priority goals for John. It is going to take John a long time to learn to master even the basic skills of tennis and softball, and exposing John to other activities would take away important instructional time (Kelly et al., 1991). However, these team sports are popular with John's peers during various seasons of the year, and it would be nice if John had at least a general understanding of the skills, rules, and flow of the game. In addition, some of John's fitness and mobility goals can easily be incorporated into these sports. The team decides that John will work on tennis during the soccer unit since it is difficult to get John up to the soccer field and move his wheelchair on the grass. However, as was the case above, the team recommended that John participate in volleyball and basketball 2 days a week and work on his targeted skills the other 3 days a week. It is understood that John will not acquire the skills for these sports, but exposing him to these sports might be of interest to him, would give him a chance to interact with his peers, would give him a chance to work on his fitness and mobility skills in a different context, and would give him a break from focusing solely on tennis and softball. Several (five to seven) of John's peers will go with John on the days he is pulled out of regular physical education. These students without disabilities are not peer tutors but friends of John who will participate alongside John in his targeted activities. Different students are picked each day to go with John and John's teacher assistant. Thus, each student would only miss one day of physical education if he or she is randomly picked. (See Figure 5.17.)

Next, daily routines in regular physical education are measured including the communication, self-help, social/emotional, and motor skills needed on a daily basis. This information will help determine what specific skills John will need to be safe and successful in regular physical education as well as suggestions for support and accommodations that John might need. Information from the ecological inventory and discrepancy analysis revealed that John can follow most routines independently. On the skills with which he has difficulty, it was determined that a peer

---

Directions: List the activities/goals targeted for the student in the left-hand column, activities that take place in regular physical education or community recreation in the middle column, and how well these activities match in the next column. (Use the key listed below.) Then provide suggestions for how the student can participate in regular physical education/community recreation.

Student's Goals	Activities in RPE/Recreation	Match	Suggestion for Placement
Tennis	Soccer	−	tennis on courts
Softball	Volleyball	−	part-time RPE, part-time wt. training
Wheelchair Mob.	Basketball	−	part-time RPE part-time commu. training
Wt. training	Softball	+	full-time RPE
	Tennis	+	full-time RPE
	Aerobics	+	full-time RPE
	Wt. Lifting	+	full-time RPE
	Golf	+/−	full-time RPE

Key for suggestions:
+   Activities directly match; regular physical education.
+/−   Activities can reasonably be modified; regular physical education.
−   Activities have no relation to student's goals; alternative activities needed in RPE.
O   Activities have no relation to student's goals; alternative activities needed outside RPE.

Figure 5.17. Comparison of student's goals to activities in RPE.

could assist John. John does have self-help problems, and he will need assistance changing into his physical education clothes. A peer can help John change his clothes in the locker room. The occupational therapist has suggested to John's parents that John wear pants with an elastic waist and pullover shirts so that he can dress faster and more independently. It does not appear that John will need more time than his peers to change into his gym clothes. The discrepancy analysis also showed that John did not have any communication problems although a peer might have to repeat more complex directions to him. John is a motivated, well-behaved learner who has no major behavior problems. (See Figure 4.3 for an example of an ecological inventory with a discrepancy analysis.)

Phase 5: Determine how to teach skills. At this point in the assessment we want to find out how to help John work on his goals and objectives. Information that is needed to make this decision includes general information about possible instructional modifications as well as specific information regarding John's communication skills, if John has any perceptual or motor problems, if John can perform the movement in the traditional way, and if John needs adapted equipment. The checklist discussed previously can help the physical educator determine how best to teach John. (See Figures 5.18–5.22 for the results of this assessment with John.) For example, John responds quite well to verbal cues and physical assistance but does not do well with demonstration. Similarly, John seems to have the range-of-motion, strength, and perceptual skills needed to respond to general instructional cues; he should be able to perform the skill the same way his peers do; however, there are modifications that seem appropriate such as using a lighter

Student's name: _John_   P.E. class/teacher: _Mrs. Smith   2nd period_

Who will implement modifications?
(RPE teacher) (Classmates)   Peer tutor   Teacher assistant   Specialist

Instructional component	Things to consider	Selected modifications/Comments
Teaching style	Command, problem-solving, discovery	none
Class format and size of group	Small/large group; stations/whole class instruction	none
Level of methodology	Verbal cues, demonstrations, physical assistance	extra physical assistance
Starting/stopping signals	Whistle, hand signals, physical assistance	none
Time of day	Early A.M., late A.M., early P.M., late P.M.	mornings better
Duration of instruction	How long will student listen to instruction?	none
Duration of expected participation	How long will student stay on task?	give extra rest in endurance activities
Order of learning	In what order will you present instruction?	none
Instructional setting	Indoors/outdoors; part of gym/whole gym	none
Eliminate distractors	Lighting, temperature, extra equipment	none
Provide structure	Set organization of instruction each day	none
Level of difficulty	Complexity of instructions/organization	make instruction and organization simpler
Levels of motivation	Make setting and activities more motivating	none

Figure 5.18. Checklist to determine instructional modifications to accommodate students with disabilities (John).

Directions: Instruct student in various situations. (See below.) Note how student responds to each type of cue or combination of cues. You may need to repeat in various instructional situations (e.g., outside versus inside; simple skills versus more complex skills).

	Responds correctly	Delayed response (5–10 seconds)	Does not respond
Verbal cues	✓		
Gestures		✓	
Demonstration		✓	
Environmental cues	✓		
Physical assistance	✓		

Situations in which this assessment was conducted (whether formally or informally):
- ✓ Inclusive physical education setting with peers without disabilities (large group)
- ____ Inclusive physical education setting with small groups (5–7 students)
- ____ Inclusive physical education setting: one-on-one instruction

Figure 5.19. Sample checklist to determine communication skills of student (John).

bat for softball, pushing his chair closer to a base, and having a peer assist him in the field. This information can be supplemented by more specific information from team members such as physical and speech therapists. In addition, John should be encouraged to try the movements in different ways to see which is best for him.

Once it has been decided whether or not John needs adaptations, the checklists shown in Figures 5.23 and 5.24 can be used to determine specific modifications. In many cases, modifications are rather simple, involving changes to equipment (e.g., lighter equipment, closer distance than peers) that really do not affect nondisabled students. Note that these checklists were filled out in general terms without any specific activities in mind. The team will want to glance over these checklists, if not actually complete them, prior to each new physical education unit.

Phase 6: Determine level of support. John will need some support in regular physical education if he is going to be successful. However, he does not have a behavior problem, and the regular physical educator and peers without disabilities feel very comfortable with John. Therefore, the team members, utilizing the checklists in Figures 5.23, 5.24, and 5.25, decide that the physical thera-

	Yes	No	Comments
Does the student appear to have typical sensory awareness?	✓		*Slower reaction*
Does the student appear to have typical body awareness?	✓		
Does the student appear to respond to specific instructional cues related to targeted skill?	✓		*except demonstrations*

Note: If the answer to some or all of the above questions is no, then the student may need to be checked for perceptual problems such as visual-motor problems or problems with body awareness. (Consult with other team members such as the occupational therapist.) If the student does have perceptual problems, he or she may need either supplemental instruction to improve these deficits or compensations to overcome these deficits.

Figure 5.20. What type of instruction does the student (John) need?

	Yes	No	Comments
Does the student have a physical disability that appears to preclude typical performance?	✓		*John's disability affects quantative performance*
Is the student having extreme difficulty performing the skill?		✓	
Is the student making little to no progress over several months or years despite instruction?		✓	
Does the student seem more comfortable and motivated using a different pattern?		✓	
Will an alternative pattern still be useful (i.e., functional) in the targeted environments?		✓	
Will the alternative pattern increase the student's ability to perform the skill?		✓	

Note: If the answer to some or all of the above questions is yes, the student may need adapted pattern.

Figure 5.21. Does the student (John) need an alternative way to perform skill?

pist and the adapted physical educator could come into regular physical education with John initially and talk with John's regular physical educator and his peers. They can provide information to the regular physical educator and peers on how to work with John, how to position him, how to help him get dressed and undressed, how to practice skills, and so forth. These specialists can then monitor how well the peers assist John, and eventually, these specialists can back off and become consultants as needed (perhaps coming in to see John and discuss his program with the regular physical educator at the beginning, middle, and end of each unit).

Phase 7: Conduct ongoing evaluation. The final phase of the assessment process is ongoing evaluation. Ongoing evaluation is critical to determine if John is making progress toward his targeted goals. If he is not making adequate progress, then ongoing evaluation can quickly discover what the problem might be. For example, John's adapted physical education teacher initially decided that a racquetball racquet was the best substitute for a tennis racquet for John. However, the regular physical educator notices that John is having problems reaching balls that are not hit

	Yes	No	Comments
Will adaptation increase the student's participation in the activity?	✓		*allows for more success*
Will it allow the student to participate in an activity that is preferred or valued by the student, friends, and family members?	✓		*popular sport that John likes*
Will it take less time to teach the student to use the adaptation than to teach the skill directly?	✓		*he may never be able to participate w/o some adaptations*
Will the team have access to the technical expertise to design, construct, adjust, and repair the adaptation?	✓		*adapted physical education specialist*
Will the adaptation maintain or enhance related motor/communication skills?	✓		*allow more interaction w/peers & more opportunities to play in game*

Note: If the answer to most of the above questions is yes, then the student may need adapted equipment.

Figure 5.22. Does the student (John) need adapted equipment?

Does the student have limited strength?

Things to consider

    Shorten distance to move or project object.

    Use lighter equipment (e.g., balls, bats).

    Use shorter striking implements.

    Allow student to sit or lie down while playing.

    Use deflated balls or suspended balls.

    Change requirements (a few jumps, then run).

Selected modifications (if any) and Comments

John can be closer than peers

Lighter, smaller bat & balls

Cut racquet / bat at handle

Sit in chair

None

Push wheelchair

Does the student have limited speed?

Things to consider

    Shorten distance (or make it longer for others).

    Change locomotor pattern (allow running v. walking).

    Make safe areas in tag games.

Selected modifications (if any) and Comments

Shorter distance for John

Push wheelchair

None

Does the student have limited endurance?

Things to consider

    Shorten distance.

    Shorten playing field.

    Allow "safe" areas in tag games.

    Decrease activity time for student.

    Allow more rest periods for student.

    Allow student to sit while playing.

Selected modifications (if any) and Comments

Push wheelchair for time, not distance

Set up John's own "special" zone

None

Extra rest as needed

None

Yes

Does the student have limited balance?

Things to consider

    Provide chair/bar for support.

    Teach balance techniques (widen base, extend arms).

    Increase width of beams to be walked.

    Use carpeted rather than slick surfaces.

    Teach student how to fall.

    Allow student to sit during activity.

    Place student near wall for support.

    Allow student to hold peer's hand.

Selected modifications (if any) and Comments

Sit in chair

None

None

None

None

Yes

None

None

Does student have limited coordination and accuracy?

Things to consider

    Use stationary balls for kicking/striking.

    Decrease distance for throwing, kicking, and shooting.

    Make targets and goals larger.

    Use larger balls for kicking and striking.

    Increase surface of the striking implements.

Selected modifications (if any) and Comments

Yes

John can stand closer

Yes

Yes

Yes (larger bat / racquet)

(continued)

Figure 5.23. Checklist to determine curricular adaptations to accommodate individuals with specific limitations (John). (Adapted from Morris & Stiehl [1989].)

Figure 5.23. (*continued*)

Use backstop.	*Tie string to chair for retrieval*
Use softer, slower balls for striking and catching.	*Nerf balls*
In bowling-type games, use lighter, less stable pins.	*None*
What can you do to maximize safety?	*Make peers aware of John, place him in skilled group who can retrieve balls.*

Note: Some or all of these modifications can be implemented. Also, these modifications can be implemented for one student, for several students, or for the entire class to make the activity more challenging and success-oriented.

directly towards him. It was decided to try a lightweight, regulation length plastic racquet, and then reevaluate how well John was doing the following week. In softball John learned how to hit a pitched Nerf ball so quickly that the regular physical education teacher has decided to work with John on hitting a pitched softball. Similarly, John has begun to demonstrate slight rotation in his trunk when he throws the ball, and his program has been adjusted so that greater rotation during throwing is targeted. (See Figure 5.26 for an example of a checklist to measure the quantitative aspects of softball.)

Things to consider	Selected modifications (if any) and Comments
Can you vary the purpose/goal of the game (e.g., some students play to learn complex strategies, others play to work on simple motor skills)?	*John will work on skill development and understanding basic rules*
Can you vary number of players (e.g., play small games such as 2 v. 2 basketball)?	*have smaller groups with John*
Can you vary movement requirements (e.g., some students walk, others run; some hit a ball off a tee, others hit pitched ball; skilled students use more complex movements, less skilled use simpler movements)?	*hit off tee, smaller basket, push chair instead of run*
Can you vary the field of play (e.g., special zones for students with less mobility; make the field narrower or wider as needed; shorten the distance for students with movement problems)?	*Special zone for John in basketball and soccer, shorter distance to 1st base*
Can you vary objects used (e.g., some students use lighter bats/larger balls; some use a lower net/basket)?	*Use lighter equipment, larger targets, closer to targets.*
Can you vary the level of organization (Vary typical organizational patterns; vary where certain students stand; vary the level of structure for certain students.)?	*John will have set position*
Can you vary the limits/expectations (Vary the number of turns each student receives; vary the rules regarding how far a student can run, hit, etc.; vary how much you will enforce certain rules for certain players.)?	*do not enforce rules with John, John gets turn every third time in basketball*

Note: Use these suggestions to modify rules for both students with and without disabilities to make the game challenging, safe, and success-oriented.

Figure 5.24. Checklist to determine curricular modifications for group games and sports (John). (Adapted from Morris & Stiehl [1989].)

	Locker room	Warm-ups	Skills	Games	General behavior
Can you handle situations on your own?	No	No	No	No	Yes
Can peers in class provide any needed as-sistance?	No	Yes	Yes	Yes	—
Does student need trained as-sistant? (Place # in box.)	Yes (3)	—	—	—	—

Comments:

APE teacher & PT will consult RPE teacher and come into RPE during first few sessions. John will have 2 teacher assistants help him in locker room.

Choices of trained assistants:
1. Different-age peer-tutor
2. Adult volunteer
3. Teacher assistant
4. Specialist/therapists
5. Adapted P.E. specialist

Figure 5.25.   Checklist for determining general supports (John).

However, John is making slower than expected progress on pushing his wheelchair to first base. Discussions with John, his peers, and his teachers as well as observations revealed that John has difficulty keeping his chair on the base path which causes him to run onto the infield grass. A peer is assigned to help John keep his chair straight, and extra practice in physical education, in the classroom, and at home is implemented to help John push his chair with greater accuracy. Finally, it is determined that John was having difficulty getting out of his chair (even with as-sistance from a peer) to do push-ups and sit-ups during warm-ups. In fact, it takes John so long to get out of his chair that he never gets a chance to do these exercises. A new modification was suggested in which John stays in his chair and works on pushing himself up out of his chair (actually, a more functional strength activity for John) and does sit-ups by isometrically contract-ing his abdominal muscles on one count and stretching his lower back by bending forward on the next count.

Softball

Days

Activities	1	2	3	4	5	6	7	8	9	10	11
Hits pitched Nerf ball	+/−	+/−	+/−	+/−	+	+	+	+			
Throws overhand 10′ with rotation	+/−	+/−	+/−	+	+	+	+	+			
Pushes wheelchair to first base in 30 seconds.	−	−	−	−	−	−	−	−			

+   = Demonstrates skill to criteria three out of four trials.
+/− = Skill is emerging or does not quite meet criteria.
−   = Cannot perform skill.

Figure 5.26. John's ongoing progress report for softball

SUMMARY

Assessment is a critical aspect of the overall physical education program. Yet, physical educators often assess their students in such a way that the information they gain does not help them decide what to teach, where to teach it, or how to teach it. What does a score of 23 on the Bruininks-Oseretsky Test of Motor Proficiency (Bruininks, 1978) tell the physical educator about how to teach a functional skill? What does a score of 56 months on the Peabody Developmental Motor Scales (Folio & DuBose, 1974) tell a teacher about what functional skills are important for a 13-year-old student with Down syndrome?

The ecological model of assessment presented here provides specific information that is relevant to teaching students with disabilities in regular physical education. The model includes seven distinct but related phases of assessment. Initial assessment information is designed to determine what skills should be targeted for instruction. This phase focuses on discussing with the student, his or her parents, peers, and the community what skills they feel are important. Targeted skills might be similar for students who have similar interests and live in similar communities. However, targeted skills might be very different for students who have different interests and abilities. The second and third phases of the model evaluate the student's present level of performance and develop the student's IEP. The fourth phase assesses the regular physical education curriculum to determine if the targeted skills match. In some cases, skills that have been targeted for students with disabilities match with the activities that take place in the regular program. In other cases, modifications can be made so that targeted goals can be effectively taught in the regular setting. On rare occasions when regular physical education activities seem inappropriate, pulling a student out of regular physical education part of the time along with several peers without disabilities might be warranted. Phase 5 determines specifically how to instruct a student, and phase 6 determines how much support a student needs. Finally, the last phase of the assessment process is ongoing evaluation in which all four previous phases are constantly evaluated to determine if the program is effective. Ongoing evaluation must be conducted on a regular basis throughout the year if we want to assure that the program we have developed for the student is working (i.e., the student is progressing).

Note that the checklists described in this chapter are not only useful for developing a program. In addition, these checklists are designed to assist the team in making informed decisions. While assessment can take the form of informal observations and discussions with team members, formal assessments should be used whenever a programmatic decision is made to ensure that the student is receiving the most appropriate program possible.

Chapter 6

Instructional and Curricular Strategies for Accommodating Students with Disabilities in Regular Physical Education

Providing support to students with disabilities as well as to regular physical educators seems to be the most important part of successful inclusion. In Honolulu, we found that many regular physical educators would not accept students with disabilities in their regular classes. In order to provide the services to our students with disabilities, we developed a program in which part-time physical education teachers provided direct adapted physical education. These services were initially conducted in self-contained settings away from regular physical education, but gradually these part-time physical educators worked with regular physical educators to bring these students into the regular setting. In several cases, regular physical educators learned how to accommodate students with disabilities and became so comfortable with these students that they no longer requested the part-time teacher. By providing support and gradually including students with disabilities rather than dumping them into the regular setting, inclusion in physical education turned out to be quite successful.

—Nathan Murata

Ming is a second-grade student who has spina bifida. She uses a wheelchair in most situations, although she is learning how to use long leg braces and crutches. Ming is fully included in a second-grade class at her elementary school, even for regular physical education. However, the regular physical educator is having difficulty figuring out how best to include Ming in regular physical education activities. Much of what takes place in second-grade physical education is locomotor movement patterns and body control activities that Ming cannot do. In addition, the regular physical educator is scared that other students will get hurt if they run into Ming's wheelchair. This teacher has gotten so frustrated that Ming no longer receives regular physical education. Rather, she receives physical therapy during this time. What can this teacher do?

Bill is a seventh grader who is visually impaired. Bill is easily accommodated in all of his seventh-grade classes through braille and taping lectures. However, Bill's physical educator has

---

Nathan Murata is an APE resource teacher for the Honolulu School District, Honolulu, Hawaii.

not figured out how to accommodate Bill in regular physical education. First, she does not know how to present information to Bill. Like many physical educators, she uses a lot of demonstrations, but Bill cannot see her demonstrations. In addition, she is concerned for Bill's safety since he cannot see balls or other students coming toward him. Right now, she has Bill do warm-up activities with the rest of the class, but during the remainder of the period she has Bill sit off to the side and listen. What can this teacher do?

Rasheed is a 10th grader who has mental retardation. Rasheed spends part of his school day in the community working on functional vocational, community, and leisure skills. The remainder of the day he takes part in regular 10th-grade classes including regular physical education. However, Rasheed's physical educator is having difficulty communicating with Rasheed in regular physical education. Rasheed does not speak or understand verbal or simple gestural cues, nor does he follow demonstrations very well. In addition, Rasheed does not know when to stop or start an activity, he tires easily and often wants to sit down, and he has an extremely short attention span. The regular physical educator has given up trying to instruct Rasheed, so she lets him run around the gym and do what he wants during regular physical education. What can this teacher do?

Students with disabilities can be safely and successfully included in regular physical education without overtly changing the program for students without disabilities or causing undue hardship for the regular physical education teacher. However, the regular physical educator (with support from the collaborative team) must be prepared to make subtle modifications to his or her program to accommodate students with disabilities. Some modifications will only affect the student with a disability (e.g., lowering a basket, making a target larger, or giving a student a peer tutor), while other modifications may affect the entire class (e.g., changing the rules of a game or changing the class format). Changes that affect the group should be implemented cautiously, since you want to avoid making changes that will negatively affect the program for the students without disabilities. However, changes that affect the entire class can be positive. For example, forcing students to pass the ball to each player on the team before shooting in a game of basketball encourages students to use teamwork and work on the skills of passing and catching. Similarly, using skill stations and individual task cards to accommodate a student with disabilities also allows students without disabilities to work on skills at their own pace.

The purpose of this chapter is to introduce a variety of techniques that can be used to accommodate students with disabilities in regular physical education. These techniques will be grouped into two major categories: 1) instructional modifications related to the teaching/learning process including how you organize the class and present information, and 2) curricular modifications including modifications to traditional games and team sports as well as the use of alternative curricular approaches such as New Games (Fluegelman, 1976; 1980). The goal of all these modifications is to allow all students, including students with disabilities, to participate in a regular physical education setting that is safe, challenging, and affords opportunities for success. Which techniques you choose to implement will depend on the particular needs of the student with disabilities, the age group with which you are working, the skills on which you are focusing, the make-up of your class, availability of equipment and facilities, availability of support personnel, and your own preferences. While specific examples are provided, it is important that you focus on the general process of how to modify your physical education programs. Once you understand the general process of creating and implementing appropriate modifications, you can apply this process to a variety of situations.

One way to decide which modification to use is to evaluate the effect that modification will have on the student with disabilities, peers without disabilities, and the regular physical educator. If the modification has a negative effect on any or all of these individuals, then it probably is not the most appropriate modification. The following four criteria should be used whenever considering a particular modification. If the modification does not meet the standards set by these criteria, then an alternative modification should be considered.

1. *Does the change allow the student with disabilities to participate successfully yet still be challenged?* For example, a student with mental retardation might not be able to hit a pitched softball when it is tossed from the regulation pitcher's mound, but this student can hit a pitched ball if the pitcher stands a little closer and tosses it right over the plate. Such a modification provides the needed accommodation for the student so that he or she will be successful. The student still will be challenged to hit a pitched ball versus hitting a ball off a tee (another accommodation that promotes success but may not be challenging).

2. *Does the modification make the setting unsafe for the student with a disability as well as for students without disabilities?* For example, you want to include a student who uses a wheelchair in a game of volleyball. You might make a rule that the student must play one of the back positions so that other students are less likely to bump into the wheelchair. In addition, you can place cones around the student's chair so that students without disabilities who get too close to the student hit the cones first rather than the wheelchair. Finally, you want to remind students without disabilities at the beginning of the class and several times during the class to be careful around the student who uses a wheelchair. Students without disabilities will quickly learn to be careful, and the student can safely participate with his or her peers.

3. *Does the change affect students without disabilities?* This point is particularly important when playing group games. For example, an elementary class might be playing a game of tag, and included in the class is a student who has autistic-like behaviors such that he is not really aware of the rules of the game. To include this student, the teacher makes a rule that, when he is the tagger, all students must sit down and let the student tag them. Obviously, the students without disabilities are not thrilled with the idea of sitting down and letting another student tag them, regardless of his disability. A better modification might be making the space smaller, eliminating "safe" places, and assisting the student to tag his peers. This way, students without disabilities are still challenged to avoid the tagger (perhaps more challenged because of the modifications), yet the student with disabilities can still be included. Similarly, it might be fun for a high school class to play "sit-down" volleyball one day to accommodate a student who uses a wheelchair or "beep softball" to accommodate a student who is blind, but such changes implemented on a regular basis would negatively affect the program for the students without disabilities.

4. *Does the change cause an undue burden on the regular physical education teacher?* For example, a student who has cerebral palsy and is learning how to walk with a walker is fully included in regular physical education. The regular physical educator wants to include this student in warm-up activities that include performing locomotor patterns in general space to music. Because this student still needs help to walk with his walker, the regular physical educator feels that it is her duty to assist this student during warm-ups. This affects her ability to attend to and instruct the other students. A better modification might be assisting this student for part of warm-ups and letting him creep on hands and knees (still his most functional way of moving) for part of the warm-ups. Or, if walking with the walker is a critical goal for this student, older peer tutors, a teacher assistant, a volunteer, or the physical therapist can come into physical education (at least during warm-ups) to assist this student.

INSTRUCTIONAL MODIFICATIONS

The first step in accommodating students with disabilities in regular physical education is to determine how you organize your class and present information (i.e., how you teach), then to determine if you can make modifications to accommodate students with disabilities. Instructional modifications can make a tremendous difference between success and failure for students with special needs, yet most modifications are relatively easy to implement. The following (adapted in part from Eichstaedt & Lavay, 1992; Seaman & DePauw, 1989; and Sherrill, 1993) provides a description of several instructional modifications and examples of how subtle changes can be implemented better to accommodate students with disabilities.

Note that in many cases you will be able to individualize your presentation to meet the unique needs of students with disabilities without changing your presentation to the rest of the class. For example, you can demonstrate a particular skill to the group and have them begin the activity. You can then provide verbal cues and physical assistance to a student who is blind so that he or she understands the task. Similarly, you can use a movement exploration approach when teaching body control skills and movement concepts to your first-grade class. At the same time, you can provide direct cues and physical assistance to a student who has severe mental retardation and autistic-like behaviors who is having difficulty exploring his or her environment independently. In this way, you are still using your typical instructional approach but making subtle additions to your instruction to accommodate the needs of students with disabilities.

One other important point is that you should utilize support personnel whenever possible when developing and implementing any modification. Chapter 3 reviewed members of the collaborative team who could be used as sources of support by regular physical educators, and Chapter 4 explained how these team members can be used to help determine which types of modifications are most appropriate for particular students. Support persons also can be used to assist the regular physical educator in implementing specific modifications. Support persons can include classmates, older peer tutors, volunteers, teacher assistants, or specialists. (See chap. 3, this volume.) All of the instructional and curricular modifications outlined below (as well as the specific modifications outlined in Chapter 7) can be more effectively implemented if support personnel are in the gymnasium to assist the regular physical educator. Even having a parent volunteer from the PTO or the custodian come in for a few minutes to help provide more individual assistance to a student with disabilities can make a tremendous difference to the student and to the regular physical educator. For example, a student who is learning how to walk with a walker might only need extra assistance to prevent him or her from falling. During warm-up activities when the class is moving about using different locomotor patterns, the custodian can come into regular physical education to assist this student. Thus, the student receives the needed one-on-one attention, yet the regular physical educator is free to focus on the larger group.

Teaching Style

The term *teaching style* refers to the learning environment, the general routine, and how the lesson is presented to the class. Mosston (1981) described six different teaching styles commonly used by physical educators. (See Table 6.1 for a summary.) Some students will respond better to certain teaching styles. For example, children who need more structure and direction to learn (such as students with attention deficit disorders or mental retardation) do better in a command style or single-task approach while students with unique movement abilities but normal intelligence may learn to compensate for their problems through guided discovery. While it may be difficult to provide different teaching styles in one class, teachers can still employ the general principles of a particular teaching style to help particular students. For example, in the context of a command style used to teach the overhand throwing pattern, a teacher could guide a student who has cerebral palsy to explore different throwing patterns (guided discovery) that meet his unique needs. Similarly, a teacher presenting body awareness concepts in a divergent style could present specific information on what to do, how to do it, and where to do it (command style) for a student with mental retardation.

Table 6.1. Mosston's teaching styles

Command—Teacher is in direct control of class, each student is given the same instructions and is expected to perform the same movements at the same pace.

Task—Student is provided a single task or series of tasks in the form of task cards or stations. All students are still expected to perform the same movements at the same pace.

Reciprocal—Two students work together with one student performing a task while the other evaluates his or her performance. Slightly more individualization, but students still must adhere to standardized performance and pace.

Individual—Program is designed to meet each student's unique needs. Goals and learning pace are individualized.

Guided discovery—Teacher provides a series of problems that students must solve. Questions are presented sequentially that lead students to a particular goal.

Divergent—A single problem with certain criteria is presented by the teacher, and students can solve the problem via any number of actions.

Class Format

The term *class format* refers to how members of the class are organized. Seaman and DePauw (1989) outlined seven different class formats that are commonly used in physical education settings: 1) one-to-one instruction (one teacher or assistant for every student), 2) small groups (3–10 students working together with a teacher or teacher assistant), 3) large group (entire class participating together as one group), 4) mixed groups (using various class formats within one class period), 5) peer teaching (using classmates without disabilities or students from other classes for teaching and assisting students with disabilities), 6) teaching stations (several areas in which smaller subsets of the class rotate through to practice skills), and 7) self-paced independent work (each student works on individual goals at his or her own pace following directions on task cards or with guidance from teacher and teacher assistants).

The format that is best for any situation will vary based on number, attitudes, and types of students with and without disabilities; type and flexibilty of facility; and availability of resources. In most situations, a combination of the above class formats is most effective. For example, a student with significant disabilities can be included in a high school physical education class during a basketball unit in which the teacher utilizes a combination of peer tutors, stations, self-paced learning, and large group instruction. Students begin the class by following the teacher through various warm-up activities (large group). The student with significant disabilities is assisted in these warm-up activities by his physical therapist who works on specific stretching and strengthening activities designed specifically for this student. Following warm-ups, students rotate through several basketball stations at their own pace, working on tasks geared to their ability levels. Students are free to choose to which station they wish to go, but they can only stay at one station for 10 minutes and no more than seven students can be at any one station at one time. Students have task cards with a hierarchy of tasks which they move through at their own pace. In order to move to the next level on a hierarchy, the student must have another student confirm that he or she can perform the skill on four out of five trials (stations/self-paced learning). The student with significant disabilities has a task card that includes tasks at the lower end of the continuum. (See Figure 6.1 for an example of an extended skill station with activities for students with more severe disabilities.)

During station work the student is assisted by a peer tutor. The culminating activity for the day is a game of basketball. Skilled students go with a "class leader" and play regulation games of 5-on-5 basketball, learning set plays and strategies (small group). Less-skilled students, includ-

Task Card

Student name:

TRIALS

_____ _____ _____ _____ _____ _____ _____ _____ drops ball into bucket with assistance

_____ _____ _____ _____ _____ _____ _____ _____ drops ball into bucket independently

_____ _____ _____ _____ _____ _____ _____ _____ tosses ball into bucket from 2′ away

_____ _____ _____ _____ _____ _____ _____ _____ tosses ball into bucket from 4′ away

_____ _____ _____ _____ _____ _____ _____ _____ tosses ball into bucket from 6′ away

_____ _____ _____ _____ _____ _____ _____ _____ steps and tosses ball into bucket 6′ away

_____ _____ _____ _____ _____ _____ _____ _____ steps and tosses ball in game situations

Key: I = independently.   + = performs skill on 3 out of 4 trials.
V = verbal cue.   +/− = performs skill, but not consistently.
P = physical assistance.   − = does not perform skill.

Figure 6.1.   Example of extended skill station for underhand throw.

ing the student with significant disabilities, go with the regular physical education teacher who organizes a modified game of basketball in which rules are changed to accommodate the needs of all these students, including the student with significant disabilities. In today's version of the modified game, the defense must play a passive zone defense (cannot steal the ball unless it is passed directly to them). In addition, every player on the offensive team must touch the ball one time before a player can shoot, and students can get points for hitting the backboard (1 point), rim (2 points), or making a basket (3 points). Students who cannot reach a 10′ basket can shoot at an 8′ target on the wall, and the student with significant disabilities can score by pushing the ball off of his lap tray into a box on the floor with assistance from a peer. The regular physical education class described above utilizes a variety of class formats during one class period which allows the teacher to accommodate the needs of all the students in her class, including a student with significant disabilities.

Two other class formats which can be used to facilitate integration are *reverse mainstreaming* and *cooperative learning*. In reverse mainstreaming, several students without disabilities are integrated into a class of children who have disabilities. These students without disabilities are not peer tutors but rather students who participate in the activity alongside students with disabilities. Students without disabilities provide good role models for students with disabilities and allow for team sports and games that require more players. For example, once a week an adapted physical education class of seven middle school students with mental retardation invite seven middle school students without disabilities to participate with them in physical education. The current unit in both adapted physical education and regular physical education is soccer. In reverse mainstreaming, all of the students begin with a warm-up activity. The students without disabilities tend to use better form in stretching, thus providing a good model for their peers with mental retardation. Similarly, the students without disabilities provide a good pace during warm-up laps for the students with mental retardation. Following warm-ups, students pair up (students with and without mental retardation paired together) to work on various soccer skills. A student without disabilities can pass the ball directly to the student with mental retardation at a slow speed so that the student with mental retardation can practice trapping the ball. (When students with mental retardation are paired together in the adapted class, they have trouble accurately passing the ball back and forth to each other.) The class culminates with a modified game of 7-on-7 soccer. (It is difficult to play soccer in the adapted class with only seven students.) The rules are modified so that both students with and without mental retardation are challenged. (Students without disabilities have to kick the ball with their nondominant foot, cannot kick the ball in the air, and cannot use their hands if they are playing goalie.) The students with mental retardation find the game more motivating and challenging when students without disabilities participate, yet they still can be successful because of the smaller game size and rules modifications.

Another class format option is *cooperative learning* in which students work together to accomplish shared goals. Group goals can only be accomplished if individual students in the group reach their shared goals (Johnson & Johnson, 1989). In cooperative learning, students are instructed to learn the assigned information and to make sure that all members of the group master the information (at their own levels). Oftentimes individuals in the group are given specific jobs/ tasks that contribute to goal attainment. Cooperative learning encourages each student to work together, help each other, and constantly evaluate each member's progress toward individual and group goals (more accountability). For cooperative learning to be effective, students must perceive that they are positively linked to other students in their group and that each member can and must contribute to the success of the group (i.e., interdependence). In addition, each member of the group must understand his or her role in the cooperative group. Less-skilled students, including students with disabilities, could be perceived to be the weak links in the group if all members perceive that they must each perform the *same* task. This will not happen if the group understands that each member has a *unique* task which maximizes his or her skills and contribution to the group goal. For example, a group of third graders are working on the skill of striking. The teacher divides the class into small groups of three or four students. The cooperative task for each group is to: 1) hit 50 paper and yarn balls across the gym, with each member hitting each ball only one time; and 2) have each student work on one key aspect of a skillful striking pattern. Since no student can hit the ball across the gym by him- or herself, only through group cooperation can the ball get across the gym (group goal). In Group A, the skilled student begins the process by hitting a pitched ball as far as possible (pitched by one of the group members). This student is working on timing and hitting the ball up into the air. The less-skilled group member then walks to where the ball lands, picks up the ball and places it on a batting tee, then hits the ball forward as far as possible. This student is working on shifting weight and stepping, and the skilled student provides feedback to the less-skilled student. Finally, the tee is moved to where the ball landed and is placed on the tee for a student who is blind. This student is working on hitting the ball off the tee with his hand using proper preparatory position, stepping, and using a level swing. Both the skilled and nonskilled students help position the student and provide him with feedback. The process is repeated until the group hits 50 balls. The group must work together to accomplish their goal, and each student must contribute in his or her own way. In addition, it benefits the group if each member improves his or her skill level. If a group member uses better form, then the ball will be hit farther and in turn help the team accomplish its goal. (See Johnson and Johnson, 1989, for an excellent review of how to use cooperative learning in integrated situations.)

Verbal Instructions

The term *verbal instructions* refers to the length and complexity of commands or verbal challenges used to convey information to the class. Students with mental retardation who cannot understand complex commands or students who have hearing impairments who cannot understand verbal commands may need to have instruction delivery modified. Seaman and DePauw (1989) suggested the following ways in which instructions can be modified for students who have difficulty understanding verbal language: 1) simplify words used; 2) use single-meaning words (e.g., "run" to the base rather than "go" to the base); 3) give only one command at a time or as many pieces of information as the student can process at once; 4) ask the student to repeat the command before performing it; and 5) say the command and then demonstrate the task and/or physically assist the student. While these modifications might be helpful for a student with a language problem, such modifications might not be needed for the majority of students in the class. These modifications can still be implemented without having a teacher change the way she delivers instruction to the rest of the students. For example, a teacher might give complex verbal directions including information about abstract strategies and team concepts to the class, then a peer could repeat key directions to the student with mental retardation. Some strategies and concepts can be demonstrated by the peer, while abstract concepts can be translated into more concrete examples or skipped altogether, depending on how much the student can understand. Similarly, a peer can demonstrate and mimic directions to a student with a hearing impairment after the teacher presents verbal directions to the class. By utilizing peers or other assistants to present directions to the special student, the teacher does not have to alter how she gives instruction to the rest of the class.

Demonstrations

Who gives demonstrations, how many are given, how often they are given, and the best location for a demonstration are all important factors in teaching style. Again, the teacher can provide a level of demonstration that is appropriate for the majority of the class while presenting extra demonstrations (or having a peer present extra demonstrations) for students with special needs. Modifications to demonstrations could be as simple as having students with poor vision stand close to the teacher while she demonstrates. For students with mental retardation, the teacher might need to highlight key aspects of the demonstration that other students might be able to pick up incidentally or have a peer repeat the demonstration several times. For example, the teacher could demonstrate the starting preparatory position, backswing, trunk rotation, and follow-through for the overhand throw to the class. For a student with mental retardation just learning to throw, the teacher (or peer) might repeat the demonstration focusing on just one aspect (stepping with opposite foot) so that this student knows on what component he should focus.

Level of Methodology

While the previous discussion reviewed how to present verbal cues or demonstration, another instructional modification is deciding whether or not you need a completely different way to communicate and instruct particular students. Thus, the term *levels of methodology* refers to the various methods a teacher can use to present information to a student. As noted in Chapter 4, levels of methodology, listed from least- to most-intrusive include: verbal instructions, gestures, demonstration, physical prompting, and physical guidance. Students with visual impairments will need verbal instruction plus physical guidance while students with hearing impairments will need more gestural prompts and demonstrations. Students with severe mental retardation often need physical guidance to understand instruction. Some students with disabilities benefit from multisensory delivery in which the physical educator uses several levels of methodology to give instructions (e.g., verbal combined with demonstration and physical assistance). Again, special instructions needed for one student do not necessarily have to change how the teacher gives instruction to the other students. For example, a teacher can give verbal instructions to the class, ask the class to begin practicing the skill, then give special verbal instructions and physical assistance to the student who is blind. Similarly, a teacher assistant, volunteer, or peer tutor can be trained in sign language to communicate with a student who has a hearing impairment or to physically guide a student with severe mental retardation.

Starting and Stopping Signals

Finding the best way to give starting and stopping commands to special students requires teacher flexibility. Students with hearing impairments may need hand signals, and students with severe mental retardation may need physical assistance to stop. The teacher can use one cue for the entire class (whistle) and still provide hand signals or physical assistance to students who need these extra cues. For example, the teacher could use a whistle to stop and start a soccer game for a high school class. When students hear the whistle, they know to locate the student with a hearing impairment and raise their hand (indicating to stop or start).

Time

The time of day or time of season that the child is going to be included is important too. Some students who receive medication (e.g., children with attention deficit disorder) do better once the medication has kicked in. They might be placed in a physical education class that meets in the afternoon. In contrast, students who tire throughout the day might be better served in a morning physical education class. Similarly, students with allergy-induced asthma might do better in a morning physical education class during pollen season since pollen is higher in the afternoon. Modifications to time should be made prior to the student's coming to school. (Utilize the collaborative team to determine what time of day is best for students with health disorders.)

Duration

How much time a student will be engaged in an activity is referred to as *duration*. Duration can include number of weeks for a particular unit, number of physical education periods per week, how long each period will be, or how long the student will be engaged in each activity during physical education. For example, a student with mental retardation might need 6 weeks to reach her goals and overlearn a skill while students without disabilities need only 3 weeks. Another student might need physical education 5 days per week to reach her goals while students without disabilities only need physical education 3 days per week. A student with an attention deficit disorder can tolerate a station or activity for 1 minute while her peers are expected to stay at a station for up to 5 minutes. In contrast, a student with mental retardation might need to stay at that same station for 10 minutes to receive an adequate amount of practice to learn a skill or concept.

Duration also refers to how long a student will stay in a game situation. A student with asthma or a heart condition who tires easily might play the game for 2 minutes then rest on the sideline for 2 minutes, or a teacher could allow for free substitution in soccer and basketball games so that students who tire easily can rest whenever necessary. While many programs are locked into daily schedules, adjustments can usually be made to accommodate students with special needs. For example, a student with mental retardation has a goal of learning the skills needed to play softball. The softball unit in regular physical education lasted 3 weeks, and now the class is playing volleyball. Volleyball is not one of the goals established for this student, and she has not acquired the targeted softball skills during the previous 3-week period. While the class moves to volleyball, this student can continue to work on softball skills with a peer who already has good volleyball skills (does not need extra practice in volleyball), with another student who also needs extra work on softball, with a different-age peer tutor, with a teacher assistant, or with a volunteer. The student can still do warm-ups with the regular class and be around her peers in regular physical education; she just practices different activities. Similarly, a student might be working on three key skills in softball while his peers are working on six skills. This student can stay at each of three stations for a longer period of time to get extra practice in the three critical skills while his peers move through all six stations. However, a student with attention deficit disorder could rotate through each of the six stations much faster than his peers, repeating each station two or three times so that he gets adequate practice trials without being forced to focus on one station for too long a period.

Order of Learning

The sequence in which you present various aspects of a particular skill is called the *order of learning*. Most teachers teach a skill such as the sidearm strike in tennis by teaching the whole task in order from first to last components (preparatory position, step, swing, and follow-through). However, a student with a learning disability might need to focus on one aspect of the movement at a time, first learning to step and swing, then learning the preparatory position, and finally learning the follow-through. Other students might benefit from breaking down the skill into even smaller steps. As was the case in several examples above, the teacher can present the whole task to the majority of the class, then change the order of learning or break down the skill more slowly (or have a peer repeat the order of learning or break down the skill) for a student with a learning disability.

Size and Nature of Group

How many students will be at a station or in a game as well as the make-up of the group (similar abilities or mixed abilities) are important factors. Students who have trouble working in large groups, such as students with autism, can be placed in a smaller group during station work. Students with mental retardation who are slower and less skilled than their peers can be placed on a team that has more players than their opponents' team so that their team will not be at a disadvantage. Similarly, teams can be selected by the teacher so that each team has an equal number of skilled, average, and unskilled players. Players of similar ability can then be paired up against each other in the game (e.g., guarding each other in a game of soccer or basketball). The teacher should select teams so that students with lower abilities (or disabilities) are not always picked last. Also, skilled students should be encouraged to use appropriate sportsmanship during the selection process (i.e., do not give funny looks when players with less ability are picked to be on their team).

Instructional Setting

The term *instructional setting* refers to all aspects related to where the class is conducted. Such factors include indoor versus outdoor, temperature, lighting, floor surface, boundaries, and markings on walls. Most teachers cannot make major changes to their instructional settings to accommodate one or two students with special needs. However, there are some simple things a teacher can do to make a setting more accommodating for students with special needs. For example, cones or bright-colored tape can be used to accentuate boundaries for students with mental retardation or students with visual impairments. Carpet squares or small tumbling mats can be placed at certain areas where students with balance problems usually stand so that there will be a cushion if they fall. Carpet squares, poly spots, or hula hoops can be used to mark off a student's personal space, and partitions such as mats stood up on end can be used to block off part of the gym for students who are easily distracted.

Elimination of Distractions

Creating an instructional setting in which extraneous noises, persons, or objects are reduced or eliminated helps the student focus on instruction. Many students with attention deficit disorders or mental retardation are easily distracted and thus have difficulty focusing on important instructional cues. For example, balloons and cones set up in the environment for a later activity might not distract most students in a class but might be extremely distracting for a student with mental retardation or attention deficit disorder. Again, the teacher should not have to make changes that negatively affect the majority of students, but there are several simple things that can be done to reduce distractors for the entire class. First, students can be positioned in such a way that they are facing away from distractors. For example, a teacher can position himself or herself so that students face the corner of the gym with their backs facing the more distracting, open part of the gym. Second, a teacher can avoid setting up equipment until the equipment is actually to be used. Pieces of equipment can be placed at stations or around the gym, but they can be put in a barrel, box, or bag or covered with a tarp until they are needed. For example, balloons placed in a large trash bag are much less distracting than having balloons placed in clear sight of the students. Third, extraneous noises, objects, or persons in the environment can be eliminated when a particular student comes to physical education. In many elementary schools the gym doubles as the cafeteria, and teachers and students walk through the gym/cafeteria in the morning to give the lunch count to cafeteria workers. Students with attention deficit disorders can be placed in a physical education class later in the day when no one walks through the gym. Similarly, some gyms have stages where music or drama classes are conducted. Schedules should be established so that no other classes are in session when the student with attention deficit disorder is in physical education. Finally, teachers can help students focus on the task at hand by providing extra cues and reinforcement to the student and by making his or her instruction more enticing. For example, using music during warm-ups can drown out the sound of noisy distractors in the environment. When the music is turned off and the environment is relatively quiet, the teacher can then give directions since his or her voice will be the most noticeable sound in the environment. Whistling and loud clapping are other ways to break a student's focus on one object and return his or her focus to the teacher.

Structure or Routine

All children learn best and are most cooperative when they know routines and what is expected of them. While most students can handle occasional changes to class structure or routines, change or the unexpected for children with autism, emotional disturbances, or mental retardation can lead to confusion, withdrawal, misbehavior, and even self-abuse. For students who do not do well with change, it is important that class structure remain as constant as possible. Structure can be as easy as having students sit on carpet squares when they enter the gym or take two or three laps, then sit against a designated wall. Even if you do not have a routine for most students, it is important to establish a set routine for the student with disabilities. For example, a physical educator may do something different for warm-ups every day. He or she can still make sure the student with autism does the same thing every day when she enters the gymnasium. (Go with the same peer to the corner of the gym and follow a certain exercise routine.) If you establish a routine for this student, she is less likely to be confused or upset and will make the transition from the classroom to the gym much more smoothly. Another time when change is inevitable is when you are going to a new unit. Carrying over previously learned activities often helps in this type of transition. For example, a basketball dribbling station (previous unit) can be added to the three volleyball skill stations (new unit).

Level of Difficulty or Complexity

The difficulty level of skills, formations, game rules, and game strategies is another factor that can be modified. Again, a teacher can vary the level of difficulty for particular students without changing the difficulty level for the rest of the students. For example, a team might play a complex zone defense in basketball, but all a student with mental retardation needs to know is to stand on a poly spot and keep his hands up. Similarly, most students can work on stepping, rotating their bodies, and lagging their arms in the overhand throw while a student just learning how to throw can work on simply getting his arm into an overhand position while throwing. Specific examples of how to modify skills and group activities will be presented later in this chapter.

Levels of Motivation

How much motivation and the type of reinforcement particular students need to be motivated to participate in physical education activities is another variable. Many students without disabilities are intrinsically motivated to participate in physical education. However, students who know that they have difficulty in physical education might need more encouragement. Extra encouragement can come in the form of verbal praise, extra privileges, free play, tokens, or even tangible reinforcers for students with more significant disabilities. For example, a student with an emotional disturbance can be reinforced for staying engaged in a physical fitness activity for 10 minutes. Reinforcement might consist of allowing the student to do an activity he or she really likes for a few minutes after the fitness activity (shooting baskets or playing catch with the teacher).

CURRICULAR MODIFICATIONS: ADAPTING THE REGULAR CURRICULUM

The previous discussion reviewed methods for modifying instruction to accommodate the needs of students with disabilities. Still, some students will need other modifications if they are to be included succesfully and challenged in regular physical education. For example, a student might understand your directions and be able to handle large group instruction, but the student may still be unsuccessful because he cannot kick a moving ball or run as fast as his peers do. This student will need specific modifications to the curriculum if he or she is going to be successful. Chapter 7 provides detailed accommodations for students who have specific problems or disabilities such as limited strength or limited balance. The following provides more general guidelines for making decisions regarding changing the curriculum to accommodate students with a wide range of disabilities. Rather than specific guidelines for specific students, the models outlined below provide the process that regular physical educators and other team members can use to accommodate students with disabilities in regular physical education. Again, once you understand the process, you can accommodate any student who enters your program.

Developmental Task Analysis

A variety of task and environmental factors influence motor performance. As explained earlier in this chapter, many of these factors can be modified by the teacher to make the activity easier or more challenging for particular students. Herkowitz's developmental task analysis (1978) is designed to identify systematically task and environmental factors which influence movement patterns. The model includes two components: 1) general task analysis (GTA), and 2) specific task analysis (STA). GTA involves outlining all the task and environmental factors which influence movements of children in general movement categories (e.g., striking, catching, jumping). These factors are then listed hierarchically in terms of levels of difficulty from simple to complex. Table 6.2 provides an example of a GTA for striking. Note how this grid provides the teacher with information on how various task factors influence specific movements and how he or she might modify these factors to make a movement simpler or more complex.

Once the teacher has a general understanding of how task and environmental factors affect movement, an STA can be developed that examines in greater detail how select factors influence a specific movement. STAs are developed by creating activities that utilize two to four factors from the GTA. Like the GTA, these factors are then broken down into levels of difficulty and listed hierarchically from simple to complex. The difference between the STA and the GTA is that levels of difficulty in STA refer to specific factors rather than general categories. Table 6.3 provides an

Table 6.2. General task analysis (GTA) for striking behavior

Factors	Size of object to be struck	Weight of object to be struck	Speed of object to be struck	Predictability of trajectory of object to be struck	Length of striking implement	Side of body to which object is traveling	Anticipatory locomotor spatial adjustments
L E Simple	Large	Light	None Slow	No movement along ground	None	Favored side	No adjustment
V E to	Medium	Moderate	Moderate	Down incline	Short	Nonfavored side	Minimal adjustment
L S Complex	Small	Heavy	Fast	In air	Long	Midline	Maximum adjustment

From Herkowitz, J. (1978). Developmental task analysis: The design of movement experiences and evaluation of motor development status. In M. Ridenour (Ed.), *Motor development: Issues and applications* (pp. 139–164). Pennington, NJ: Princeton Book Co.; reprinted by permission.

Table 6.3.   Specific task analysis (STA) for striking behavior

Factors influencing student performance	Factors influencing student performance		
	Size of ball	Length of striking implement	Predictability of trajectory of ball
L Simple	S1 12″ ball	L1 hand	P1 rolled along ground
E V to E	S2 9″ ball	L2 ping-pong paddle	P2 bounced along ground
L S Complex	S3 4″ ball	L3 18″ dowel rod	P3 aerial ball
	S4 tennis ball	L4 36″ plastic bat	

From Herkowitz, J. (1978). Developmental task analysis: The design of movement experiences and evaluation of motor development status. In M. Ridenour (Ed.), *Motor development: Issues and applications* (pp.139–164). Pennington, NJ: Princeton Book Co.; reprinted by permission.

example of an STA for striking. Note how more specific, observable information is provided in this STA. The teacher can quickly evaluate how specific levels of difficulty in various factors influence movement performance in various students. The goal is to get the student to perform the task under the most complex circumstances, in this case using a 36″ plastic bat to strike a tennis ball that is tossed. STAs also can be used to help less-skilled students and students with disabilities be more successful in a particular task. In striking, a student who has limited strength could use an 18″ wooden dowel rather than a 36″ plastic bat, or a student who has difficulty contacting a tennis ball can hit a 9″ Nerf ball rather than a tennis ball. Limitations such as strength and visual-motor coordination can mask a student's ability to perform a task using a more skillful pattern. By simply altering task and environmental demands, these students might be able to demonstrate more skillful patterns. Teachers also can use STAs to evaluate a student's present level of performance (circumstances under which a student can perform a given task) as well as progress the student is making (do these circumstances change over time?). (See Herkowitz, 1978, for examples of STA evaluation grids.)

Ecological Task Analysis

Davis and Burton (1991) recently developed a new type of task analysis that extends Morris's task complexity model (described later in this chapter) and Herkowitz's developmental task analysis. They noted that, while a great beginning in skill analysis, both Morris's and Herkowitz's models have several flaws. The two greatest flaws are the fact that neither Morris's nor Herkowitz's models consider the goal of the given task or the attributes of the mover.

The goal of the task can have a tremendous influence on the movement pattern a mover might display. For example, a mover might throw using what appears to be a very inefficient movement pattern (not stepping or stepping homolaterally, not extending his arm in backswing, and having very little follow-through). If the goal of the task was to throw a dart at a dart board from 10′ away, the movement pattern described above might be very appropriate. Similarly, a student might perceive the goal of a task to be different than the goal the teacher wants. In such situations, the student might appear to be displaying movement patterns that are different than those the teacher wants. For example, a student might demonstrate a chopping movement with very little bat motion in his striking pattern because he wants to hit the pitched ball (goal is perceived as hitting ball), while the teacher was hoping that the student would take a full, horizontal swing at the ball including rotating the body (goal is perceived as using a certain striking pattern). The intended goal of the task is critical to eventual peformance of the movement, yet the goal of the task is not discussed in either Morris's or Herkowitz's models.

The second weakness noted by Davis and Burton is the absence of the person in the task analysis equation. Task analyses such as those developed by Morris and Herkowitz focus on the characteristics of the task rather than the characteristics of the mover. Yet movers with different capabilities and physical characteristics will respond quite differently to changes in task factors. For example, Herkowitz lists ball size and balance requirements of the task as factors that can affect throwing performance. However, the size of a mover's hand and his or her own innate balance abilities will affect exactly how much ball size and balance requirements affect performance. For some children with large hands, subtle changes in ball size might not affect throwing performance. In contrast, a slightly larger ball presented to a student with Down syndrome who has a smaller hand compared to his or her age peers will change his or her throwing pattern from one-handed to two-handed (Block & Provis, 1992). Similarly, balance requirements in the task might not negatively affect a student who has good balance, yet such requirements could have a dramatic effect on a student with ataxic cerebral palsy who has difficulty with even simple balance tasks. Performer characteristics, like the goal of the task, are critical determinants to performance, yet performer characteristics are absent from previous task analysis models.

In an effort to correct flaws found in Morris's and Herkowitz's models, Davis and Burton proposed the "ecological task analysis" model (ETA). The major tenets of ETA are as follows:

1. *Actions are the result of the complex relationship between the task goal, the performer, and the environment.* ETA includes a description of the task goal and the performer as critical factors in movement outcome.

2. *Tasks should be categorized by function and intention rather than movement pattern or mechanism of performance.* The same function can be achieved through very different movement patterns. While a particular pattern might be most efficient for a group of movers who have similar abilities and physical characteristics, other movers with different abilities and characteristics might find a different movement pattern more efficient. This is particularly true for students with disabilities who often have very unique abilities and characteristics. Rather than describing a movement pattern such as skipping or throwing, ETA utilizes a functional task category that describes the general intent of the movement. Skipping thus becomes one form of the function: *locomotion*—to move from one place to another, and throwing becomes one form of the function: *propulsion*—to propel a stationary or moving object or person. Within each functional task category are criteria for performance. For example, under locomotion (to move from one place to another), criteria include to move with efficiency, precision, accuracy, speed, and/or distance. Each mover might use a different pattern to accomplish a given function and criteria.

3. *Invariant features of a task and variations within a task may be defined in terms of essential and nonessential variables, respectively.* Essential variables describe the invariant characteristics of the movement. Basically, essential variables refer to the underlying patterns that organize and define a movement. Relative timing between the two lower limbs in walking or galloping are examples of an essential variable. For practical purposes, broader descriptors of patterns of coordination such as arm action in throwing also can be viewed as an essential variable. Nonessential variables refer to dimensions or control parameters that, when scaled up or down, may cause the mover to change to a new, qualitatively different pattern of coordination (new essential variable). These control variables can include physical dimensions of the mover such as limb length or weight, body proportions, or postural control; or they can refer to task factors such as ball size, weight of striking implement, or size of target. For example, throwing a ball at a wall from 5' away would result in the student displaying a pattern of coordination (essential variable) that is characterized by no stepping, no preparatory backswing, and no trunk rotation. As we ask the student to move away from the wall (scale up the nonessential variable of distance to throw), his or her throwing pattern will stay intact up to a critical distance. At that critical distance (given that the student has the underlying ability to display a different throwing

pattern), the student's pattern will abruptly change to a qualitatively different throwing pattern, stepping with opposition, trunk rotation, and preparatory backswing.

4. *A direct link should be established between the task goal and the constraints of the mover and environment.* In traditional task analyses, we measure the environment (ball size) without reference to the mover's characteristics (hand size). ETA uses a "performer-scaled" measure that links the dimensions of the environment and the mover. What results is a specific boundary condition in which the mover–environment relationship affords one type of movement but not another. For example, we can measure ball size as a ratio of a mover's hand size. The mover-ball size ratio for a mover who has a hand span of $8''$ and a ball size of $9''$ would be equal to $9''/8'' = 1.125$ performer-scaled ratio. Recent research suggests that when the ball-to-hand size ratio is slightly greater than 1.0 (ball is slightly larger than person's hand size), the student will change to a different throwing pattern (Burton, Greer, & Wiese, 1992). While this change is somewhat subtle in students without disabilities (change from level III to level II in arm and trunk action), it can be quite dramatic in students with Down syndrome (change from one-hand to two-hand throwing) (Block & Provis, 1992).

To conduct an ETA, the four steps below should be followed:

1. *Select and present the task goal* (one of the functional movement categories)—For young children or students with disabilities, you may have to structure the environment and provide verbal and other cues to the student that allow understanding of the task goal.
2. *Provide choices*—have the student practice the task, allowing him or her to choose the skill and the movement form (e.g., task is to locomote; skill is to gallop; and movement form is quality of galloping). Observe and record the skill choice and movement form in qualitative measures and the performance outcome in quantitative measures. (This gives a baseline of performance.) For example, you might observe that the student galloped by leading with right foot, exhibiting minimal flight phase, and not using arm swing (qualitative measure), and that the student galloped a distance of $15'$ in 10 seconds (quantitative measure).
3. *Identify relevant task dimensions and performer variables*—Manipulate one or two task dimensions to find optimal performance level. Observe skill choice, movement form, and performance outcome in qualitative and quantitative measures, and then compare results with previous measures. For example, obstacles in environment and regularity of support surface (gym floor versus grass) are two task variables that might affect galloping performance. The student is observed attempting to gallop on the gym floor versus grass, in an uncluttered environment versus one with obstacles, and then a combination of the two—on grass going around obstacles. Record the student's behavior in both qualitative and quantitative terms and compare with baseline measures.
4. *Provide direct instruction in skill selection and movement form*—Manipulate task variables to challenge student and perhaps help student perform skill at a higher level. Observe skill choice, movement form, and performance outcome in qualitative and quantitative measures, and compare with previous results.

According to Davis and Burton, some of the advantages of using the ETA are that a teacher can more accurately determine: 1) under which set of conditions the student is able to achieve the task; 2) which set of conditions elicits the most efficient and effective pattern (optimal performance); and 3) the dimension values at which the student chooses to use a different skill to perform a skill (e.g., changes from galloping to running). ETA appears to be a viable approach to understanding how a mover prefers to move and how changes in task variables affect movement.

CURRICULAR MODIFICATIONS: MODELS FOR CHANGING GAMES/SPORTS

Group games and team sports are popular activities in physical education. When used properly, group games and team sports can facilitate skill development as well as promote an understanding of rules, strategies, and concepts. Some group games also can be designed to promote sportsmanship, cooperation, and teamwork. Unfortunately, group games and team sports are often conducted in such a way that they promote competition and adherence to rules designed for very skilled athletes. For example, it is not unusual to see upper level elementary school physical education students playing regulation basketball games in which 10′ baskets are used and professional rules are strictly followed even though most students at this age cannot reach a 10′ basket or follow the rules of the game. Skilled students might enjoy these games, but the majority of students quickly get frustrated and take on roles of passive, unhappy participants. And what of students with disabilities? Many regular physical educators assume that group games and team sports are beyond the skill level or cognitive ability of students with disabilities, so these students are relegated to watching from the sideline, keeping score, or keeping time. When allowed to participate in the game, they rarely have success because they cannot perform the skills as quickly or as accurately as their peers.

Fortunately, many physical educators modify games and team sports so that all students can successfully participate. These modifications can be implemented without changing the general format of the game or forcing skilled students to play at a lower level. Rather, modifications can make the game challenging for all students while allowing students with lower ability opportunities for success. Several models for modifying group games (or activities in general) have been developed over the years. General concepts from these models can be applied to integrating students with disabilities into group games and team sports. The following section describes six models of how to modify group games systematically and team sports or alternative games that can be used in regular physical education.

Games Design Model

Morris and Stiehl (1989) developed a systematic approach for analyzing and then changing group games. Their approach uses the following three basic steps:

Step 1. Understanding any game's basic structure Various aspects of games can be altered to include students with varying abilities. Key aspects of any game can be analyzed and then modified to accommodate the needs of students of varying abilities. Table 6.4 outlines how Morris and Stiehl conceptualized six major aspects of games and variations, which can change the nature of a game. These include the following:

Purposes of games can vary from one simple focus (e.g., improving one motor skill) to expecting students to acquire a variety of skills, concepts, and behaviors. Not all students in-

Table 6.4. Games design model

Purposes	Players	Movement	Object	Organization	Limits
Develop motor skills	Individuals	Types	Types/uses	Types	Performance
Enhance self-worth	Groups	Location	Quantity	Location	Environment
Improve fitness, enjoyment	Numbers	Quality	Location	Quantity	
Satisfaction		Relationships			
Develop cognitive skills		Quantity			
		Sequence			

From Morris, G.S.D., & Stiehl, J. (1989). *Changing kids' games*. Champaign, IL: Human Kinetics Publishers. Copyright © 1989 by Gordon S. Morris and Jim Stiehl. Reprinted by permission.

volved in a game necessarily have to work on the same goals. For example, a locomotor game played by all students in a kindergarten physical education class could have different goals for different students, including improving walking gait for a student with cerebral palsy, improving hopping skills for students with limited locomotor abilities, and improving skipping in skilled students. Similarly, goals for a game of soccer played by all students in 10th grade physical education could include improving cardiovascular fitness for a student with Down syndrome, improving range of motion for a student with cerebral palsy, developing basic skills and understanding of the rules of the game for students with lower ability, and using various strategies for skilled students.

Players involved in the game can vary in two major ways: 1) how the players are grouped, and 2) the number of players involved in the game. Players can be grouped homogeneously by gender, size, or skill level; players can be grouped heterogeneously so that each team has an equal representation of skilled/unskilled players; or players can be randomly assigned to groups. The number of players involved in a game can vary by having more than, less than, or the same number of players that a particular game calls for. Group size can be varied so that a particular team might have more or fewer players than other teams. How players are selected for a particular group as well as the number of players involved in a game will have a profound effect on how successfully a student with disabilities is included. For example, a teacher needs to break down her seventh-grade physical education class into four teams for a modified game of volleyball. The class includes a student named Bill who has muscular dystrophy (MD), uses an electric wheelchair, and has limited strength and mobility in his upper body. The teacher decides to group the teams by skill level with each team having skilled players, average players, and unskilled players. The student with MD is assigned to team A. Teams B, C, and D also have unskilled players, so the addition of the student with MD should not be an unfair disadvantage to Team A. The teacher also could have divided the class so that some teams (probably the one with Bill) had more players than teams that had more skilled players.

Movement refers to the types of movement involved in a particular game and how these movements are used. Types of movement include different types of locomotor, nonlocomotor, manipulative, and body awareness skills. Type of movements can be varied so that skilled students work on one skill during the game (e.g., skipping, throwing with a skillful pattern), other students work on different skills (e.g., galloping, throwing with a basic overhand pattern), and a student with disabilities might work on even different skills (e.g., on pushing his wheelchair forward, grasping and releasing). Other ways in which Morris and Stiehl suggested that movements could be modified included locations of movement (personal space, general space, following certain directions, levels, or pathways), quality of movement (variations in force, flow, and speed requirements), quantity of movement (several repetitions, a few repetitions), variations in relationships (moving with or without object or other players), and sequences (following a particular sequence or having no sequence). Modification in movement dimension is one of the best ways to ensure that students with disabilities are appropriately and successfully engaged in regular physical education activities. For example, Susie is a third grader who has mental retardation and autistic-like behaviors. Susie's class is working on the ball skills of dribbling and passing a playground ball, skills that Susie does not do independently. The class consists of 25 students who have varying abilities, so the teacher has modified the movement requirements so that all students are challenged yet successful in the activity. More-skilled students are working on dribbling the ball while running in and out of cones and on passing by playing a game of keep-away (with one person in the middle trying to steal the pass from two players who pass the ball back and forth using different passing patterns). Students who can dribble and pass but who still need practice are working on dribbling the ball while jogging forward and passing the ball back and forth with a peer from various distances, depending on each student's strength. Students who are just learning how to dribble and pass are working on dribbling a ball while standing in one place and passing a ball so that it hits a large target on the wall. Finally, Susie is working on dribbling by dropping the ball and catching it before it bounces again (with assistance from different peers in her class). Susie works on passing by handing the ball to a peer upon a verbal request. During relay races at the end of class, each student uses the skills he or she has been working on. That is, some students have to dribble between cones, some students have to dribble while jogging forward, some students have to dribble the ball 10 times, and Susie has to drop and catch the ball with assistance. The basic movements are similar, but how these movements are operationalized during practice as well as during the game varies from student to student depending on abilities.

Object refers to any equipment used during practice or during a game. Objects can vary in terms of how a student moves in relation to the object (e.g., going under, over, or through hoops; catching, kicking, or throwing a ball), how the object moves a student (e.g., scooterboards, skates, tricycles), how an object is used to send other objects away (bats, hockey sticks, racquets, feet or hands), or how objects are used to gather other objects in (e.g., gloves, hands, lacrosse sticks, milk cartons). In addition, the number and placement of objects in the environment can vary depending on the needs of each student. For example, some students might use regulation-size bats to send objects away from their bodies (i.e., batting), other students might use slightly larger bats, while still other students might use very large bats to hit very large balls. Varying the objects will ensure that each student is working at a level that meets his or her unique needs.

Organization refers to decisions regarding the patterns, structure, and location of players. Some games might have very strict patterns to follow (e.g., relay races in which students are expected to line up behind each other or dodgeball that is played in a circle). In contrast, the structure can be undefined so that players are allowed to move anywhere they wish in the environment (with or without set boundaries). Another decision is the location of players and objects within the boundaries. Are players going to be in close proximity to each other or are they going to be spread out? For a student with limited mobility or strength, a fair accommodation would be to have other students stand near him when it is his turn to toss a ball to them or to tag them. However, if the student were hitting a ball off a tee in a game of softball, it would be reasonable to have the defensive team stand far away from him. Similarly, how far each student has to run in a relay race could vary based on individual abilities.

Limits refers to the general rules we force on players. Some games might have movements that are deemed acceptable or unacceptable or necessary or unnecessary. For example, it might be necessary for a skilled student to dribble through several cones while this rule is not necessary for lesser-skilled students. It might be unacceptable for skilled students to spike a volleyball unless it goes into a certain zone. (If the ball is spiked and it does not go into the zone, the other team gets the ball.) Limits also refers to the physical aspects of the environment and activity conditions. Physical aspects of the environment can vary in terms of how wide the field is, if there are special zones for students with disabilities, size and type of equipment, and number of players in the game. Activity conditions can vary in terms of how long the game is, how long a particular student gets a turn, scoring, or rules. For example, a skilled student might get one pitch to hit in a softball game, a less-skilled student gets three pitches, and a student with disabilities gets to hit the ball off the tee. In terms of scoring, the skilled student would be safe if he or she made it all the way to second base before the other team could retrieve the ball, the less-skilled student would run to the regulation first base, and the student with disabilities would go to a first base which is only 10' from home plate.

Step 2. Modifying a game's basic structure This level of game analysis involves applying the components outlined in the first step to specific games. That is, games will be devised and modified based on how you answer questions such as: what is the purpose of the game, how many players will be involved, what are the movements, and what objects will be used?

Modifying a game's basic structure can take two distinct forms. First, you can manipulate the components in Step 1 to make up a completely new game. For example, if your purpose is to help students develop and improve kicking skills (Purpose/Movement components), you can make up a game that works on these skills by manipulating the game components. One game could consist of equal teams of three players per team (Players component). Each team is given one large box to kick (Object component) (boxes for washing machines or refrigerators work very well), and the object of the game is to kick the box across the gym. The rules are that each player on the team must kick the box at the same time (count 1, 2, 3, kick) and that players cannot touch or kick anyone else's box (Organization/Limits components). This novel game ensures that teammates work together and that each player gets many turns to practice the skill of forceful kicking.

A second way of manipulating game components is to modify traditional games. Traditional games of soccer, basketball, or volleyball often are dominated by one or two skilled players. Game analysis can be used to modify traditional sports so that everyone gets opportunities to participate, improve skills, and contribute in the game. For example, basketball can be changed so that the focus of the game is on improving passing skills and teamwork (Purpose/Movement components). Six teams of five players are selected by the teacher so that each team has an equal representation of skilled and nonskilled players (Players component). Rules are modified to encouraging passing and teamwork by changing how teams can score points. Points can be scored by making baskets, but a team that passes the ball to each player before someone shoots gets double points for every basket made (Limits component). In addition, every time a different player makes a basket, the team gets five bonus points. This would encourage teammates to pass the ball before shooting and to make sure everyone on the team shot the ball at least once during the game. In addition, some players must shoot at a 10′ basket while other players can shoot at an 8′ basket (Objects component). Manipulating game components is an easy way to ensure that the class is focused on specific goals and that maximum participation and practice is afforded to each student.

Step 3. Managing a game's degree of difficulty   This level of analysis is probably the most important in terms of accommodating students with disabilities. This step involves analyzing each of the game components and then creating a continuum from easy to difficult. The continuum can then be used to make a game or skill easier or more difficult for particular students. Skilled students can be challenged by making the activity more difficult, and students with lower abilities or specific disabilities can become more successful by making the activity easier. Morris and Stiehl outlined the following strategy for identifying degree of difficulty.

Action 1: Identify factors that may limit a player's performance   List the various aspects of the task that can be manipulated. External factors such as ball size, size of targets, and speed of objects should be the focus at this level. The authors note that a student's personal abilities such as visual perception or strength should not be considered at this level of analysis since these factors cannot be influenced directly by game analysis. However, personal limitations can be accommodated by making simple changes in task complexity. For example, a larger, slower-moving ball can be used for kicking or striking for a student who has a visual perception problem or a visual impairment.

Action 2: Diagram the task complexity spectrum   Factors identified in Action 1 can now be sequenced along a continuum from less difficult to more difficult. For example, the factor "ball speed" in kicking might be listed as follows:

Task	Task complexity	Ball speed
Kicking	Easy	Stationary
		Slow-moving
	Difficult	Fast-moving

All of the factors related to targeted skills should be sequenced as in the above example. These sequences will begin to help you understand how to modify activities to accommodate varying abilities.

Action 3: Begin to create tasks that vary in difficulty The final action is to take all of the factors and the sequences you have developed and compile them into a *task complexity (TC) spectrum* for a particular skill. An example of one of Morris and Stiehl's TC spectrums is presented in Table 6.5. Game categories (e.g., limits, players) also can be modified to make a particular game easier or more difficult for a group of students. For example, having four teams going at four separate goals in soccer would make the game more difficult, while having two teams of just three players on each team would make the game easier. Similarly, having a smaller playing field would make soccer easier for players with limited endurance, but a smaller tennis court would make the game more difficult for a skilled player. The TC spectrum shows in one schematic how several factors can be manipulated to accommodate a student with disabilities, make a task slightly less difficult for a student just learning a skill, or make an activity more challenging for a skilled player.

In summary, Morris and Stiehl's Games Design model involves three basic stages: understanding the basic structure of the game in general, modifying that structure for a specific game, and altering the game's degree of difficulty. Systematic analysis of games will assist the physical education teacher in making good decisions on how to integrate students with disabilities successfully into regular physical education activities.

Project Adventure

A second example of how activities can be modified to include students with disabilities is Project Adventure (Rohnke, 1977). Project Adventure applies the concepts of Outward Bound to public education. The program focuses on outdoor "adventure-type" activities for teaching physical education. The goals of adventure programs are as follows:

1. To increase the participant's sense of personal confidence
2. To increase mutual support within a group
3. To develop an increased level of agility and physical coordination
4. To develop an increased joy in one's physical self and in being with others
5. To develop an increased familiarity and identification with the natural world

The program incorporates ropes-course activities and initiative/cooperative games to achieve these goals. Some physical educators use the adventure program as the basis for their entire physical education program, while others incorporate some of the key concepts into traditional physical education programs. This latter application is most useful for including children with disabilities in regular physical education activities.

One of best aspects of the adventure program and the one that is most reproducible in schools is "group initiative activities." Group initiative activities are designed "to increase a student's

Table 6.5. Task complexity: Balance factors

TC	Size of support base	Center of gravity	Speed	Time
Easy	Eight body parts	Directly over and close to base of support	Slow	8 seconds
	Four body parts	Slightly off center and above base of support	Fast	18 seconds
Difficult	One body part	Moderately off center and far above base of support	Faster	30 seconds

From Morris, G.S.D., & Stiehl, J. (1989). *Changing kids' games.* Champaign, IL: Human Kinetics Publishers. Copyright © 1989 by Gordon S. Morris and Jim Stiehl. Reprinted by permission.

ability to be an active member of a group which has a problem to solve. . . . This problem-oriented approach can be useful in developing each student's awareness of decision-making, leadership, and the obligation of each member within a group" (Rohnke, 1977, p. 65). In terms of including students with disabilities, group initiative activities can be used to highlight the importance of having all students in the class work together to achieve a team goal. The rules of the game do not permit exclusion of any participants, forcing the team to figure out how to safely and meaningfully include all participants. In fact, initiative games help team members focus on each person's strengths and how he or she can best contribute to the solution to the problem. Students can then apply cooperative problem-solving skills learned in initiative games to include students with disabilities in more traditional team sports.

An example of a simple initiative game is Reach for the Sky (Rohnke, 1977). The object of the game is to place a piece of tape as high as possible on a wall. Teams of as few as three and as many as 15–20 players work together to build a human tower to place the tape. Groups quickly realize that heavier students should be on the bottom supporting smaller players. A person who uses a wheelchair can be a good support on the bottom of the tower, using his wheechair as a base and using his arms to help hold a person in place. Smaller students such as those with fetal alcohol syndrome (FAS) can be used near the top of the tower. Thus, a person's strengths are highlighted rather than his or her weaknesses, and students without disabilities learn to appreciate how each person can contribute to team efforts despite having a disability.

Tranferring this concept to traditional games, students without disabilities can focus on both a student's strengths and weaknesses when modifying the game. For example, in a game of basketball, a student who uses a wheelchair can be seen as a tough obstacle to get around as a point guard positioned in a 2–1–2 defense alignment (typical zone defense alignment in which two players guard the area near the foul line, one player guards the middle, and the last two players guard the area close to the basket). The student with FAS who may be hyperactive might be used as a chaser while playing defense, chasing the ball and harrassing any player who has the ball. In a game of football, the student who uses a wheelchair can be used as an offensive lineman protecting the quarterback by moving his wheelchair so that oncoming rushers must run around him. Similarly, the student with FAS can be a rusher who enjoys chasing other players. Obviously, including students who use wheelchairs or other students who use adapted equipment can be dangerous. Make sure that you talk to the group about safety, especially being aware of the student who uses a wheelchair. In addition, you might want to make special rules for the student who uses a wheelchair, limiting the range in which he or she can move so that the students without disabilities know where "safe" areas are. Students will learn quickly if they are given proper instruction.

One of the nice aspects of group initiative games is that there are no set solutions or answers to the problems presented by the leader. Solutions will depend on the unique characteristics of each member and how these characteristics interact with the characteristics of other group members. This fact should be pointed out to the group at the end of each initiative game or at the end of a class that included several initiative games. Group discussions are a critical part of the adventure project, and participants are encouraged to share their thoughts on how they solved problems during the activity. Group discussion is a good place to help focus on how each member of the team contributed to the group goal. Group discussions also can be used to guide students to think of how children with different disabilities/abilities can be included in an activity and contribute to the team. For example, the leader can ask a group how they completed the task with John (the student who uses a wheelchair). The leader could then ask the group how they would achieve the goals of the task if a student who was blind or a student with cerebral palsy were included in the activity. The group could then learn about and discuss the various disabilities and abilities of individuals who are blind or who have cerebral palsy and how best to modify activities to include them safely and successfully in the activities.

Cooperative Games

Cooperative sports and games (Orlick, 1978) are designed to help students play with one another and work together to overcome challenges rather than against one another to overcome other people. The major goal of cooperative games is to create an environment that helps students "play together for common ends rather than against one another for mutually exclusive ends. In the process, they [students] learn in a fun way how to become more considerate of one another, more aware of how other people are feeling, and more willing to operate in one another's best interests" (Orlick, 1982, p. 4). Obviously, the atmosphere created by cooperative sports is conducive to including students with disabilities in regular physical education.

The major difference between traditional games and cooperative games is the focus and structure. As Orlick explained, traditional games such as King of the Mountain have one person as king while all others are to be pushed down the mountain. Players are compelled to work against each other, and only one player can achieve the goal of the game. Thus, the game has an inherent competitive focus and structure. In contrast, a cooperative version of the same game, People of the Mountain, has a completely different focus in which the objective is to get as many people as possible to the top of the mountain, forcing children to work together rather than compete against each other. The focus of the game is inherently cooperative and encourages classmates to help and support each other. In addition, everyone is a winner in this game as opposed to one winner in the competitive version of the game.

Many physical education programs, while focusing on skill development, present skill development through competitive activities. While fun and motivating for skilled students who can win competitive games, students with less ability, including students with disabilities, rarely have an opportunity to win. In addition, competitive team sports force skilled players to pressure less-skilled players. Mistakes are more glaring, and what often happens is that more-skilled players dominate the game and block out less-skilled players. Less-skilled players lose confidence and self-esteem and even learn how to avoid fully participating in the game. For example, after mis-kicking a soccer ball during a soccer game and being ridiculed by her teammates and teased by her opponents, it is easy for this less-skilled player to avoid kicking the ball by positioning herself away from the action for the remainder of the game. Is this what we want for our physical education programs? Is this student going to improve her soccer skills? If this happens to less-skilled students without disabilities what would happen to students with disabilities who were included in such an atmosphere?

An alternative to competition in physical education is cooperation. Cooperative games can be implemented at various levels. One level is to play only cooperative games such as People of the Mountain. This approach is most appropriate for elementary children who are learning how to work together and who have not been exposed to traditional sports. A second level is introduced cooperation within traditional competitive activities. For example, the focus of the game of volleyball can be how many different players on a team can hit the ball before it is hit over the net rather than which team scores the most points. Such an approach is appropriate for students just learning skills of games who need practice in a game atmosphere without the added pressure of competition. A third level is to include self-paced activities that are not assessed or scored. For example, Clean Out Your Backyard, a fun throwing game for young children, can be played without highlighting which team has fewer balls on their side. For older students, a basketball game can be less competitive by simply not keeping score. Finally, the fourth level includes goal-oriented play in some situations and lighthearted play in other situations. For example, some days the class can work on basketball following traditional rules while on other days the focus can be on which team passes the ball the most before shooting and which team has the most players score.

Most traditional physical education activities including group games and team sports can easily become more cooperative by making just a few changes. *The Cooperative Sports and Games Book* (Orlick, 1978) and *The Second Cooperative Sports and Games Book* (1982) present several suggestions for making traditional competitive games cooperative. For example, Musical Hoops is a cooperative version of Musical Chairs. In traditional Musical Chairs, chairs are taken away and children fight against each other for a chair in which to sit. The quickest children usually get to sit in the remaining chairs while less-skilled players, including students with disabilities, are the first to be eliminated. In Musical Hoops, when the music stops and hoops are taken away, players must share the remaining hoop. Imagine an entire class of kindergartners, including a student who is blind and another with cerebral palsy who is much slower than his peers, working together to fit into one hoop! Another example is Alaskan Rules Baseball. One of the problems in traditional baseball is that players in the field stand around waiting for the ball to be hit to them. Even if a ball is hit to a less-skilled player or a player with a disability, chances are that a more-skilled player will run over and try to field the ball. What results is skilled players getting more turns and becoming more skilled while less-skilled players and players with disabilities get fewer practice turns and grow bored. In Alaskan Rules Baseball, all players in the field must touch the ball before a player is out. The first player who gets the ball picks it up and all other players on the team line up behind that player. The ball is then passed (or tossed) from player to player. When the last player has the ball, he yells "stop," at which time the player's turn is over. The batter gets one run for every base he touches.

New Games

New Games (Fluegelman, 1976; 1980) are games that allow persons of all ages and abilities to play in an atmosphere where fun and creativity are the goals. The following are the major philosophies of New Games:

1. Individuals choose games and make changes to rules as needed so that everyone can be involved.
2. Modifications can occur at any time during the game (even in the middle of the game).
3. Everyone should enjoy the activities. If everyone is not having fun, then modifications are probably needed.
4. Fair, fun competition is important, but winning is deemphasized.

The New Games Book and *More New Games* have descriptions of hundreds of games that can be played by as few as two players and as many as 100 players. Games are also categorized by how active the participants are. New Games lend themselves nicely to including students with disabilities and can be a fun rainy day activity for students without disabilities. The following are two examples of New Games that can easily accommodate students with varying abilities:

- *People to People*—Students are paired up and stand in a circle facing one player who is the leader. The leader calls a name of one or two body parts, for example "back" to "back," and the partners must touch their backs together. When everyone is touching backs, the leader then calls two more body parts, for example "head" to "knee," and each partner must touch his or her head to the partner's knee. The game continues this way until the leader says, "People to People," at which time everyone (including the leader) tries to find a new partner. Whomever is left without a partner is the new leader.
- *Amoeba Tag*—Players scatter about the playing area, and one player is designated "it." Players move about the playing area while "it" tries to tag a player (every so often you can

change the way players move, such as galloping, skipping, jumping, hopping, traveling at different levels, or following different pathways). When a player is tagged, he or she holds "its" hand and both players become "it." When another player is tagged, he or she holds hands with the two-person "it" to form a three-person "it." As new persons are tagged, they join the ever increasing "it." Eventually, all but one player is "it."

SUMMARY

Students with disabilities often have difficulty performing typical physical education activities as well as their peers. However, simple modifications may allow students with disabilities to participate in typical physical education activities with more success. This chapter has outlined two major categories that, when modified, can facilitate the performance of students with disabilities. These categories include: 1) instructional modifications that relate to the general organization of the class as well as how the teacher presents information, and 2) curricular modifications including general ways to modify skills as well as general ways to modify group games and team sports. In addition, alternative games and activities were introduced including Adventure programs, New Games, and cooperative games. Many of these modifications can be implemented without drastically changing the game for students without disabilities. In addition, many of these changes would benefit students without disabilities who have lower abilities than their peers. However, remember that any changes that are made to accommodate a student with a disability should be viewed cautiously and should meet the four criteria outlined earlier in this chapter. As a reminder, these criteria include:

1. Does the change allow the student with disabilities to participate successfully yet still be challenged?
2. Does the modification make the setting unsafe for the student with a disability or for students without disabilities?
3. Does the change affect students without disabilities?
4. Does the change cause an undue burden on the regular physical education teacher?

Chapter 7

Modifications for Specific Disabilities

What I have been most amazed at is how children without disabilities who have been in inclusive physical education settings have learned to accept diversity, and beyond that, how they have learned how to see similarities rather than differences. For example, I have included several students with physical disabilities into regular physical education. Initially, most of my students without disabilities assumed that students who used walkers or wheelchairs could not do regular physical education activities. But after several weeks of inclusion, students without disabilities realized that these students could do a lot of things they could do. All that was needed was some minor modifications to the activities such as allowing students who used wheelchairs to shoot into a lower basket during basketball or allowing students who used walkers to move a shorter distance in relay races. Acceptance of students with disabilities became second nature. In fact, we found that inclusion carried over to the playground where students without disabilities continued to adapt recreation activities so that all students could participate. They really wanted to get everyone involved, so they started to figure out their own adaptations that made games truly inclusive.

—Phyllis Cranfield

Jacob is a 9-year-old student who has muscular dystrophy. Although he still can walk independently, he is getting progressively weaker. Jacob's third-grade class is presently in a unit that includes playing tag and doing relay races. Unfortunately, Jacob can no longer run, and his walk is very slow. The physical educator wants to accommodate Jacob's limited strength, but she does not want to change the tag games or relay races so much that it negatively affects her students without disabilities. What should this teacher do?

Kristen is a seventh grader who has athetoid cerebral palsy. She can walk and run and perform most manipulative skills, and she understands the rules of all the lead-up sports that her teacher has been presenting. Still, Kristen has a problem with accuracy. She has difficulty controlling her body so that she can toss a ball accurately to a peer or hold the bat steady enough to hit a pitched ball. Her favorite activity is volleyball, and even though she has the strength to hit the ball over the net or to a peer, she does not have the ability to pass the ball accurately. Kristen's physical educator wants to help Kristen participate more successfully in seventh-grade physical education, but she just doesn't know how to help her. What should this teacher do?

Phyllis Cranfield is a physical educator for Adams County School District No. 14, Commerce City, Colorado.

José is an 11th grader who is blind. The regular 11th-grade physical education curriculum focuses on a variety of individual and team sports, many of which require the ability to follow a moving ball. José is interested in playing traditional sports with his peers or at least in gaining a better understanding of what basketball, soccer, football, and baseball are like when he goes to high school games or when he listens to games on television. The teacher wants to help him, but he cannot figure out how to modify traditional sports for a student who is blind. What should this teacher do?

The previous chapter provided instructional and curricular modifications that could facilitate the successful inclusion of students with disabilities into regular physical education. In particular, several models described the process of making curricular modifications so that physical educators can begin to make their own modifications tailored to meet the unique needs of their students. However, some physical educators feel more comfortable if they have specific suggestions on how to accommodate students with distinct deficits or disabilities. Others want specific modifications to the traditional individual and team sports that make up the bulk of their curriculum. These modifications can then be quickly plugged into existing programs to meet the needs of students with disabilities.

The purpose of this chapter is to review modifications designed to accommodate students with specific disabilities as well as specific suggestions for accommodating traditional sports. This chapter is organized as follows: 1) accommodations for students with specific deficits such as problems with endurance or accuracy, 2) accommodations for students with specific types of disabilities such as cerebral palsy or visual impairment, and 3) accommodations to traditional individual and team sports with suggestions for students with specific disabilities. Although it is difficult to generalize modifications across categories, the specific modifications reviewed in this chapter should give physical educators and other team members ideas on how to modify activities for students with specific types of problems or disabilities.

One final note before introducing specific accommodations. While ideas to accommodate students with specific disabilities are provided (e.g., mental retardation, orthopedic disability), you should focus on the functional strengths and weaknesses of your particular students rather than their diagnostic labels. For example, it is difficult to generalize modifications for all students who have cerebral palsy. Functionally, students with cerebral palsy can be quite different. Some may have problems with coordination, while others may have problems with strength. Thus, accommodations should be different for each individual student based on functional needs as opposed to a label. As you read this chapter, and particularly the section on specific disabilities, try to think of the functional deficits that your students have. Then go back to the introductory section on specific functional deficits to cross-reference the best possible accommodation. As always, utilize the collaborative team members to provide more specific information regarding functional abilities of particular students.

ACCOMMODATIONS FOR STUDENTS WITH SPECIFIC FUNCTIONAL DEFICITS

Some students with disabilities have specific problems that affect the ability to perform at a level equal to their peers. Such deficits can become very frustrating for these students, eventually causing them to dislike physical education and physical activity altogether. Some deficits, such as problems with strength or endurance, often can be remediated so that the student can perform the skill at a higher level. However, structural deficits such as extreme short stature (dwarfism), visual impairments, or a physical disability cannot be remediated. In these situations, modifications to activities can be introduced that allow the student to perform the skill more successfully. Most of these changes do not have to affect other students, although you may want to use some of these techniques to accommodate students without disabilities who are having difficulty with specific tasks. The following (adapted from Arbogast & Lavay, 1986, Herkowitz, 1978, and Sherrill, 1993) outline some general factors which can be manipulated to accommodate students with specific deficits.

Adaptations for Students with Deficits in Strength, Speed, and Endurance

1. *Lower targets.* Students who do not have the strength to get an object to a target can have the target lowered. For example, a student who cannot reach a 10' basket in basketball can shoot at a 6' or 8' basket. Similarly, a student who cannot hit a ball over a regulation volleyball or badminton net can have the net lowered. By lowering the target, students will have a greater opportunity for success which in turn will encourage them to continue to practice the skill. Targets set at reasonable heights also facilitate the desired movement pattern. For example, students who cannot reach a 10' basket with a basketball using a "typical" shooting pattern often resort to different, less effective shooting patterns (e.g., sidearm hurl, underhand, tossed backward over their head). However, they will use a more standard pattern when the basket is lowered.

2. *Reduce distance/playing field.* Many physical education activities require students to throw, pass, serve, or shoot a ball a certain distance or require students to run a certain distance. For example, shooting a free throw must be from behind the free throw line, serving a volleyball must be from behind the back line, and running to first base must be from home to first base. These distances, while necessary when playing intramural or interscholastic games, can be altered when teaching skills or playing lead-up or recreational games in physical education. Distances can be reduced so students with disabilities can be successful. For example, a student could push his wheelchair to a first base that is half the distance to the regular first base to accommodate his limited speed. Similarly, a student who can serve a ball only 10' can be allowed to serve from 8' away from the net rather than from the back line. Such accommodations do not give either team any advantage, yet allow the student with disabilities an opportunity to be successful. For games that require running up and down an entire floor or field (e.g., basketball or soccer), games can be played using the width of the field rather than the length, or half-court games can be played. Another modification that would not affect the entire class is allowing a particular student to play in just half the field (just play defense or offense) or placing the student in a position that requires less movement (playing defender in soccer rather than midfielder; playing lineman in football rather than wide receiver).

3. *Reduce weight and/or size of striking implements, balls, or projectiles.* Students with limited arm or grip strength or who have smaller-than-normal hand size may have difficulty holding large or heavy striking implements or balls. For example, a regulation-size tennis racquet might be too long and heavy for a student with muscular dystrophy who is very weak in her upper body. Allowing this student to use a racquetball racquet or badminton racquet or a tennis racquet with the handle cut off would enable this student to have more success. Some students with more subtle strength problems might need to simply be encouraged to choke up on the racquet. Similarly, a student with a small hand (e.g., a student with Down syndrome) might have difficulty gripping a softball with one hand. The student thus resorts to throwing the softball with two hands when he could demonstrate a one-handed throwing pattern if given a tennis ball. Finally, some balls are too heavy for students to handle or may even scare students. Balloons, beach balls, or Nerf balls can be good substitutes for a volleyball or basketball that is too heavy or too intimidating for a student.

4. *Allow the student to sit or lie down while playing.* Activities played while lying or sitting demand less fitness than games played while standing or moving. Students with limited strength and endurance (e.g., students with cystic fibrosis or asthma) can be allowed to sit down when the ball is at the other end of the playing field in soccer or sit while playing in the outfield. These

students also can be allowed to sit while practicing some skills during part of physical education and move while practicing other skills. For example, a student with a heart condition who tires easily can warm up with the class by performing every other locomotor pattern the class performs. The student can be allowed to sit down when he is not performing a locomotor pattern.

5.   *Use partially deflated balls or suspended balls.* By their nature, balls tend to roll when put in motion. While most young children enjoy chasing balls, students who fatigue easily may use up all their energy chasing the ball after every turn, thus missing out on important practice trials. Balls that are partially deflated or paper balls (crumpled up piece of paper wrapped with a few pieces of masking tape) do not roll away as easily as regular balls. Also, balls suspended from a basket or ceiling or balls tied to a student's wheelchair are easy to retrieve.

6.   *Decrease activity time/increase rest time.* Games and practice sessions can be shortened for students who fatigue easily. Students can be allowed to play for 5 minutes, then rest for 5 minutes; periods could be shortened so that all students play for 3 minutes then rotate to an activity that requires less endurance; or the number of points needed to win a game can be reduced. For example, a game of sideline basketball could be played in which three players from each team play for 3 minutes while the other players on each team stand on opposite sidelines prepared to assist their teammates. Such a game would allow a student to be active for 3 minutes, then rest for 3 minutes. Another possibility is to allow free substitutions in a game. For example, a student with asthma can come out of a soccer game every 2–3 minutes to make sure he does not have an asthmatic episode; he would not have to wait until the ball went over the end line or sideline to be substituted.

7.   *Reduce speed of game/increase distance for players without disabilities.* Many games can move quite quickly, leaving slower players and players with limited endurance behind. It only takes a few times of finishing last to begin to dislike yourself and physical activity. Modifications can be made so that races and games are fairer for students with limits in speed and endurance. For example, slower students in a relay race need only go up and back one time while more skilled students need to go up and back two times. Similarly, a special zone in soccer can be marked off for a student who has limited speed. When the ball goes into the zone, this student is the only one who can kick the ball.

Specific Adaptations for Students with Limited Balance

1.   *Lower center of gravity.* Allow the student to perform activities while sitting down or on hands and knees. Also, encourage the student to bend his or her knees while moving, stopping, and standing. For example, a student should be encouraged to land with feet apart when jumping down from a box. When performing locomotor patterns, students should be encouraged to perform animal walks that lower the center of gravity (crawling, creeping, bear-walking) or to move with knees bent when performing locomotor patterns such as running and jumping.

2.   *Keep as much of the body in contact with the surface as possible.* Allow students with balance problems to walk or run flat-footed rather than on tiptoes, or allow students to perform balance activities on three or four body parts rather than on one or two body parts. For example, when working on locomotor patterns, allow a student with balance problems to jump on two feet while her classmates hop on one foot.

3.   *Widen base of support.* Encourage students to stand with feet farther apart to provide more stability. For example, students should be encouraged to stand with feet apart while preparing to catch a ball. Similarly, students can be allowed to walk or run with feet apart until they develop more postural control.

4.   *Increase width of beams to be walked.* Students should be allowed to walk on the floor or on wider beams until they develop more postural control. For example, a balance station could

have 2″ × 4″, 2″ × 6″, 2″ × 8″, and 2″ × 10″ beams so that each student is challenged at his or her own level of ability. In addition, a hierarchy of challenges can be set up, beginning with walking with one foot on and one foot off the beam, using a shuffle step across the beam, walking across the beam holding on to the wall or a peer's hand, and finally increasing number of independent steps taken.

5. *Extend arms for balance.* Encourage students to hold their arms out to the side when performing balance activities. For example, have a student hold arms out to the side while walking on a beam or when learning how to walk, run, jump, or hop.

6. *Use carpeted rather than slick surfaces.* When possible, provide surfaces that increase friction. For example, learning how to roller skate on a tumbling mat or carpeted surface is easier than learning how to skate on a gym floor. Similarly, it is easier to perform various locomotor patterns on a carpeted surface as opposed to a slick surface. Finally, encourage students to wear rubber-soled footwear rather than shoes with slick bottoms.

7. *Teach students how to fall.* Students who have postural control problems that are not easily remediated (e.g., student with ataxic cerebral palsy) will fall often. While teaching these students how to compensate for balance problems (e.g., widen base of support, keep arms out), also teach students how to fall safely by practicing how to fall on mats. You can even make a game of falling that all children can play. For example, a simple game like Ring Around the Rosy requires all students to fall at the end of the song. During the game students can practice falling forward, backward, and sideward.

8. *Provide a bar to assist with stability.* During activities that require balance, allow the student to hold on to a wall, bar, chair, or table for extra stability. For example, allow the student to hold on to a wall as he or she walks across a beam, or allow the student to hold on to a chair while practicing the leg action in kicking. Allowing a student to use balance aids while learning motor skills such as throwing and kicking may enable a student to exhibit more advanced motor patterns. For example, a student who has difficulty stepping and throwing because of balance problems might be able to demonstrate a step and throw if allowed to hold on to a chair while throwing. The chair can then be gradually faded away as the skill becomes more ingrained.

9. *Teach the student to use eyes optimally.* Vision plays a critical role in postural control. Teach students how to use their vision to facilitate balance. For example, the student can be taught to focus his or her vision on a stationary object on a wall while walking a beam or while performing standing balance activities.

10. *Determine whether balance problems are related to health problems.* Balance problems may be related to health problems such as inner ear infections. For example, children with chronic inner ear infections often walk later than children with no inner ear problems. Talk to the student's special education teacher, parent, or physician to determine if there are any health problems that might negatively affect balance. In addition, find out if the student is taking any medication that might affect balance. Balance difficulties caused by health problems or medication might be acute in nature, in which case you might want to have the student avoid activities that require balance. If the problem is more chronic or will last for several weeks or months, then you want to implement some of the modifications described above.

Specific Adaptations for Students with Problems of Coordination and Accuracy

1. *For catching and striking activities, use larger, lighter, softer balls.* Larger balls are easier to catch and strike than smaller balls. However, larger balls may promote an immature catching pattern (scooping into body rather than using hands). If a student is unsuccessful or frightened of smaller, harder balls (e.g., softballs), then the use of a larger Nerf ball, balloon, or punch ball is appropriate. Gradually introduce a smaller ball to elicit a more skillful pattern. In

addition, balls tossed directly to a student are easier to catch than balls tossed to a student's side, while balls tossed to a student's side are easier to strike than balls tossed directly at a student.

2. *Decrease distance the ball is thrown and reduce speed.* The distance the ball is tossed should be reduced for students who have difficulty tracking balls. For example, one student might be allowed to hit a ball pitched from 10′ away in a game of softball while other students are expected to hit a ball pitched from 20′. Similarly, a ball can be tossed slowly for some students, faster for others, and still faster for more skilled students. Ideally, the teacher will vary distance and speed so that each student is challenged at his or her level, yet has an opportunity to succeed.

3. *For throwing activities, use smaller balls.* Some students might have trouble gripping a ball (e.g., students with spastic cerebral palsy). Allow these students to use smaller balls or balls that are more graspable such as yarn balls, Koosh balls, paper balls, or bean bags. Again, the teacher should have a variety of balls available for students to choose from so that each student is challenged yet successful.

4. *In striking and kicking, use a stationary ball before trying a moving ball.* Allow students who have coordination problems to kick a stationary ball or strike a ball on a tee before practicing with to a moving ball. Suspended balls that move at slower speeds and on a known trajectory are also easier to kick/strike than moving balls. Again, allow the student to be successful and demonstrate skillful patterns with adaptations; then gradually fade away adaptations as student gains confidence and skill.

5. *Increase the surface of the striking implement.* Allow students to use lighter bats with a larger striking surface (e.g., plastic bat) or a racquet with a larger striking surface. Again, have a variety of striking implements from which students may choose.

6. *Use a backstop.* Students who miss the ball often may spend most of their time retrieving the ball rather than practicing the skill. This does not promote good use of practice time, and it can become very frustrating for the student. When working on striking, kicking, or catching activities in which students may miss the ball several times, have a backdrop, backstop, nets, or rebounder available. You can also attach a string to the ball and then to a student's wheelchair for ease of recovery.

7. *Increase size of target.* Allow students to throw or kick to larger targets, or allow students to shoot at larger baskets. In addition, give points for coming close to targets, such as points for hitting the rim or backboard in basketball or points for throwing a ball that hits the side of the target but not the middle. Less-skilled students can be allowed to stand closer to the target in order to promote initial success, then gradually move back.

8. *In bowling-type games, use lighter, less stable pins.* In games or activities in which the goal is to knock something down, use lighter objects (e.g., milk cartons, aluminum cans) so that any contact with the object will result in success. In addition, use more pins and spread them out farther than normal so that tosses or kicks that would normally miss the target still result in success.

9. *Concentrate on safety.* Students who have problems with coordination are more prone to injury, especially in activities that involve moving balls. Students who are prone to injury should be allowed to wear eyeglass protectors, shin guards, helmets, and face masks. When necessary, provide a peer tutor who can protect the student from errant balls.

ADAPTATIONS FOR CHILDREN WITH SPECIFIC DISABILITIES

The following provides information regarding adaptations for students who have specific disabilities. This discussion includes: 1) students with physical disabilities, 2) students with mental retardation, 3) students with hearing impairments, 4) students with visual impairments, 5) students with emotional disturbances, and 6) students with health disorders. For more information about the medical and/or motor characteristics of any of these disabilities, refer to most adapted physical education texts or medical texts. As noted earlier in this chapter, diagnostic results do not provide much information about a student's functional abilities. As you think of your particular students, cross-reference the modifications presented in this section with modifications outlined in the previous section on functional deficits. Also, you will see some redundancy between the suggestions in this section and the previous section.

Students with Physical Disabilities

1. *Confer with the collaborative team to determine the exact nature of disability*. Make sure you get medical information from the student's physician and physical therapist including contraindicated activities, activities that need modifications, and precautions for safety. Adhere to these restrictions. For example, a student's physical therapist can provide you with information regarding a student's range of motion in various joints as well as best position for functional movement.

2. *Prepare students without disabilities*. Provide them with general information about physical disabilities as well as specific information about the particular student to be included. Talk about wheelchairs. (Allow students without disabilities to sit in and move a wheelchair to see what it is like.) Talk about ways students without disabilities can informally help the student who uses a wheelchair. For example, students without disabilities can retrieve errant balls or help push a student to a station. Students without disabilities also can be a special student's partner in group activities. In general, students without disabilities should be encouraged to welcome the student with disabilities into their class.

3. *Think safety*. Students without disabilities should be aware of the other student's wheelchair or crutches when moving about the environment. Cones could be set up around a student who uses a wheelchair as a buffer to warn students that they are getting close to the student who uses a wheelchair. For example, in a game of soccer, a peer can be assigned to retrieve the ball for a student with a disability who is in a special zone. This peer also can protect the student from errant balls and warn other students when they are getting too close to the zone.

4. *Allow students with physical disabilities to be included in decision processes* regarding adaptations for certain activities. The student probably knows better than anyone else his or her movement capabilities and how best to accommodate his or her abilities and limitations. For example, if you are working on locomotor patterns, a student who uses a wheelchair can decide how he or she is going to move his or her chair to simulate hopping (using one arm), skipping (moving arms rhythmically), or how best to throw a ball (maybe backward over his or her head rather than the traditional forward way).

5. *Make accommodations for limited strength, endurance, and flexibility*. Simple modification that helps a student overcome problems with physical fitness (see previous section, this chapter) can improve a student's success and ability to participate with peers in a variety of group games and sports. Encourage students to find their own modifications to accommodate their limitations.

6. *Make accommodations for limited coordination and reaction speed*. For example, utilize Herkowitz's developmental task analysis or Morris's task complexity model to determine how you might modify such task factors as size of the ball, speed of the ball, or trajectory of the ball (see chap. 6, this volume, for more detail).

7. *Use rebounders or tie balls to a student's wheelchair* so that the student does not have to spend a lot of time retrieving balls. For example, a student can practice throwing a ball that is tied to his or her chair with a 20' string. After the throw, the student simply pulls the string to retrieve the ball.

8. *Reduce playing area for the student in a wheelchair.* While students without disabilities can be allowed to use the whole field or court, a student who is learning how to push his or her wheelchair can be allowed to move in a smaller space.

9. *Use "game analysis" techniques* to determine best ways to accommodate students who use wheelchairs in traditional games and sports. Allow students without disabilities to participate in the decision process so that they feel the modifications are not dictated to them. Use cooperative and initiative games and encourage the group to figure out ways to include the student who uses a wheelchair safely (see chap. 6, this volume, for more detail).

10. *Utilize sports rules* from the National Wheelchair Athletic Association (NWAA), United States Cerebral Palsy Athletic Association (USCPAA), National Amputee Athletic Association (NAAA), or Les Autres Athletic Association (LAAA). Each of these sports associations has specific rule modifications for various sports that can be utilized by persons with physical disabilities. For example, in tennis a person who uses a wheelchair is allowed two bounces before he or she must hit a ball, and in basketball a person who uses a wheelchair can dribble by pushing his or her wheelchair while keeping the ball on his or her lap.

Students with Mental Retardation

1. *Confer with the collaborative team* regarding a student's cognitive abilities and limitations. Information from the student's special education teacher regarding his or her ability to comprehend verbal cues will be important. The special education teacher and the speech therapist can give you vital information regarding how best to communicate with the student. Also, find out if the student has any behavior problems and what behavior management techniques are used when the student does misbehave.

2. *Prepare students without disabilities.* Provide information in general about mental retardation and specifically about the student who will be included in their class. Encourage students without disabilities to help students with mental retardation in terms of understanding directions, understanding where to go and where to stand in activities and games, and how to practice skills correctly. Also, encourage students to invite the student to join their stations or groups. Praise students without disabilities for befriending the student with mental retardation, and sternly reprimand students who tease, ridicule, or take advantage of the student with mental retardation. Students without disabilities should realize that the student with mental retardation wants to do well in physical education and wants to be friends with other students. However, he or she may be shy or uncomfortable at first. Students without disabilities can help the student feel more comfortable by simply befriending the student during early physical education sessions.

3. *Do not underestimate the abilities of students with mental retardation.* Given enough instruction, practice, and time, many students with mental retardation can learn skillful movement patterns. For example, most persons with mental retardation, particularly students with less severe mental retardation, should be expected to demonstrate skillful throwing, striking, and catching patterns that would allow them to be more successful in a game of softball. Only after exhaustive efforts should you accept less-skillful movement patterns (e.g., hitting a ball off a tee, throwing without rotating the trunk). Many students with mental retardation also can learn to follow the basic rules of individual and group games and sports. There are many examples of Special Olympics athletes playing team sports such as basketball, volleyball, softball, and soccer. These players not only adhere to the rules of the game without any special modifications but use complex strategies and team concepts such as zone defenses in basketball and set dead-ball plays in soccer. Again, more instruction, practice, and time may be needed for these students to learn rules and concepts, but every effort should be made to give them an opportunity to learn how to play the game the correct way. Then and only then will these students have an opportunity to participate in integrated, community sport programs.

4. *Select activities based on chronological age* rather than mental age of skill development. This is particularly true for older students (middle school and older). While students with mental retardation may be delayed by 2 years or more in mental and skill development compared to their peers without disabilities, it is important that you teach skills that will allow these students to interact with their peers and develop recreation fitness skills for postschool life. For example, a high school student with severe mental retardation has the mental abilities and motor skills of a 5-year-old. While it may seem reasonable to work with this student on activities appropriate for a 5-year-old (e.g., learning basic locomotor and manipulative patterns), such activities will not help this student participate in activities his high school peers play or help him acquire skills necessary to participate independently in recreation activities as an adult. Realistically, you may have to work on two or three targeted activities rather than all the activities typically conducted in regular physical education. For example, you may want to work only on softball, basketball, weight training, and aerobic dance with a high school student who has severe mental retardation since it will take this student a long time to learn the basics of these four activities (see Block, 1992, for more information on working with students with severe mental retardation).

5. *Think safety.* Students with mental retardation often cannot anticipate potential dangerous situations such as walking in front of a soccer goal when other students are shooting or moving in front of a target toward which students are throwing objects. Remind students with mental retardation of the safety rules (as well as students without disabilities), and tell students without disabilities to be extra cautious of students with mental retardation (and other students in general).

6. *Provide direct instruction on how to play* with toys and physical education equipment (i.e., actually show students how to play with equipment such as throwing bean bags, walking on beams, tossing and catching balloons). Students with mental retardation may not understand how to play with toys and equipment or how to interact with peers or teammates. Have other students act as role models for appropriate play, and encourage other students to invite students with mental retardation to play with them. For example, if you are playing a cooperative game such as Musical Hoops, have other students in the class invite the student with mental retardation to share their hoop.

7. *Keep verbal directions to a minimum and use extra demonstration and physical assistance* when providing instruction. Many students with mental retardation do not understand verbal directions as well as their peers without disabilities, and they may miss key points in demonstrations. Help students focus on critical aspects of a movement by giving extra, specific verbal cues, demonstrating key movement aspects, and even physically assisting students to perform the movement correctly. Even if you are using a movement exploration approach, you may need to provide some physical assistance to a student with mental retardation to help get the student "in the ballpark" of the movement.

8. *Break skills down into smaller components.* For example, if you are working on the task of hopping with a class of kindergartners, most students can learn the skill by breaking it down into three or four critical steps: preparatory position, place arms out to side, bend knee, simultaneously extend knee and hip to lift body up. For students with mental retardation, you may need to extend this task analysis into 10 steps.

9. *Measure progress and reinforce skill development in smaller increments.* Students with mental retardation will learn, but their progress will be much slower than their peers without disabilities. Use various ways of detecting and reinforcing progress. For example, progress can include less-intrusive levels of assistance (going from physical assistance to demonstration), throwing a ball farther or with more accuracy measured in inches rather than feet, or noting use of one or two more components in the overall locomotor or manipulative pattern.

10. *Be aware of limited motivation*, particularly in activities that require physical fitness. Plan on providing external reinforcers (tokens, primary reinforcers, free play) to encourage stu-

dents with mental retardation to perform activities that are difficult such as running, sit-ups and push-ups, and practicing the correct pattern for throwing.

11.   *Let students with mental retardation know that they will not be ridiculed* for performing a movement or activity incorrectly or more slowly than their peers. Encourage students without disabilities to be patient with the student with mental retardation and to reinforce him or her for trying difficult activities.

12.   *Plan to help students maintain and generalize skills.* For maintenance, you will need to give the student many extra trials after he or she acquires a skill to help him or her overlearn the skill. Similarly, students will not generalize skills from one environment to another. That is, if a student is taught how to bowl in the gym, he or she may not be able to perform this skill at a bowling alley. Therefore, you may need to teach critical lifetime skills in the actual environment where they will take place. This is especially true for high school students who will soon graduate from school and will be using their motor skills in community recreation settings (see Krebs & Block, 1992, for more detail).

13.   *Be prepared to provide compensations for processing problems*, perceptual problems, and fitness problems. Students with mental retardation may not be able to process complex verbal instruction as quickly as their peers. Give them extra time to process information, and be prepared to repeat directions at a later time. Ask the student to repeat key parts of the verbal cues to make sure he or she understands what to do. Similarly, some students with mental retardation may have problems taking in visual or auditory information or they may have problems with spatial awareness. Actually set up activities in which the student can work on improving perception. For example, an activity at one station can include practicing going over, under, and between obstacles without touching them. A peer at the station can change the heights of obstacles to encourage the student to practice making correct decisions (e.g., when should she go over versus under). In terms of physical fitness, allow the student to do fewer repetitions or run fewer laps at a slower pace than peers. Encourage the student to try to improve his or her fitness by gradually increasing fitness demands, but be sure to reinforce even small amounts of progress. For example, most of the students do 20 sit-ups as a warm-up activity, but the student with mental retardation works on doing five sit-ups. Encourage the student to do six, then seven, then eight, as the year progresses.

Students with Hearing Impairments

1.   *Confer with the collaborative team* regarding the student's specific hearing impairment and any residual hearing. Obtain specific information from the student's audiologist and speech teacher. Ask how the student communicates and how best to communicate with the student. While learning sign language may be difficult for most teachers, learning a few key signs will help you convey instructional and management cues to the student more effectively. For example, simple signs such as *stop, go, sit, stand up, run, walk, line up, copy me* are relatively easy to learn. Most students do well with a good demonstration.

2.   *Prepare students without disabilities.* Give them general information about hearing impairments and specific information about the student who will be included. Explain the best way to communicate with the student, and encourage students to learn a little sign language so they can communicate with the student. Also, encourage students without disabilities to interact with the student who has a hearing impairment and to invite him or her to join their stations or groups. Encourage students to offer to be a buddy to the student in terms of repeating directions, providing extra demonstrations, and generally watching out for the student if he or she looks confused.

3.   *Position the student in front of the class* and as close to you as possible when giving instructions. If the student has residual hearing, you may want him or her to actually stand next to

you. If the student is trying to read your lips, he or she should have a good view from the front of the class. Do not speak any more slowly or more exaggeratedly than normal, and remember, even good lipreaders understand only about 30% of what the speaker is saying. Be prepared to repeat verbal directions to the student off to the side after you have given directions to the entire class.

4.   Be prepared to *provide extra demonstrations* after you have given verbal cues to the class. After you present information to the class, pull the student with a hearing impairment off to the side and give him or her a brief demonstration, focusing on the exact component of the skill on which you want the student to focus. For example, you might give a second demonstration in which you focus on the preparatory position for catching. Have the student repeat the demonstration to make sure he or she understands what to work on.

5.   *Use extra visual cues* such as written directions or pictures to describe exactly what you want the student to do. For example, you can have a picture of the correct throwing pattern taped to the wall of a station. Point to the particular aspect of the movement on which you want the student to focus. Also, give the student written information regarding rules and strategies that other students get verbally.

6.   *Make sure the learning environment has adequate lighting.* When outside, do not have the student face the sun since this will make it difficult to read lips and see demonstrations. In the gymnasium, make sure the janitor fixes all lights and that stations are set up where lighting is the best.

7.   For students who use hearing aids, *encourage use of residual hearing.* Discuss the student's hearing ability with the collaborative team, and determine how much residual hearing the student has. Also determine if one ear hears more than the other, and if speaking into that ear would be helpful.

8.   *Avoid excessive noise in the environment* so that students can focus on key verbal cues and directions. Physical education classes tend to be noisy, but you can ask for quiet during critical instruction time. Again, if the environment is too noisy when you are relaying information to the class, repeat the directions (using demonstrations and gestures as needed) off to the side in a quieter setting.

9.   *Be cautious of the student's hearing aids.* (Remove hearing aids when going swimming.) Students should be encouraged to wear their hearing aids during physical education to assist them in picking up verbal cues and sounds, but they should be aware of these aids in contact activities. Removal of aids in combative activities such as wrestling, karate, and football is probably appropriate, but check with the student's audiologist or physician.

10.   *Utilize peer tutors to repeat directions*, give extra demonstrations, and to help the student understand what to do and where to go. For example, if the teacher gives complex directions regarding to which station to go and how to perform an activity, a peer can repeat the information to the student with a hearing impairment via gestures and demonstrations. Some students without disabilities enjoy learning sign language and may be able to learn enough to communicate more explicit cues to the student.

Students with Visual Impairments

1.   *Confer with the collaborative team* regarding the student's visual impairment and any residual vision, any other disabilities he or she may have, and any specific safety considerations or contraindications. Obtain information from the student's ophthalmologist and vision specialist. For example, a student with a detached retina can lose the little vision he or she has with a direct blow to the head. Caution should be taken when exposing these students with detached retinas to activities using balls, and most combative-type activities (e.g., wrestling, karate, football) will be contraindicated for these students.

2. *Always think safety.* If a student wears glasses, consider having him or her wear eye protectors during activities in which balls will be used. Adhere to recommendations given by the collaborative team regarding safety precautions and contraindicated activities. When you are not sure that a student can protect himself or herself in an activity (e.g., playing outfield in softball or wing fullback in soccer, or performing a locomotor pattern in a scattered formation), assign a peer to work with the student. For example, a student with a visual impairment can play deep center field in softball with a peer playing short center field who can protect the student from line drives and hard-hit balls. When possible, replace hard balls with Nerf balls so that if the student does get hit, it will not cause injury. There are new, firmer sponge balls that have the bounce and feel of softballs, basketballs, and soccer balls that can be used by the class without affecting the game. (This would make the game safer for all students, including students without disabilities who have less ability than their peers.)

3. *Do not assume that all students with visual impairments will only like to play stereo-typical activities* that are popular among persons who are blind. For example, while gymnastics, swimming, and bowling are relatively easy activities for students who are blind to learn, many students who are blind will want to participate in the same activities as their peers. With modifications and extra assistance from a peer, these students can participate in volleyball, softball, basketball, and soccer, team sports that are not usually played by persons who have visual impairments. While students who are blind might not be able to play these sports independently, they can learn the rules of these sports and gain a better understanding of the various positions and strategies used in the game. This will enhance their enjoyment when listening to high school, college, or professional games, and many students may learn to enjoy working on the skills used in the game such as shooting baskets, hitting a softball off a tee, or hitting a tennis ball using verbal cues.

4. *Assist students who are blind in moving safely and independently* in the gym environment. Have a peer take the student through the locker to show him or her where the bathrooms, showers, and lockers are. Also, take the person around the gym to show the boundaries and where equipment is located. Pay particular attention to stored equipment into which the student might walk. When changing the environment so that new equipment is placed around the gym, take time to show the student where the equipment is, what it is used for, and how it feels. Encourage the student to explore balls, bats, and other pieces of equipment tactually in order to better understand their use.

5. *"Anchor" the student to the play area.* Anchoring means telling the student who is sitting next to him or her in the gym. This can be as easy as having the student sit next to the same students every time he or she comes to gym (e.g., in the same squad). If students sit randomly, have students without disabilities next to the student who is blind introduce themselves so that the student knows who is sitting nearby.

6. *Prepare students without disabilities.* Students without disabilities should know a little about visual impairments in general and about the specific visual skills of the student being included. They should be encouraged to assist the student informally and to be his or her friend during physical education. Provide simple ways in which students without disabilities can provide informal assistance, such as retrieving errant balls, helping the student find stations or positions on the field, and helping the student perform movement correctly. Also, encourage students without disabilities to talk with the student who is visually impaired, share team strategies, and help the student understand where other students are positioned around the playing area.

7. *Use brightly colored objects and objects that contrast with the surrounding environment* to encourage students to use their residual vision. For example, use yellow balls when playing outside on grass, or use blue balls when playing inside on an orange gym floor. Use brightly colored cones or tape to mark boundaries.

8. *Use tactile or auditory boundaries.* For example, use cones or changes of the surface (from grass to gravel) to indicate a boundary. Hang crepe paper from the ceiling for boundaries or mark the floor with tape that the student can feel with toes or hands. Use beeper cones or music (a tape player works well) to indicate where a target is. For example, placing a tape player under the basket helps a student locate which direction to shoot a basketball.

9. *Be prepared to use very specific verbal directions and physical assistance* when giving instruction and feedback. For example, you will have to tell a student (or have a peer tell a student) exactly how he or she missed the target ("You missed the target by throwing the ball 1' too high and 6" to the left"). You will also have to give explicit feedback regarding a student's movement pattern (e.g., "Bend your elbow so that it is at 90°") when getting into backswing position of backhand in tennis). In most cases, students with visual impairments will learn best if you provide them with physical assistance. You can physically assist the student through appropriate patterns so that the student "gets a feel" for how to move, or you can have the student hold on to you while you perform the movement. This later technique (called *reverse manual assistance*) works well as a supplement to more traditional physical assistance and explicit verbal cues. Auxter and Pyfer (1989) noted that you can present a demonstration to the class by using the student with a visual impairment as an assistant. You demonstrate the movement and physically assist the student who is blind. This way you are giving direct tactile feedback to the student who is blind without taking time away from the rest of the class.

10. *Allow the student to use special equipment* as needed to ensure success. For example, bowling guides that are placed parallel to the student allow him or her to know where the side boundary is while taking the approach. This device could be used in similar situations when side boundaries are needed. Another simple modification is to attach a string to balls and to the student's hand so that balls do not get away so easily. In throwing, for example, sighted students can see where their balls go and can easily retrieve them. For students who are blind, they can throw the ball, then retrieve it by pulling the string toward them. Other simple adaptations are having a guide rope when running to first base, running sprints, or swimming; using beep cones to indicate where to run; using foot markers for proper stance when batting; or dangling crepe paper as reference points throughout the gym to mark certain critical points.

11. *Have the vision specialist braille all handouts* and cognitive concepts such as rules of games, strategies, and names of equipment. For example, have the vision specialist braille a diagram of a baseball diamond with the names of all the positions. Students who are blind also should be allowed to take written tests orally. (Have someone read questions and allow him or her to answer verbally.)

12. *Utilize rules from the United States Association for Blind Athletes* (USABA). This sports-governing body, specifically for athletes who are visually impaired, has a variety of suggestions for modifying traditional sports such as swimming, track and field, and gymnastics. The suggested modifications can assist you when including a student who is visually impaired in regular physical education. For example, one of the rules for wrestling is that students must remain in contact at all times. This could be a fair compensation to which a student without disabilities wrestling a student who is blind should adhere. In addition, the association offers information and rules for unique sports designed specifically for students who are visually impaired such as Beep Baseball and Goal Ball. While designed specifically for students who are blind, they can be fun games to introduce to blindfolded students without disabilities to show them what it is like to have a visual impairment.

Students with Emotional Disturbances

1. *Confer with the collaborative team* to determine the student's specific behavioral problems and what other team members do to prevent or deal with behaviors. Discuss any activities

that might "set the student off" or make the student feel uncomfortable, and discuss simple ways that such situations can be modified. Determine which activities, teaching methods, instructional formats, or pieces of equipment (if any) should be avoided for particular students. For example, some students might fear loud sounds such as balloons popping. If you are planning to use balloons with a first grade class, this student might work at stations away from the balloons or in the hallway with a teacher assistant during this particular activity. Similarly, some students do not do well in large class formats (too much noise and stimulation). These students might be integrated slowly (part of the class during small group work or stations, but removed during group games). Finally, some students are "tactually defensive" (do not like being touched). These students should be given directions verbally and through demonstration. Physical assistance can be provided in small doses, and the student should be told ahead of time that you will be touching him or her for a few seconds.

2. *Prepare students without disabilities.* They should know a little about emotional disturbances and how this particular student behaves in certain situations. They should be encouraged to interact with the student, but they should also learn when to back off from the student who is having a difficult time. For whatever reason, some students will set off students with emotional disturbances. You may need to hand-pick groups so that students who set each other off are separated.

3. *Provide activities that ensure success.* This will help the student feel good about himself or herself and about physical education. As the student feels comfortable with you and the class structure, you can begin to introduce more challenges, which may result in occasional failures. For example, initially you can have the student shoot at a lower basket in basketball to ensure success. Later, you can introduce shooting at a higher basket for part of the class, reinforcing the student for good efforts as well as successful baskets. You may even want to set up a scoring system that reinforces good efforts. For example, a student can be reinforced for touching a ball with his or her hands when practicing catching (not just being able to catch the ball).

4. *Actually teach the student that it is all right to fail and how to accept failure or loss.* Spend some early sessions with the class so that everyone learns appropriate sportsmanship. Set up structured situations in which one team will lose. Warn them ahead of time and explain how to lose properly. Also, play more cooperative and initiative games as well as competitive games that deemphasize winning and losing. For example, play games in which points are scored by passing the ball to teammates, or play a tag game in which players tagged do five jumping jacks and then can go back into the game.

5. *Provide a release for students who are aggressive.* If a student is prone to hitting others or throwing things when he or she is angry, have a special station set up to which to go and throw bean bags at a target. Explain to the student that it is all right to get angry and mad, but throwing bean bags at a target is more appropriate than hitting. Encourage the student to think of other more appropriate ways to vent anger and frustration.

6. *Provide extra stimulus to help students focus on relevant information.* Many students with emotional disturbances (especially those with related attention deficit disorders) have difficulty focusing on the targeted activities. If you make the activities more fun and reinforcing, students will be more apt to pay attention and stay on task. For example, having a student hit balls off a tee against a wall is not as stimulating as hitting empty soda cans off a tee against the wall. (Soda cans make a lot more noise.)

7. *Provide more external reinforcers for students.* Some students with emotional disturbances (like many students without disabilities) are not intrinsically reinforced by physical education activities. Be prepared to provide extra reinforcers for these students to help motivate them to try new and challenging physical education activities. While not bribing them, use a simple "Premack principle" (e.g., "If you do a good job with this activity, then you can have a few minutes of

free play"). Another technique that works is using a token system in which students receive tokens for good behavior, following directions, or good effort. Students can then trade in tokens at the end of the day, week, or month for something they want to do (e.g., playing a special game, using a special piece of equipment, or playing with a special partner). Discuss possible behavioral programs with the student's special education teacher.

8. *Clearly state consequences for misbehavior and follow through when the student misbehaves.* Students need to know exactly what will happen when they perform the desired activities and when they misbehave. Describe in detail both positive and negative consequences to students *prior to* implementing the program. You may want to practice the consequences one or two times in a nonthreatening way so that the students clearly understand. Once the students know the program and the consequences, make sure you follow through with these consequences when a student misbehaves. Do not give warnings unless they are part of the behavior program. Students will test the program in its early stages, and if you waiver in your delivery of consequences, a student will think he or she can get away with misbehavior. Again, confer with the collaborative team regarding specific behavior management techniques.

9. *Allow some flexibility in behavior.* Some students will come to your gym with a "chip on the shoulder" from something that happened at home or in the classroom. The student is in no mood for physical education, and if you insist on participation, you will no doubt have to deal with a major behavior problem. Let the student know that you realize he or she is having a hard time today, and that he or she can choose to participate with the group or sit out. Point out that this is a special situation and that normally he or she would be expected to participate or face the consequences.

Students with Health Disorders

1. *Confer with the collaborative team* to determine specific precautions, modifications, and contraindications to physical activity. Particularly important is information from the student's physician. Adhere to these guidelines when planning and implementing your program. For example, a student with a congenital heart defect might be able to participate in all physical education activities except those that raise his heart rate over a long period of time. Examples of activities that would be restricted include long distance running, basketball, and soccer. However, the student might be allowed to play basketball and soccer if he only plays for 2-minute periods, rests for 5 minutes or works on skills, then plays another 2 minutes. Again, any modifications should be approved by the student's physician.

2. *Prepare students without disabilities.* Give students without disabilities general information about health disorders and specific information about the student who is being included. (Do not give information that will affect the student's right to privacy or cause him or her ridicule.) For example, the class should understand why a student who has a seizure disorder must wear a helmet to physical education. They should be told that there is no need to be scared, and they should be encouraged to interact with the student and invite him or her to participate with them in their stations or on their teams. Right to privacy is a tricky situation, particularly for students with acquired immune deficiency syndrome (AIDS), so you will need to confer with the collaborative team as to how much information you can give to the students without disabilities.

3. *Think safety.* While integrating the student is important, it is of utmost importance that the student participates safely. Modifications can be made so that students with health disorders can participate in regular physical education activities. However, care should be taken so that participation will not jeopardize the student's health and safety. For example, a student who has a seizure disorder should not be allowed to participate in climbing activities, but the student can participate in low ropes or low gymnastic activities with spotters and mats. Similarly, this student

can participate in swimming activities with peers if he or she has a one-on-one assistant. Again, safe modifications should be a collaborative team decision. Students with health disorders should not be immediately dismissed from physical education nor should they be tossed in without considering their individual condition. Students with AIDS or hepatitis pose a unique health risk to the teacher and other students in the class. Utilize universal precautions in situations in which injuries causing cuts or scrapes may occur. For example, use gloves when treating bloody injuries, and do not allow other students near the student who is bleeding. You will probably want to confer with the school nurse for specific procedures for when a student with AIDS or hepatitis incurs an injury.

  4. *Be aware of the effects of medication.* Some students who have health disorders take medication that has side effects that can affect their physical abilities. For example, some seizure medications can make a person's gums weak and prone to bleeding. These students can still participate in physical activity, but they may need to be extra careful not to take a blow to the face. Similarly, some medications may affect a person's balance. Such persons should be given a balance aid (as simple as a chair) or an assistant (could be a peer) in activities in which balance is needed. A student might need to wear a helmet during physical education if a seizure disorder is not under control or if medication causes problems in balance.

  5. *Be aware how time of day or seasons affect particular students.* Some students do better once their medication has taken effect (e.g., after a student with attention deficit disorder takes Ritalin). Other students (some students with heart defects) gradually tire throughout the day and can hardly walk, let alone participate in physical activity, by seventh period. Still other students might be affected by the season (e.g., students with allergy-induced asthma). Whenever possible, accommodations should be made to have the student come to physical education earlier or later in the day depending on his or her condition. Similarly, students with allergy-induced asthma might receive physical education indoors during particularly bad pollen days in the fall and spring. Again, confer with the team as to the best time for the student to receive physical education and when alternatives to regular physical education are warranted.

SPECIFIC MODIFICATIONS TO TEAM AND INDIVIDUAL SPORTS

Many physical educators, particularly those in middle school and high school, think in terms of the traditional sports that they present to their students rather than the specific functional needs of particular students. The appendix to this chapter provides information on specific ways to modify selected individual and team sports to meet the needs of students with disabilities. Information, written in outline form, includes: 1) general suggestions for modifying skill work, 2) general suggestions for modifying games, and 3) modifications for students with specific disabilities. This is not intended to be a comprehensive list but rather general suggestions for modifying sports. As you begin to learn more about the functional skills of your students, as well as how to utilize these modifications, you will quickly begin to incorporate your own modifications that meet the needs of your particular students.

  Again, try to focus on the functional requirements of a particular sport skill and how they relate to the functional abilities of your students. For example, running to first base in a game of softball requires a certain amount of balance and the ability to run (or move) a certain distance. How do these requirements match the particular balance and running abilities of students with disabilities? Similarly, the functional requirements for hitting a tennis ball are strength and coordination. How do these requirements match the particular strength and coordination abilities of students with disabilities? As you review the specific suggestions in the appendix at the end of this chapter, go back to the previous section on accommodating students with specific functional deficits as a cross-reference to modifications.

SUMMARY

Students with disabilities usually will need some accommodations to the regular program if they are going to be included successfully and meaningfully in regular physical education. These accommodations can be as simple as giving the student a lighter racquet in tennis or slightly shortening the base in softball. However, modifications can include specific changes to rules of games, such as giving students free passes in basketball or setting up special zones in soccer. In all of these cases, these accommodations can mean the difference between successful inclusion and frustration for students with disabilities.

This chapter has outlined modifications to physical education activities for students with specific functional deficits, specific diagnostic labels, and specific individual and team sports. These modifications are not meant to be an exhaustive list but rather to help physical educators and other team members begin to think of simple, yet innovative ways to include students with disabilities safely and successfully in regular physical education. As noted throughout this chapter, your focus should be on the functional abilities and deficits exhibited by your students as opposed to more general diagnostic labels. Therefore, much of the information in this chapter is redundant and cross-referenced.

As noted in the previous chapter, the specific accommodations you implement should meet four specific criteria. If your modifications do not meet these criteria, you should seriously think of choosing a different modification. As a reminder, these four criteria include:

1. Does the change allow the student with disabilities to participate successfully yet still be challenged?
2. Do the modifications make the setting unsafe for the student with a disability or for students without disabilities?
3. Does the change affect students without disabilities?
4. Does the change cause an undue burden on the regular physical education teacher?

Accommodations to Individual and Team Sports for Students with Disabilities

TEAM SPORTS

Basketball Skills

Dribbling

General
- Use larger or smaller balls.
- Use playground balls, Nerf balls, or punch balls (large balloons).
- Vary distance required to travel.
- Vary speed required.
- Only use dominant hand.

Students who use wheelchairs (normal upper body strength)
- Hold ball on lap and push wheelchair.
- Push wheelchair a few rotations, bounce ball one time, then push wheelchair again.

Students who use wheelchairs (limited upper body strength and control)
- Have peer push wheelchair while student holds ball in lap or in hands.
- Have peer physically assist student in bouncing ball.
- Have student repeatedly hit ball when it sits on lap tray while being pushed.

Students with visual impairments
- Allow student to dribble in place.
- Allow student to use two hands to dribble.
- Allow student to dribble in place a few times, then walk forward toward sound of peer.
- Allow student to walk forward while dropping and catching ball for dribbling.
- Attach string to ball and to student's wrist so that ball is easy to retrieve.
- Have student stand in corner of gym while dribbling so that ball is less likely to bounce away.
- Put bell or beeper in ball so that student can retrieve it when it bounces away.
- Have peers assist student by giving verbal cues for direction and by retrieving balls that get away from student.

Students with mental retardation/learning disabilities
- Allow student to walk while dribbling.
- Allow student to stand, bounce, and catch ball.
- Allow student to walk while holding ball.
- Allow student to use two hands to dribble.
- Allow student to walk forward while dropping and catching ball for dribbling.
- Encourage proper technique.

Passing and Catching

General

- Use suspended balls.
- Use larger or smaller balls.
- Use textured balls.
- Use playground balls, Nerf balls, or punch balls (large balloons).
- Vary distance required to pass (have peers stand closer).
- Toss ball more slowly than required.
- Toss ball at known trajectory.

Students who use wheelchairs (normal upper body strength)

- Encourage student to find best way to pass (overhead v. chest v. sidearm).
- Use soft ball (Nerf ball) for safety as needed.

Students who use wheelchairs (limited upper body strength and control)

- Use soft ball (Nerf ball) for safety.
- Push ball down ramp.
- Push ball off lap.
- Swing arm and hit ball held by peer.
- Kick ball if legs have more control than arms.
- Hit ball off tee (or held by peer) with head.

Students with visual impairments

- Use soft ball (Nerf ball) for safety.
- Use verbal cues (tell student when ball is released for catching; tell student where to pass).
- Use bounce pass (ball makes sound).
- Put bells or beeper in ball.
- Use physical assistance to instruct student.

Students with mental retardation/learning disabilities

- Use soft ball (Nerf ball) for safety.
- Start with a balloon and gradually work toward faster-moving balls.
- Use suspended balls.
- Use physical assistance when teaching skill.
- Encourage proper technique.

Shooting

General

- Use larger or smaller balls.
- Use playground balls, Nerf balls, or punch balls (large balloons).
- Vary distance required to shoot.
- Vary height of basket.
- Vary size of basket (use large box for basket or hang hula hoop on wall).

Students who use wheelchairs (normal upper body strength)

- Encourage student to find best way to shoot (overhead v. chest v. sidearm).
- Use soft ball (Nerf ball) for safety as needed.

Students who use wheelchairs (limited upper body strength and control)

- Use soft ball (Nerf ball) for safety.
- Push ball down ramp into box.
- Push ball off lap into box.
- Swing arm and hit ball held by peer into box.
- Kick ball into box if legs have more control than arms.
- Hit ball off tee (or held by peer) with head into box.

Students with visual impairments
- Use soft ball (Nerf ball) for safety.
- Use verbal cues to tell student where to shoot.
- Give student specific verbal feedback to tell him or her how close his or her shot was to the basket.
- Use physical assistance to instruct student.
- Tie string to ball and to student's wrist so that ball is easy to retrieve.
- Place radio under basket to cue student.
- Put bells or beeper in ball.

Students with mental retardation/learning disabilities
- Use soft ball (Nerf ball) for safety.
- Use physical assistance when teaching skill.
- Place handprints on ball to show proper technique.
- Encourage proper technique.

Basketball game

General
- Encourage students without disabilities to develop modified rules that will be fair for everyone, including student with disabilities.
- Allow student to shoot at lower basket.
- Allow student to use different ball when it is his or her turn to dribble or shoot.
- Make rule that no student can steal ball when student is dribbling.
- Make rule that no student can block or interfere with student's pass.
- Have student play a zone position away from the basket.
- Match student with disability against lower-ability student without disabilities.
- Give student a peer to assist him or her during game.
- Allow free substitution for student if he or she tires easily.
- Give student's team extra player (6 v. 5 game).
- Allow student to play only offense or defense if he or she has limited mobility.
- Split the class and allow skilled students to play competitive, full-court games while allowing less-skilled players (including student with disabilities) to play slower, less competitive games (half-court, 3 v. 3, run set plays).
- Play lead-up basketball games such as half-court basketball, horse, relays.

Students who use wheelchairs (normal upper body strength)
- Caution peers about wheelchair.
- Have student play away from basket on defense and offense for safety.

Students who use wheelchairs (limited upper body strength and control)
- Provide student with peer to assist him or her.
- Allow student to use adapted equipment practiced during skills (e.g., ramps).
- Bring basket (can be box or trash can) to student.

Students with visual impairments
- Have peer guide student around court.
- Have a guide rope across gym so student can move up and down court.
- Place carpet square on floor to mark where student should stand for defense and offense.
- Have teammates give extra verbal cues to student to describe where he or she is, where teammates are, and where opponents are.
- Use ball with bell.
- Place radio under basket.
- Have teammates wear brightly colored pinnies.
- Use brightly colored ball.
- Put brightly colored ribbons or streamers on basket.

Students with mental retardation/learning disabilities
- Give student peer to assist him or her during game.
- Give student extra time to pass and shoot without being defended.
- Give student free shot at basket.

Soccer Skills
Dribbling
General
- Use larger or smaller balls.
- Use playground balls, Nerf balls, or punch balls (large balloons).
- Vary distance required to travel.
- Vary speed required (allow student to walk).
- Only use dominant foot.

Students who use wheelchairs (normal upper body strength)
- Hold ball on lap and push wheelchair.

Students who use wheelchairs (limited upper body strength and control)
- Have peer push wheelchair while student holds ball in lap or in hands.
- Have peer physically assist student in moving foot to kick ball.
- Have student repeatedly hit ball when it sits on lap tray while being pushed.

Students with visual impairments
- Tie string to ball and to foot so that ball can be retrieved.
- Give student peer to guide him or her in correct direction.
- Put bells or beeper in ball.
- Dribble toward sound of peers.
- Use deflated ball.
- Place student along wall or fence so that he or she can place hand against wall for balance and for reference.

Students with mental retardation/learning disabilities
- Allow student to walk while dribbling.
- Allow student to use deflated ball.
- Tie ball to student's foot so that ball does not get away.
- Practice on grass (ball moves more slowly).
- Have peer assist student (extra verbal and physical cues).
- Encourage proper technique.

Passing and trapping
General
- Use suspended balls.
- Use larger or smaller balls.
- Use playground balls, Nerf balls, or punch balls (large balloons).
- Vary distance required to pass (have peers stand closer).
- Pass balls more slowly as required.
- Try to pass ball directly to student.

Students who use wheelchairs (normal upper body)
- Allow student to throw or roll ball for passing.
- Encourage student to find best way to pass (overhead v. chest v. sidearm).
- Use soft ball (Nerf ball) for safety as needed.

Students who use wheelchairs (limited upper body strength and control)
- Use soft ball (Nerf ball) for safety.
- Kick (push with foot) ball down ramp.
- Kick ball held by peer.

- Push ball off lap.
- Hit ball off tee (or held by peer) with head.

Students with visual impairments
- Use soft ball (Nerf ball) for safety.
- Use verbal cues to help student stand in correct direction.
- Use verbal cues (tell student when ball is released for trapping; tell student where to pass).
- Put bells or beeper in ball.
- Use physical assistance to instruct student.

Students with mental retardation/learning disabilities
- Use soft ball (Nerf ball) for safety.
- Start with a balloon and gradually work toward faster-moving balls.
- Use suspended balls.
- Use physical assistance when teaching skill.
- Encourage proper technique.

Shooting

General
- Use larger or smaller balls.
- Use playground balls, Nerf balls, or punch balls (large balloons).
- Use balls with varying texture.
- Vary distance required to shoot (allow student to stand closer).
- Vary size of goal (larger for less skilled students).

Students who use wheelchairs (normal upper body strength)
- Allow student to substitute throwing for shooting.
- Encourage student to find best way to shoot (overhead v. chest v. sidearm).
- Use softball (Nerf ball) for safety as needed.

Students who use wheelchairs (limited upper body strength and control)
- Use soft ball (Nerf ball) for safety.
- Kick ball or push ball down ramp toward goal.
- Push ball off lap toward goal.
- Kick or swing arm and hit ball held by peer toward goal.
- Hit ball off tee (or held by peer) with head toward goal.
- Allow student to kick or strike ball into box next to chair as goal.

Students with visual impairments
- Use soft ball (Nerf ball) for safety.
- Use verbal cues (goalie) to tell student where to shoot.
- Give student specific verbal feedback to tell him or her how close his or her shot was to goal.
- Use physical assistance to instruct student.
- Place radio in middle of goal to cue student.
- Put bells or beeper in ball.
- Use target that makes noise when hit.

Students with mental retardation/learning disabilities
- Use soft ball (Nerf ball) for safety.
- Use overinflated playground balls (travel farther with less strength).
- Use physical assistance when teaching skill.
- Encourage proper technique.

Soccer game
General
- Encourage students without disabilities to develop modified rules that will be fair for everyone, including student with disabilities.
- Set up special zone for student where only he or she can play ball.
- Allow student to shoot at wider goal.
- Allow student to use different ball when it is his or her turn to dribble or shoot.
- Make rule that no student can steal ball when student is dribbling.
- Make rule that no student can block or interfere with student's pass.
- Have student play a wing position away from fastest action.
- Match student with disability against lower-ability student without disabilities.
- Give student a peer to assist him or her during game.
- Allow free substitution for student if he or she tires easily.
- Give student's team extra player (12 v. 11 game).
- Allow student to play only offense or defense if he or she has limited mobility.
- Split the class and allow skilled students to play competitive, full-field games while allowing less-skilled players (including student with disabilities) to play slower, less competitive games (half-field, 6 v. 6, keep-away games, cooperative games).
- Play lead-up soccer games.

Students who use wheelchairs (normal upper body strength)
- Caution peers about wheelchair
- Have student play goalie (requires less mobility) and make rule that skilled students cannot shoot from closer than 20 yards out.

Students who use wheelchairs (limited upper body strength and control)
- Provide student with peer to assist him or her.
- Allow student to use adapted equipment practiced during skills (e.g., ramps).
- Allow student free shot at goal from close distance.

Students with visual impairments
- Have peer guide student around field.
- Have special zone for student marked with rope or cones where only he or she can play ball (make rule that ball should be played into zone every 2–3 minutes).
- Have teammates give extra verbal cues to student to describe where he or she is, where teammates are, and where opponents are.
- Use ball with bell.
- Use brightly colored ball.
- Place radio in goal.
- Have teammates wear brightly colored pinnies.
- Allow student free shot from penalty line at least once during game.

Students with mental retardation/learning disabilities
- Provide student with peer to assist him or her.
- Give student extra time to pass and shoot without being defended.
- Give student occasional free shot at goal.

Softball Skills

Throwing/catching/fielding
General
- Use suspended balls.
- Use Velcro balls and Velcro mitts.

- Use larger or smaller balls.
- Use playground balls, Nerf balls, or punch balls (large balloons).
- Vary distance required to throw (have peers stand closer).
- Throw balls more slowly than required.

Students who use wheelchairs (normal upper body strength)
- Encourage student to find best way to throw (overhead v. sidearm).
- Use soft ball (Nerf ball) for safety as needed.

Students who use wheelchairs (limited upper body strength and control)
- Use soft ball (Nerf ball) for safety.
- Push ball down ramp, then have peer throw it rest of way.
- Push ball held by peer, then have peer throw it rest of way.
- Push ball off lap, then have peer throw it rest of way.
- Hit ball off tee (or held by peer) with head; then have peer throw it rest of way.
- Use legs and kick ball if student has more control over legs.

Students with visual impairments
- Use soft ball (Nerf ball) for safety.
- Use suspended ball.
- Use verbal cues to help student stand facing correct direction.
- Use verbal cues (tell student when ball is released for catching; tell student where to throw).
- Put bells or beeper in ball.
- Use physical assistance to instruct student.

Students with mental retardation/learning disabilities
- Use soft ball (Nerf ball) for safety.
- Start with a balloon and gradually work toward faster-moving balls.
- Use suspended balls.
- Use physical assistance when teaching skill.
- Encourage proper technique.

Batting

General
- Use larger or smaller balls.
- Use playground balls, Nerf balls, or punch balls (large balloons).
- Use larger or smaller striking implements.
- Use lighter striking implements.
- Hit ball off tee.
- Vary distance ball is pitched.

Students who use wheelchairs (normal upper body strength)
- Encourage student to find best way to position chair for batting.

Students who use wheelchairs (limited upper body strength and control)
- Use soft ball (Nerf ball) for safety.
- Hit ball off tee with hand.
- Strap small striking implement to hand for striking.
- Push ball down ramp.
- Push ball off lap.
- Swing arm or use head to hit ball held by peer.
- Kick ball if legs have more control than arms.

Students with visual impairments
- Use verbal cues to tell student when ball is pitched.
- Give student specific verbal feedback to tell student how close he or she was to hitting ball.

- Use physical assistance to instruct and help student.
- Put bells or beeper in ball.
- Hit ball rolled across table.

Students with mental retardation/learning disabilities
- Use physical assistance when teaching skill.
- Encourage proper technique.
- Hit ball rolled across table.

Base running

General
- Vary distance to first base.
- Vary width of base path.

Students who use wheelchairs (normal upper body strength)
- Allow student to push wheelchair.

Students who use wheelchairs (limited upper body strength and control)
- Have peer push chair while student tries to keep arms up.
- Have peer push chair while student tries to keep head up and look at first base.

Students with visual impairments
- Use verbal cues to tell student where to run (first baseman).
- Use physical assistance to instruct and help student.
- Put bells or beeper at first base.
- Put radio by first base.
- Have rope between home plate and first base to guide student's path.

Students with mental retardation/learning disabilities
- Use physical assistance as needed.
- Encourage proper running technique.

Softball game

General
- Encourage students without disabilities to develop modified rules that will be fair for everyone, including student with disabilities.
- Establish special rules, such as ground rule double when ball is hit to student with disabilities.
- Give student extra strikes.
- Allow student to hit ball off tee.
- Allow pitcher to stand closer to player and pitch ball more slowly.
- Allow student to use larger ball when it is his or her turn to bat.
- Allow student to use lighter, larger bat (even racquet) when batting.
- Have student play outfield with peer assistant.
- Have student play catcher (requires less mobility).
- Place first base closer to home for student.
- Give student a peer to assist him or her during game.
- Allow student to play only offense or play every other inning if he or she tires easily.
- Give student's team extra player (11 v. 10 game).
- Split the class and allow skilled students to play competitive, regulation game while allowing less-skilled players (including student with disabilities) to play slower, less competitive games with modified game (e.g., cooperative game).
- Play lead-up softball games.

Students who use wheelchairs (normal upper body strength)
- Caution peers about wheelchair.
- Have student play catcher or first base (requires less mobility).

Students who use wheelchairs (limited upper body strength and control)
- Provide student with peer to assist him or her.
- Allow student to use adapted equipment practiced during skills (e.g., ramps).
- Force player without disabilities to play "regular depth" on defense to give student fair chance to make it to first base.
- Make different rules for scoring (if student hits ball a certain distance, he or she gets a single, double, triple, or home run).

Students with visual impairments
- Have peer assist student in field.
- Have teammates give extra verbal cues to student to describe where he or she is and where teammates are.
- Use ball with bell or beeper and first base with beeper.
- Place radio at first base.
- Use brightly colored ball.
- Make first base brightly colored.
- Make different rules for scoring (if student hits ball a certain distance, he or she gets a single, double, triple, or home run).

Students with mental retardation/learning disabilities
- Provide student with peer to assist him or her.
- Have student play catcher or outfield (less mobility and skill needed).

Volleyball Skills

Setting/passing

General
- Use larger or smaller balls.
- Use lighter and softer balls (Nerf balls, balloons, beach balls, volley trainers).
- Vary distance requirements (stand closer to net).
- Vary speed required (slow down the ball).
- Lower the net.

Students who use wheelchairs (normal upper body strength)
- No modifications needed.

Students who use wheelchairs (limited upper body strength and control)
- Hit suspended ball.
- Push ball held by peer, then have peer pick up ball and pass it to other teammates.
- Push ball off lap tray, then have peer pick up ball and pass it to other teammates.
- Push ball down ramp or across table; then have peer pick up ball and pass it to other teammates.
- Use legs or head if student has better control with these body parts; then have peer pick up ball and pass it to other teammates.
- Provide physical assistance as needed.
- Allow student to touch ball; then have peer pick it up and pass it to other teammates.

Students with visual impairments
- Use brightly colored balls.
- Have peers tell student in which direction to stand and where to pass.
- Put bells or beeper in ball.
- Hold ball for student and let him or her hit it out of your hands.
- Allow student to self-toss and then set ball.

Students with mental retardation/learning disabilities
- Allow students with limited coordination to toss ball rather than hit it.

- Have peer assist student (extra verbal and physical cues).
- Encourage proper techniques.

Bumping
General
- Use larger or smaller balls.
- Use lighter and softer balls (Nerf balls, balloons, beach balls, volley trainers).
- Vary distance requirements (stand closer to net).
- Vary speed required (slow down the ball).
- Lower the net.

Students who use wheelchairs (normal upper body strength)
- Encourage student to lean forward to bump or bump to side of chair.
- Allow overhead passing to be used as substitute for bumping.

Students who use wheelchairs (limited upper body strength and control)
- Hit suspended ball.
- Push ball held by peer, then have peer pick up ball and bump it to other teammates.
- Push ball off lap tray, then have peer pick up ball and bump it to other teammates.
- Push ball down ramp or across table; then have peer pick up ball and bump it to other teammates.
- Use legs or head if student has better control with these body parts; then have peer pick up ball and bump it to other teammates.
- Provide physical assistance as needed.
- Allow student to touch ball; then have peer pick it up and bump it to other teammates.

Students with visual impairments
- Use brightly colored ball.
- Have peers tell student in which direction to stand and where to bump ball.
- Provide physical assistance as needed.
- Put bells or beeper in ball.
- Hold ball for student and let him or her bump it out of your hands.
- Allow student to self-toss and then bump ball.

Students with mental retardation/learning disabilities
- Allow students with limited coordination to toss ball rather than bump ball.
- Have peer assist student (extra verbal and physical cues).
- Encourage proper technique.

Serving
General
- Use larger or smaller balls.
- Use lighter and softer balls (Nerf balls, balloons, beach balls, volley trainers).
- Vary distance requirements (stand closer to net).
- Lower the net.

Students who use wheelchairs (normal upper body strength)
- Encourage student to find best way to serve (overhand v. sidearm).

Students who use wheelchairs (limited upper body strength and control)
- Hit suspended ball.
- Push ball held by peer, then have peer pick up ball and serve it over net.
- Push ball off lap tray, then have peer pick up ball and serve it over net.
- Push ball down ramp or across table, then have peer pick up ball and serve it over net.
- Use legs or head if student has better control with these body parts; then have peer pick up ball and serve it over net.
- Provide physical assistance as needed.
- Allow student to touch ball; then have peer pick it up and serve it over net.

Students with visual impairments
- Use brightly colored balls.
- Have peers tell student in which direction to stand and where to serve.
- Provide physical assistance as needed.
- Put bells or beeper in ball.
- Put radio under net to help student locate net.

Students with mental retardation/learning disabilities
- Allow students with limited coordination to throw ball rather than serve it.
- Have peer assist student (extra verbal and physical cues).
- Encourage proper technique.

Volleyball game

General
- Encourage students without disabilities to develop modified rules that will be fair for everyone, including student with disabilities.
- Set up special zone for student where only he or she can play ball.
- Have student play back and outside positions for safety.
- Allow student to throw ball rather than hit it.
- Allow student to use different ball when it is his or her turn to dribble or shoot.
- Make rule that student's team gets an extra hit.
- Make rule that no student can block or interfere with student's pass.
- Match student with disability against lower-ability student without disabilities.
- Give student a peer to assist him or her during game.
- Allow free substitution for student if he or she tires easily.
- Give student's team extra player (7 v. 6 game).
- Split the class and allow skilled students to play competitive, regulation games while allowing less-skilled players (including student with disabilities) to play slower, less-competitive games (e.g., cooperative games).
- Play lead-up games.

Students who use wheelchairs (normal upper body strength)
- Caution peers about wheelchair.
- Have student play back and side position only.

Students who use wheelchairs (limited upper body strength and control)
- Provide student with peer to assist him or her.
- Allow student to use adapted equipment practiced during skills (e.g., ramps).

Students with visual impairments
- Have peer guide/assist student during game.
- Mark floor with carpet squares to help student find position.
- Have teammates give extra verbal cues to student to describe where he or she is, where teammates are, and where opponents are.
- Use brightly colored ball.
- Put brightly colored ribbons or streamers on net.
- Use ball with bell.
- Place radio under net.
- Have teammates wear brightly colored pinnies.
- Allow student to hit ball held by peer.

Students with mental retardation/learning disabilities
- Provide student with peer to assist him or her.
- Give student extra time to pass and shoot without being defended.
- Allow student to hit ball held by peer.

INDIVIDUAL SPORTS

Tennis Skills

Forehand

General
- Use larger or smaller balls.
- Use lighter and softer balls (Nerf balls, balloons, beach balls, volley trainers).
- Use shorter, lighter racquets (racquetball racquet, panty-hose racquet).
- Use racquets with larger heads.
- Vary distance requirements (stand closer to net).
- Vary speed required (slow down the ball).
- Lower the net or do not use net.

Students who use wheelchairs (normal upper body strength)
- Encourage student to find best position to hit forehand.
- Hit ball off tee.
- Encourage student to work on maneuvering wheelchair and then hitting ball.

Students who use wheelchairs (limited upper body strength and control)
- Use strap or Velcro to attach racquet or striking implement to student's hand.
- Hit suspended ball.
- Hit or push ball held by peer, then have peer pick up ball and hit over net.
- Hit or push ball off lap tray, then have peer pick up ball and hit it over net.
- Hit or push ball down ramp or across table, then have peer pick up ball and hit it over net.
- Use legs or head if student has better control with these body parts; then have peer pick up ball and hit it over net.
- Provide physical assistance as needed.
- Allow student to touch ball; then have peer pick it up and hit it to other teammates.

Students with visual impairments
- Use brightly colored balls.
- Have peers tell student in which direction to stand and where to hit ball.
- Provide physical assistance as needed.
- Put bells or beeper in ball.
- Put radio by net for direction.
- Hold ball for student and let him or her hit it out of your hands.
- Allow student to self toss and then hit ball.
- Attach string to student and to ball so that student can quickly retrieve ball.

Students with mental retardation/learning disabilities
- Allow student with limited coordination to hit suspended ball.
- Allow student with limited coordination to hit ball off tee.
- Have peer assist student (extra verbal and physical cues).
- Encourage proper technique.

Backhand

General
- Use larger or smaller balls.
- Use lighter and softer balls (Nerf balls, balloons, beach balls, volley trainers).
- Use shorter, lighter racquets (racquetball racquet, panty-hose racquet).
- Use racquets with larger heads.
- Vary distance requirements (stand closer to net).
- Vary speed required (slow down the ball).
- Lower the net or do not use net.

Students who use wheelchairs (normal upper body strength)
- Encourage student to find best positions to hit forehand.
- Hit ball off tee.
- Encourage student to work on maneuvering wheelchair and then hitting ball.

Students who use wheelchairs (limited upper body strength and control)
- Hit suspended ball.
- Hit or push ball held by peer; then have peer pick up ball and hit it over net.
- Hit or push ball down ramp or across table, then have peer pick up ball and hit it over net.
- Use legs or head if student has better control with these body parts; then have peer pick up ball and hit it over net.
- Provide physical assistance as needed.
- Allow student to touch ball; then have peer pick it up and hit it to other teammates.

Students with visual impairments
- Use brightly colored balls.
- Have peers tell student in which direction to stand and where to hit ball.
- Provide physical assistance as needed.
- Put bells or beeper in ball.
- Put radio by net for direction.
- Hold ball for student and let him hit it out of your hands.
- Allow student to self-toss and then hit ball.
- Attach string to student and to ball so that student can quickly retrieve ball.

Students with mental retardation/learning disabilities
- Allow students with limited coordination to hit suspended ball.
- Allow student with limited coordination to hit ball off tee.
- Have peer assist student (extra verbal and physical cues).
- Encourage proper technique.

Serving

General
- Use larger or smaller balls.
- Use lighter and softer balls (Nerf balls, balloons, beach balls, volley trainers).
- Use shorter, lighter racquets (racquetball racquet, panty-hose racquet).
- Use racquets with larger heads.
- Vary distance requirements (stand closer to net).
- Lower the net or do not use net.

Students who use wheelchairs (normal upper body strength)
- Encourage student to find best way to serve (overhand, sidearm).
- Serve ball off tee or have ball tossed to person to serve.

Students who use wheelchairs (limited upper body strength and control)
- Hit or push ball held by peer, then have peer pick up ball and hit it over net.
- Hit or push ball off lap tray, then have peer pick up ball and hit it over net.
- Hit or push ball down ramp or across table, then have peer pick up ball and hit it over net.
- Use legs or head if student has better control with these body parts, then have peer pick up ball and hit it over net.
- Provide physical assistance as needed.
- Allow student to touch ball, then have peer pick it up and hit it to other teammates.

Students with visual impairments
- Use brightly colored balls.
- Have peers tell student which direction to stand and where to hit ball.
- Provide physical assistance as needed.

- Put bells or beeper in ball.
- Put radio by net for direction.
- Allow student to hit ball off of tee.
- Allow student to bounce ball then hit it.

Students with mental retardation/learning disabilities
- Allow students with limited coordination to hit ball off tee.
- Toss the ball to student if this is easier for him or her.
- Have peer assist student (extra verbal and physical cues).
- Encourage proper technique.

Tennis game

General
- Allow student to hit ball after two to three bounces.
- Allow student to hit to doubles lines while opponent hits to singles line.
- Match student with less-skilled student without disabilities.
- Play lead-up games rather than regulation games.
- Play game without net.
- Play doubles and allow team with student to have extra player (3 v. 2).
- Play modified or lead-up games.

Students who use wheelchairs (normal upper body strength)
- Allow student to serve ball off tee or have ball tossed to person to serve.

Students who use wheelchairs (limited upper body strength and control)
- Give peer assistant.
- Make special rules that if ball is hit a certain distance, it counts as over the net. Then, peer assistant can hit ball over net to opponent.
- Allow student to use adapted equipment.

Students with visual impairments
- Use brightly colored balls.
- Have textured markers on court or guide wires so that student knows where he is on court.
- Have peers tell student in which direction to stand and where to hit ball.
- Provide physical assistance as needed.
- Put bells or beeper in ball.
- Put radio by net for direction.
- Allow student to hit ball off of tee for serving.
- Allow student to bounce ball, then serve it.

Students with mental retardation/learning disabilities
- Allow students with limited coordination to hit ball off tee for serving.
- Toss the ball to student if this is easier for him or her when serving.
- Have peer assist student.

Golf Skills

Hitting ball

General
- Use larger balls.
- Use lighter balls.
- Use shorter, lighter clubs (junior clubs or children's plastic clubs).
- Make club with a larger head.
- Vary distance requirements (allow student to hit it shorter than peers).
- Always put ball on tee.

Students who use wheelchairs (normal upper body strength)
- Encourage student to find best way to hit ball.

Students who use wheelchairs (limited upper body strength and control)
- Hit or push ball held by peer.
- Hit or push ball off lap tray.
- Hit or push ball down ramp or across table.
- Use legs or head if student has better control with these body parts.
- Provide physical assistance as needed.
- Use switch that activates machine that hits ball off tee.

Students with visual impairments
- Use brightly colored balls.
- Have peers tell student which direction to stand and in which direction to hit ball.
- Provide physical assistance as needed.
- Put bells or beeper in ball.
- Put radio out in field for target.

Students with mental retardation/learning disabilities
- Have peer assist student (extra verbal and physical cues).
- Encourage proper technique.

Archery Skills[1]

Shooting

General
- Use shorter arrows.
- Use lighter bows.
- Use shorter, smaller, lighter bows.
- Vary distance requirements (allow student to shoot it a shorter distance than peers).
- Make target larger.

Students who use wheelchairs (normal upper body strength)
- Encourage student to find best way to shoot with bow.
- Allow use of adapted release cuffs.
- Use adapted archery bow.

Students who use wheelchairs (limited upper body strength and control)
- Use crossbow with adapted trigger device.
- Use adapted archery bow.
- Shoot with physical assistance.

Students with visual impairments
- Use brightly colored arrows and targets.
- Have peers tell student in which direction to stand and in which direction to shoot.
- Provide physical assistance as needed.
- Put bells or beeper in target.
- Put radio in front of target.
- Have target make sounds if it is hit.
- Use special auditory device for lining up shot.

Students with mental retardation/learning disabilities
- Use crossbow with adapted trigger device if strength is a problem.
- Use adapted archery bow if coordination is a problem.

---

[1]For more information on the crossbow with adapted trigger, adapted archery bow, adapted release cuff, or other unique adaptations of archery to meet the needs of individuals with specific disabilities, see Adams, R., & McCubbin, J. (1991). *Games, sports, and exercises for the physically disabled* (4th ed.). Philadelphia: Lea & Febiger.

- Shoot with physical assistance.
- Encourage proper technique.

Badminton Skills[2]

Forehand
General
- Use larger birdies.
- Use lighter and softer birdies (Nerf balls, balloons).
- Use shorter, lighter racquets (panty-hose racquet).
- Use racquets with larger heads.
- Vary distance requirements (stand closer to net).
- Vary speed required (slow down the birdie).
- Lower the net or do not use net.
- Practice with suspended ball.

Students who use wheelchairs (normal upper body strength)
- Encourage student to find best position to hit forehand.
- Hit birdie off tee.
- Encourage student to work on maneuvering wheelchair and then hitting birdie.

Students who use wheelchairs (limited upper body strength and control)
- Strap racquet to player's hand.
- Hit or push birdie held by peer, then have peer pick up birdie and hit it over net.
- Hit or push birdie off lap tray, then have peer pick up birdie and hit it over net.
- Hit or push birdie down ramp or across table, then have peer pick up birdie and hit it over net.
- Use legs or head if student has better control with these body parts, then have peer pick up birdie and hit it over net.
- Provide physical assistance as needed.
- Allow student to touch birdie, then have peer pick it up and hit it to other teammates.

Students with visual impairments
- Use brightly colored birdies.
- Have peers tell student which direction to stand and where to hit birdie.
- Provide physical assistance as needed.
- Put bells or beeper in birdie.
- Put radio by net for direction.
- Suspend birdie from string with Velcro so that birdie releases when hit.
- Place birdie on tee.
- Allow student to self-toss and then hit birdie.
- Attach string to student and to birdie so that student can quickly retrieve birdie.

Students with mental retardation/learning disabilities
- Allow students with limited coordination to hit suspended birdie.
- Allow student with limited coordination to hit birdie off tee.
- Have peer assist student (extra verbal and physical cues).
- Encourage proper technique.

Serving
General
- Use larger birdies.
- Use lighter and softer birdies (Nerf balls, balloons).

[2]For more information on unique adaptations of badminton to meet the needs of individuals with specific disabilities, see Adams, R., & McCubbin, J. (1991). *Games, sports, and exercises for the physically disabled* (4th ed.). Philadelphia: Lea & Febiger.

- Use shorter, lighter racquets (panty-hose racquet).
- Use racquets with larger heads.
- Vary distance requirements (stand closer to net).
- Lower the net or do not use net.

Students who use wheelchairs (normal upper body strength)
- Encourage student to find best way to serve (overhand, sidearm).
- Serve birdie off tee or have birdie tossed to person to serve.

Students who use wheelchairs (limited upper body strength and control)
- Strap racquet to player's hand.
- Hit or push ball held by peer, then have peer pick up birdie and hit it over net.
- Hit or push ball off lap tray, then have peer pick up birdie and hit it over net.
- Hit or push ball down ramp or across table, then have peer pick up birdie and hit it over net.
- Use legs or head if student has better control with these body parts, then have peer pick up birdie and hit it over net.
- Provide physical assistance as needed.
- Allow student to touch birdie, then have peer pick it up and hit it to other teammates.

Students with visual impairments
- Use brightly colored birdie.
- Have peers tell student which direction to stand and where to hit birdie.
- Provide physical assistance as needed.
- Put bells or beeper in birdie.
- Put radio by net for direction.
- Allow student to hit birdie off of tree.

Students with mental retardation/learning disabilities
- Allow students with limited coordination to hit birdie off tee.
- Toss the birdie to student if this is easier for him or her.
- Have peer assist student (extra verbal and physical cues).
- Encourage proper technique.

Badminton game

General
- Allow student to hit to wider court while opponent hits to narrower court.
- Match student with less-skilled student without disabilities.
- Play lead-up games rather than regulation games.
- Lower net or play game without net.
- Play doubles and allow team with student to have extra player (3 v. 2).
- Play modified or lead-up games.

Students who use wheelchairs (normal upper body strength)
- Allow student to serve ball off tee or have ball tossed to person to serve.

Students who use wheelchairs (limited upper body strength and control)
- Give peer assistant.
- Make special rules that if birdie is hit a certain distance, it counts as over the net. Then, peer assistant can hit birdie over net to opponent.
- Allow student to use adapted equipment.

Students with visual impairments
- Use brightly colored birdies.
- Have textured markers on court or guide wires so that student knows where he or she is on court.
- Have peers tell student in which direction to stand and where to hit birdie.

- Provide physical assistance as needed.
- Put bells or beeper in birdie.
- Put radio by net for direction.
- Allow student to hit birdie off tee for serving.
- Allow student to bounce birdie then hit it.

Students with mental retardation/learning disabilities
- Allow students with limited coordination to hit birdie off tee for serving.
- Toss the birdie to student if this is easier for him or her when serving.
- Have peer assist student.

Dancing Skills

General
- Use colored markers or cones on floor for direction.
- Use colored markers on hands and feet for left and right.
- Practice small portions of dance and gradually add more steps.
- Slow down music.

Students who use wheelchairs (normal upper body strength)
- Substitute arm movements for leg movements.
- Allow partner to push person's wheelchair as needed.

Students who use wheelchairs (limited upper body strength and control)
- Substitute any controllable movements the student has for more traditional movements.
- Allow peers to assist students in movements.
- Allow students to push wheelchair.
- Encourage student to maintain proper posture and to focus eyes on partner.

Students with visual impairments
- Use brightly colored markers on floor.
- Have partner wear brightly colored pinny or shirt.
- Have partner wear bells on wrist.
- Have partner tell student in which direction to stand and where to move.
- Have partner provide physical assistance as needed.

Students with mental retardation/learning disabilities
- Have peers assist student (extra verbal and physical cues).
- Encourage proper technique.

IMPLEMENTING AN INCLUSIVE PHYSICAL EDUCATION PROGRAM

Chapter 8

Including Preschool Students with Disabilities in Regular Physical Education

I teach my students with physical disabilities in both a segregated and an inclusive setting. I find that I push my students more when they are included in regular physical education. I guess I have higher expectations for them, and I tend to challenge them more. In regular physical education, I know the standards for the children without disabilities, and in turn I can set my expectations for my students more realistically. I find that my students with disabilities push themselves more when they are included in regular physical education. It seems to mean more to them to succeed in regular physical education than in smaller, separate classes.

—Cathy Bryan

Nick is a bright, active little 3-year-old boy who loves balls and trucks and aggravating his 6-year-old sister. Nick also has cerebral palsy, which makes it difficult for him to control his body. He cannot walk yet, although he can roll and crawl on his stomach. He also has difficulty grasping and releasing objects, but he loves to push balls back and forth with friends. His speech is difficult to understand, but he seems to get his message across fairly well. Because of Nick's disabilities, he qualified for special education services, and an individualized education program (IEP) has been developed for him. While Nick could have been placed in a special preschool class for children with disabilities, his collaborative team decided that his IEP could be implemented in a regular childcare center around the corner from his house. Thus, a special education teacher has been assigned to Nick (as well as several other preschoolers who are fully included in other childcare centers around the town), and she comes to visit Nick and his teachers once a week. In addition, there is a part-time assistant who helps Nick and the other preschoolers in his class in the mornings, and Nick's physical and occupational therapists come to work with Nick once a week.

Nick is doing quite well in the childcare center, and he seems to be well accepted by the regular childcare staff as well as his peers without disabilities. One problem the childcare teacher has noticed is during recess. While the other children are able to run around, ride tricycles, and climb on the playground equipment, Nick can only crawl around or participate with a great deal of assistance. In addition, there is special motor time in the afternoon in which children listen and move to movement records (e.g., Hokey-Pokey; Head, Shoulders, Knees, and Toes; animal walks

Cathy Bryan is an APE specialist at Fairhill School in Fairfax, Virginia.

to music). While Nick tries to move to the directions, he has difficulty keeping up with the group and making the movements as accurately as his peers. What can this teacher do to help Nick during recess and during movement activities?

Many childcare centers and early childhood programs are beginning to accept students like Nick who have disabilities (Folsom-Meeks, 1992; Strain, 1991). In addition, community motor development programs such as Gymboree and Little Steps accept preschool children with mild disabilities under certain circumstances (e.g., if they are accompanied by a parent or special assistant). Finally, self-contained preschool programs for children with disabilities are often placed in included regular elementary schools, and older preschool students are frequently included in regular kindergarten classes for part of the day, including during physical education. Thus, programs designed for children without disabilities (and staff who are trained to work with preschoolers without disabilities) are faced with the dilemma of how to accommodate children with special needs. These regular preschool programs want to make sure that children with disabilities receive a quality program that meets their individual needs. However, these programs also must be concerned that including children with disabilities does not affect the safety or quality of programming afforded to their children without disabilities. Accommodating the needs of students with disabilities in regular preschool motor programs can be difficult, but it can be done.

The purpose of this chapter is to suggest ways in which children with disabilities can be safely and meaningfully included in regular preschool movement programs without presenting undue hardship on the regular staff or children. This chapter contains the following information: 1) description of typical movement programs offered in childcare centers and community motor development programs, 2) outline of how to include preschoolers in typical movement programs following the programming model in Chapter 4, and 3) specific examples of how Nick and other children with disabilities can be successfully included in typical, preschool movement programs.

PRESCHOOL MOVEMENT PROGRAM

Movement Programs at Childcare Centers

There are three basic types of gross motor movement activities offered at typical childcare centers. First, most childcare centers use "center-based" or "activity-based" programming in which the room is set up in various activity centers such as art (coloring, painting, cutting, pasting, Play-Doh), library (looking at books, puzzles), make-believe (dressing up using various clothes), construction (building blocks, Legos, Tinker toys), housekeeping (kitchen set, brooms, house), and dolls (dollhouse and dolls, castle and dolls) (Bricker & Cripe, 1992). Some centers lend themselves to gross motor movement activities such as housekeeping and make-believe. Movements in these centers include walking, lifting, bending, twisting, directions, and levels (high, medium, low). Some programs even offer a movement center which allows children the opportunity to perform various locomotor and manipulative movements such as jumping, galloping, hopping, skipping, throwing, kicking, and catching. A second type of gross motor movement activity that is offered at childcare centers is music and movement time. Typically, a teacher brings the children together to listen to various movement-oriented records or tapes such as Hap Palmer records, which instruct children to move their bodies in various ways. For example, one song instructs students to move like animals while another song instructs children to move fast or slow. A variety of locomotor and nonlocomotor movements can be included in these activities. Finally, gross-motor movement is afforded when students are allowed to go outside to the playground. While playgrounds vary from center to center, typical equipment includes slides, climbing equipment, swings, sandboxes, tricycles, and balls. Children can be extremely active on the playground and can explore a variety of movements.

Community-Based Movement Programs

Many communities offer movement programs for preschool children. These programs tend to provide a more structured and comprehensive movement program than childcare centers. Additionally, these programs are usually conducted by trained movement specialists (usually someone with a physical education degree). Community motor programs usually follow one of two formats. Some motor programs follow a fairly structured routine that includes an introductory activity, a skill or theme focus, and a concluding activity that incorporates the skill focus. Introductory activities usually include moving body parts to music, doing simple stretches and movements in self-space, doing simple finger plays and songs that incorporate movement, and performing animal walks or locomotor patterns around the play area. Skill activities, presented in a movement exploration format, focus on teaching students specific body management, locomotor, non-locomotor, or manipulative skills. Table 8.1 provides an example of the content typically covered in a preschool motor program. Activities are usually presented in a play or exploratory format guided by the instructor. The concluding activity usually involves a fun game that incorporates some of the skills worked on during the skill focus. For example, if the skill focus for the day was learning the movement concepts of fast/slow, high/low, and forward/backward/sideways, the con-

Table 8.1.   Typical content covered in preschool/kindergarten motor development program

BODY AWARENESS	
Body Parts Identification	Effort Qualities
Body Awareness	Time/speed (slow, fast)
Bending	Force (strong, light)
Stretching	Flow (free-flowing, bound)
Curling	Relationships
Twisting	Of body parts (round, narrow, wide, twisted,
Space Awareness	symmetrical)
Self-space (standing in own space and moving	To objects (over, under, on, off, in front, behind,
body parts)	through, around, near, far)
General space (moving around gym without	To people (leading, following, mirroring, match-
touching peers)	ing, unison, contrast, between groups, group
Levels (high, medium, low)	partners, solo, alone in mass)
Directions (forward, backward, sideways, up,	
down)	
Pathways (straight, zigzag, curvy)	
LOCOMOTOR SKILLS	
Crawling	Galloping
Creeping	Sliding
Rolling	Hopping
Walking	Dodging
Running	Chasing
Jumping	Fleeing
NONLOCOMOTOR SKILLS	
Turning	Stretching
Twisting	Jumping and Landing
Balancing	Transferring Weight
Curling	Stopping and Starting
MANIPULATIVE SKILLS	
Overhand Throw	Catching
Underhand Throw	Kicking
Underhand Roll	

Adapted from Graham, Holt/Hale, & Parker (1993).

cluding activity might be a game of tag in which children are asked to incorporate these movements as they play the game.

A second format of community motor programs involves less structured movement exploration activities. Typically, a variety of toys and equipment are set up around the play area. Equipment is specifically designed to encourage children to move in certain ways and improve specific movement skills. For example, climbing equipment encourages children to climb up and down and move over and through various surfaces. These activities promote body and spatial awareness, agility, flexibility, and strength. The teacher acts as a facilitator who assists, reinforces, guides, and challenges children on the various pieces of equipment. The equipment is often changed each day or after several days to encourage different movements.

Kindergarten Physical Education

Kindergarten offers two types of movement opportunities: recess/free play and organized physical education. Similar to childcare programs, recess/free play involves children going out to the playground and playing on playground equipment, playing with balls, playing with jump ropes, and playing simple sidewalk games such as Four-Square or Hopscotch. Children usually choose with whom and what they want to play, and the kindergarten teacher usually takes the role of a supervisor overseeing the entire playground and making sure children are playing safely. Physical education in kindergarten varies from teacher to teacher, but most programs are similar to the one described in the structured community preschool movement program (i.e., introduction, skill focus using movement exploration, and reinforcing activity). Activities focus on body management and movement concepts, locomotor and nonlocomotor patterns, manipulative patterns, and simple rhythms. (See Table 8.1.)

INCLUDING STUDENTS WITH DISABILITIES
IN REGULAR PRESCHOOL MOTOR PROGRAMS

Childcare Programs

1. Determine What to Teach   Following the model in Chapter 4, the first step in including students with disabilities in regular childcare movement activities is to determine what critical motor skills the student needs to be successful in his or her current (childcare center) and future (elementary physical education) placements. Information at this level should include a list of the motor skills needed in the childcare center, his or her interests as well as his or her parents' interests, and what his or her peers do now for recreation as well as what they will do when they go to elementary school. Much of this information can be collected during the initial collaborative team meeting by asking the childcare center teachers and the child's parents. This information can then be listed as specific skills that in turn form the reference for later assessment. That is, assessment of the child's present level of performance (strengths and weaknesses) will be referenced to what behaviors are expected of typical preschool children. (See chap. 4, this volume, for more detail.)

For example, Nick's collaborative team determined which motor skills were critical for Nick to be successful in his childcare center as well as at home. (See Table 8.2 for a listing of Nick's present abilities and targeted functional skills.) Skills focused on motor activities that were typically used by preschoolers without disabilities throughout the day. Nick's parents concurred that similar skills were needed at home. In addition, Nick's parents had just bought an adapted tricycle for Nick since many children in Nick's neighborhood ride tricycles. They were hoping that he could learn how to ride the adapted tricycle independently. Now, Nick can be evaluated on these critical skills, skills that are meaningful to Nick at childcare and at home. Results of this type of assessment provide the team with information that is directly related to the real-life, everyday skills Nick needs to be more successful in childcare and at home. (See Table 8.2.)

Table 8.2.   Nick's present level of performance, referenced to functional activities needed in his childcare center

Functional motor skill	Nick's present abilities
Locomote from one part of room to another.	Nick moves slowly by crawling on his stomach. He can move approximately 10' in 2 minutes before he needs to rest. Nick crawls by pulling with his arms (simultaneously) and by dragging his legs. He can roll short distances (2'–3' in less than 1 minute), and he is learning how to walk with a walker.
Stand/sit at center or during group activities.	Nick cannot sit independently because of poor postural control and poor balance. However, he can sit independently in a Tumbleform chair or if a teacher sits behind him. He can stand in a prone stander or if a teacher supports him.
Manipulate toys and materials.	Nick can grasp most objects at the various centers. He does have difficulty releasing objects, and he has difficulty controlling objects (i.e., putting things in, doing puzzles, drawing). His grasp pattern is a slow movement with limited range of motion in his fingers, and his grasp is still a rather crude palmar grasp.
Climb up playground structure (stairs and ladder).	Nick cannot climb up stairs or up the ladder on the playground. Someone usually places him up on the main platform. Even when assisted, he does not have the range of motion in his knees or hips to bend his legs enough to clear even low steps.
Ride tricycle.	Nick can sit on adapted tricycle that has support for his trunk as well as Velcro straps for his feet. He can pedal with assistance (someone pushing him from behind), and he can independently hold onto the handlebars. He still has difficulty keeping his knees in proper alignment. (They tend to bow in and touch when he pedals, and he does not have the strength to pedal fully with any speed.)
Perform movements to movement records.	Nick seems to be aware of the required movements on the records, but he cannot coordinate his movements quickly enough to keep up with the tapes (e.g., he can identify his body parts during Head, Shoulders, Knees, and Toes, but he cannot keep up with the speed of the song). In addition, he does not have the range of motion to do any of the movements fully. He does seem to understand the concepts of high/low, over/under, forward/backward, and fast/slow. He just cannot get his body to do these movements as quickly or as accurately as needed to keep up with the other children.

Once the child has been evaluated on functional skills, the team should develop a top-down, long-term plan for the child. In essence, the long-term plan reflects what global goals the team would like to see the child achieve either at the end of significant periods of time (e.g., end of childcare, end of elementary school, end of high school) or at the culmination of formal schooling (i.e., graduation from school [Kelly et al., 1991]). For older students who do not have as much time before they graduate from school, the team might want to have a long-term plan that culminates with graduation. For example, a middle school–age student with mental retardation might have a long-term plan that states that the student will be able to participate independently in two defined lifetime leisure skills in the community upon graduation from school. In the case of Nick and other preschoolers, it might be more realistic to have a long-term plan that culminates with graduation from childcare rather than upon completion of school. While a top-down plan for preschoolers will eventually lead to the development of lifetime leisure skills upon graduation from school, sometimes such a long-term plan is difficult to apply to preschool children who are not going to graduate for another 16–19 years and who may change drastically in their abilities and rate of skill development. New long-term plans can then be developed as needed for elementary school and high school based on any progress (or lack of progress) a particular student has made. (See Table 8.3 for an example of Nick's long-term plan.)

Once a long-term plan is in place, the team can then develop the child's IEP. Recall from Chapter 4 that the IEP should include long-term goals or annual goals (should take approximately

Table 8.3. Nick's long-term plan, including long-term goals and short-term instructional objectives

LONG-TERM PLAN: Nick will demonstrate the ability to participate independently in 90% of the movement-based activities in his childcare center and at home.

Long-Term Goal 1: Nick will demonstrate the ability to walk independently and safely with a rolling walker throughout his childcare room and at home.

Short-Term Instructional Objectives

1. Nick will walk forward using a rolling walker with assistance for balance a distance of 10' in 1 minute or less, three out of four trials.
2. Nick will walk forward using a rolling walker independently a distance of 5' in 1 minute or less, three out of four trials.
3. Nick will walk forward using a rolling walker independently a distance of 10' in 1 minute or less, three out of four trials.
4. Nick will walk forward as well as around obstacles using a rolling walker independently throughout his childcare classroom without running into obstacles or peers 100% of the time, three out of four trials.

Long-Term Goal 2: Nick will pedal an adapted tricycle independently for increasing distances.

Short-Term Instructional Objectives

1. Nick will pedal adapted tricycle with assistance in pushing down on pedals and for steering a distance of 10' in 1 minute or less, three out of four trials.
2. Nick will pedal adapted tricycle independently with assistance for steering as needed a distance of 5' in 1 minute or less, three out of four trials.
3. Nick will pedal adapted tricycle independently with assistance for steering as needed a distance of 10' in 1 minute or less, three out of four trials.
4. Nick will pedal adapted tricycle independently including steering a distance of 10' in 1 minute or less, three out of four trials.

Long-Term Goal 3: Nick will sit independently demonstrating proper body alignment for up to 5 minutes while playing at a center.

Short-Term Instructional Objectives

1. Nick will sit on floor with assistance for balance for 3 minutes, three out of four trials.
2. Nick will sit on floor without assistance for up to 30 seconds, then with minimal assistance for an additional 3 minutes, three out of four trials.
3. Nick will sit on floor without assistance for up to 1 minute, then with minimal assistance for an additional 2 minutes, three out of four trials.
4. Nick will sit on floor without assistance for up to 2 minutes, then with minimal assistance for an additional 2 minutes, three out of four trials.

Long-Term Goal 4: Nick will demonstrate improved general body control as exhibited by maintaining balance and improving functional manipulation skills.

Short-Term Instructional Objectives

1. Nick will take off coat with minimal assistance getting arms out of sleeves in 2 minutes or less, three out of four trials.
2. Nick will take off coat independently in 2 minutes or less, three out of four trials.
3. Nick will pick up finger foods and use adapted spoon and cup independently without spilling or losing food 100% of the time during lunch and snack, three out of four trials.
4. Nick will manipulate body to go over, under, and through objects and obstacles in the room and on the playground without touching object or obstacles 100% of the time, three out of four trials.

one year to achieve) and short-term instructional objectives (should take anywhere from a few weeks to several months to achieve). These goals will help a student move toward the global goals outlined in the long-term plan. Table 8.3 lists Nick's IEP goals and objectives. Note how these goals and objectives are directly related to the overall long-term plan as well as Nick's present level of performance.

2. Analyze the Regular Routines   The next step is to determine what specific activities take place in the childcare center and how (if at all) each of the above goals can be incorporated into these activities. A simple Daily Routines Chart can be developed by the student's therapist, adapted physical education specialist, or special education teacher (in conjunction with the childcare staff) that highlights the typical routine of the day and where this child's motor goals can be incorporated. (See Table 8.4 for an example of Nick's program.) In most cases, the child's specific goals can easily be incorporated in the daily routine of the childcare center. For example, Nick's goal of learning how to walk with a rolling walker can be incorporated during transitions from one activity to another, and sitting independently can be incorporated into activities that require sitting, such as at centers or during group activities. Thus, the motor goals are not worked on in isolation but rather throughout the day when the skills are actually used. This makes practice more meaningful and motivating for Nick. For example, it is more motivating for Nick to practice walking with his walker when training takes place during the transition from indoors to the playground (he cannot wait to get out to the playground) rather than simply walking the halls just for the sake of walking with a therapist or teacher.

   3. *Determine Modifications Needed*   Now that we know what the child's goals and objectives are and where they can be incorporated in the regular childcare routine, the next step is to determine what specific modifications will be needed for the child. That is, a plan should be developed that specifies how each of the child's IEP objectives is going to be presented to the child. As outlined in Chapter 4, there are five major questions to answer that can help guide this process. First, how often will the child receive instruction? For some students, direct instruction can be incorporated during the normal daily routines of the day. For example, one of the childcare teachers can provide direct instruction to Nick in using his walker when it is time to transition between centers or when transitioning from playing indoors to outdoors. However, some children might need extra instruction above and beyond what is available during daily routines. In such cases, usually children with more significant disabilities, a therapist can come in and provide the extra assistance. For example, a physical therapist comes into the childcare center to work with Nick once a week on proper sitting mechanics and on stretching tight muscles and strengthening weak muscles. This way, Nick gets extra instruction to meet his unique needs.

   The next question to ask is, where will the student receive instruction? In the case of most inclusive childcare programs, direct instruction will occur in the regular setting during regular routines. As explained above with Nick, he will work on his specific IEP objectives at times when they can be easily incorporated into the daily routine. Even when therapists come to work with Nick, they work with him at centers, during lunch, or while he is out on the playground. Some students may need to be pulled out on occasion for special therapy. For example, a vision therapist

Table 8.4.   Nick's Daily Routines Chart (arrival through lunch), with motor goals embedded

Time	Activity	Embedded goals
8:15– 8:45	Arrival/Free play	Walking (walking with parent to room), body management (taking off jacket)
8:45– 9:00	Breakfast	Walking (from play area to breakfast table)
9:00– 9:30	Circle/Story	Walking (from table to floor), sitting (during circle and story time)
9:30–10:30	Centers	Body management (putting on pretend clothes, moving in and out of house), walking (from station to station), upper body strength (picking up objects in various centers, Play-Doh), sitting (at centers while playing)
10:30–11:00	Playground	Walking (from room to playground), riding tricycle, body management (moving in, on, over, and through equipment with assistance), sitting (in sandbox, on swing, on trike)
11:00–11:15	Clean-up	Walking (from playground to room), body management (taking off jacket, washing hands), posture (standing and washing hands)
11:15–11:45	Lunch	Walking (from room to table), body management (picking up utensils and food), sitting (sitting in chair)

could conceivably pull out a preschooler who has a visual impairment to work on vision training. Still, most therapies can usually be administered within the regular setting at times when such therapy is most meaningful for the student. For example, an adapted physical education specialist or can come and assist Nick in riding his adapted tricycle and in using playground equipment such as climbing the stairs and going down the slide when Nick's class is on the playground.

The next question to ask is, how will the student be prepared for instruction? Remember from Chapter 4 that preparation for instruction includes physical preparation for children with physical disabilities and instructional preparation for children with behavioral problems. Many students will need no special preparation to receive instruction. For example, a student who has a visual impairment may not need special physical or instructional preparation prior to receiving vision therapy at a home-living station. In contrast, a student like Nick may need some relaxation and range-of-motion exercises prior to using his walker or tricycle if he is going to benefit from these adapted pieces of equipment. Physical or occupational therapists can provide such preparation, or more likely, they could provide childcare staff with instructions on how to stretch Nick's legs so that he will have more success on the tricycle. Figure 8.1 provides an example of a stretching routine that can be adapted for Nick and implemented by the childcare staff for 5–10 minutes just prior to Nick using his tricycle.

Students with behavior problems or autistic-like behaviors may need some extra preparation prior to receiving direct instruction. These students often have difficulty making a transition from one activity to another or from one adult to another. In such cases, the childcare staff or the therapist might give the student extra cues that a transition will take place. For example, Chrissy, a 4-year-old with autistic-like behaviors, has difficulty leaving the "library center" and moving to the playground. The childcare teacher knows to cue Chrissy several times while Chrissy is in the library center that the next activity is the playground. In addition, a routine has been established in which the lights are turned out for a minute or two to accentuate the end of center time and the beginning of outdoor play. While such extra cues are not needed by the other children, these cues certainly do not detract from their program. However, such cues seem to make it easier for Chrissy to make the transition.

The next question to ask is, what system and types of cues and prompts will be used to elicit desired performance? Recall from Chapter 4 that types of cues or prompts include natural or environmental cues, verbal cues, pointing/gesturing, picture cards, demonstrating, physical prompting, and physical assistance. Ideally, students learn to respond to natural cues in the environment (e.g., pick up and read a book at the library center without any extra cues) or verbal cues (e.g., put away toys at one center and move to another center upon verbal cue: "Please clean up your center and find a new center"). However, some students will need extra cues to respond successfully in various activities. Team members can observe and work with the student with disabilities and make a determination as to what types of cues he or she needs. For example, Nick needs physical assistance to sit independently and to manipulate toys at several stations; thus, the team notes that he needs physical assistance. In contrast, Marquetta, who has a hearing impairment, needs extra visual cues to know when to move from center to center. These cues usually consist of turning the lights on and off one or two times or pointing to the next activity area. Similarly, J.R., who has a visual impairment, needs extra verbal cues and someone to walk with him (usually another student) to move to a new center and to interact with peers and with toys at various centers. Again, the amount and type of cuing a particular student will need should be a team decision and will vary based on each student's unique abilities.

Finally, the last question to ask is, what specific adaptations and/or adapted equipment will be used to enhance a student's inclusion and performance? Table 4.15 in Chapter 4 contains a checklist that can be helpful in determining if a particular adaptation is appropriate, and Chapters

6 and 7 provide specific examples of adaptations that can be used with students to enhance their motor performance. While these chapters can provide the team with some good general information and guidelines, specific adaptations should be determined after several team members have had the opportunity to observe carefully and work with the student. For example, the team was concerned that Nick was having difficulty crawling on his stomach with any speed. In addition, his peers were upright most of the day, and they thought it would be better if Nick could be upright as well. After careful observation and evaluation by the adapted physical education specialist, special education teacher, physical therapist, and occupational therapist, it was decided that Nick could learn how to walk using a rolling walker. This became a goal on his IEP, and the physical and occupational therapists wrote a program for the childcare staff that included a picture, specific teaching methods, and hints on teaching Nick how to walk. (See Table 8.5 for an example of Nick's program.) In addition, the physical and occupational therapists trained the regular childcare staff in how to assist Nick on the walker, and these therapists came into the childcare center once a week to work with Nick on the walker and talk with the childcare staff. Other simple modifications for Nick included a special Tumbleform chair to sit in at lunch and at the library center, an adapted tricycle for the playground as well as physical assistance on the climbing apparatus, and special utensils for lunch and snacks. In addition, while listening to a song that asks the children to move like various animals, Nick is encouraged to move around in his walker in various directions, at various speeds, and at various levels. When following songs such as "The Hokey-Pokey," Nick is encouraged to move his hands near his body parts rather than touching them so that he can keep up with the group yet still follow the directions. (See Figure 8.2 for a checklist to determine if a child needs an alternative way to perform a skill in an activity a group is performing.)

4. *Determine Support the Student Will Need* The next step in the model is to determine who will be responsible for directly implementing the program. Most childcare centers follow state guidelines for teacher/student ratios. For example, in Virginia the teacher–student ratio for 3-year-olds is one teacher for every eight children. (Most 3-year-old classes have two teachers and 14–16 children.) It is difficult enough for the childcare staff to watch and tend the children without disabilities, let alone work one-on-one with a student who has special needs. While childcare staff can implement part of a child's program without disrupting or taking away from other children, they will no doubt need some extra support to implement the entire program successfully. Again, the amount of support a child will need should be a team decision based on the child's goals and how much assistance he or she needs to perform these goals and other daily activities, the number of other children in the class, the number of staff in the class, and the general set-up of the class. For example, a child like Nick will need quite a bit of support because he needs assistance in walking and sitting, his class has 15 children without disabilities with only two staff members, and the classroom is quite large and spread out so it will take a long time for Nick to get from one part of the room to another. In Nick's case, the team came up with some creative ways to provide support for Nick (and the two classroom teachers). First, an older child in the childcare center was given the job of pushing the lunch cart from the kitchen to the 3-year-old classroom which freed up one staff member to assist Nick in walking to the bathroom, in the bathroom, and then walking back to the lunch table. In addition, the director of the childcare center was scheduled to go to the 3-year-old room from 10:30 A.M. to 10:40 A.M. to assist the children out to the playground while one of Nick's classroom teachers assisted Nick with his walker from the room to the playground. Similarly, the childcare center's cook helped Nick's class move to the playground from 3:30 P.M. to 3:40 P.M., so that one of Nick's teachers can help him walk to the playground. Such "shuffling" of childcare staff to fill in for each other is common in most childcare centers and should pose only slight scheduling problems. Other available support often available at childcare centers include

Decreasing Spasticity

Spasticity can be inhibited or decreased by holding the spastic body part in patterns opposite to those of the dominating spastic patterns. In the flexor pattern, spasticity pulls the shoulder back and the elbow and wrist into flexion. To counteract the flexor pattern, put your hand behind the shoulder and bring it forward. Then gently and slowly straighten the elbow and bring the arm out and away from the body with the wrist and hand facing up.

In the extensor pattern, the legs are extended at the hip, knee, and ankle. To help break up this spastic pattern, flex the hip and knee. Control of the head is often a problem for individuals with cerebral palsy. The neck can thrust the head back into extension or make the head fall forward into flexion. Be certain when positioning or moving your clients that their heads are well supported and not allowed to fall forward or backward or to the side.

The more normal you can make a movement feel for the person you care for, the better the individual will be able to reproduce that movement independently. Normal movement patterns experienced again and again inhibit spastic, hypertonic muscles and make functional, directed movement more likely.

Rolling movement of the lower part of the body near the hips is called *rotation*. Rotation tends to be relaxing and has the effect of reducing spasticity. The relaxation technique illustrated makes use of rotation and can be incorporated into your daily routine with hypertonic individuals.

Relaxation Technique Using Rotation

1. With the individual in back lying, slowly and gently bend the hips and knees toward the body. Keep the client's head in the center or midline of the body. Your hands should be on the knees, guiding the movement and keeping the knees apart.

2. Then slowly and gently move both legs as a unit to the left, and then to the right. Repeat this until you feel the legs and body relax.

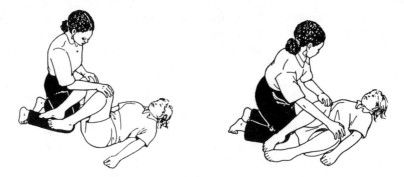

These two illustrations show the rotation technique.

Range of Motion for the Legs

The Hip

The hip joint is capable of six movements: flexion, extension, abduction, adduction, internal rotation, and external rotation. In spasticity, the muscles that bend (flex) the hip and the muscles that pull the leg in toward the midline of the body (adduct) are often tight. The following hip exercises work best with the individual in back lying. Placing the person in the stomach lying position, though, is useful for passively stretching the hip joint into extension, especially for individuals who spend much of their day in a wheelchair.

To flex the hip, put one hand on the front of the knee with the other hand cupping the heel. The ankle should be at a right angle to the lower leg. Don't allow the knee to pull in (adduct). Bend the hip so the knee comes up toward the chest. To extend the hip, reverse the movement, straightening the hip and knee.

(continued)

Figure 8.1. Example of a therapeutic stretching program that can be adapted for Nick (to be carried out by childcare staff). (From French, C., Gonzalez, R.T., & Tronson-Simpson, J. [1991]. *Caring for people with multiple disabilities: An interdisciplinary guide for caregivers,* pp. 13–15. Tucson, AZ: Therapy Skill Builders, 3830 Bellevue, P.O. Box 42050, Tucson, AZ 85733; reprinted by permission.)

Figure 8.1. (*continued*)

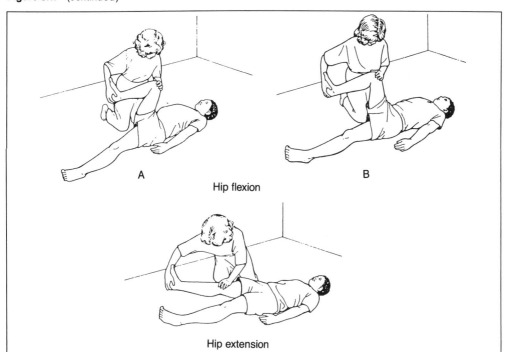

A   B

Hip flexion

Hip extension

To abduct the hip, move the leg away from the midline of the body by placing one hand on the top and inside of the knee and the other hand on the top and outside of the hip. The muscles on the inside of the leg are often tight. Hold the leg in this position to stretch these muscles. Adduct—that is, move the leg back—just to the midpoint of the body.

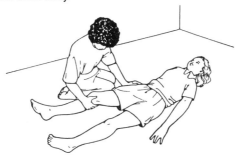

Hip abduction

To externally rotate the hip joint, place one hand on the top and inside of the knee and the other hand on the top and outside of the hip. The knee should be slightly flexed. Rotate the upper leg by moving the knee so it faces away from the body. Internally rotate the hip back to the starting position until the knee points straight up.

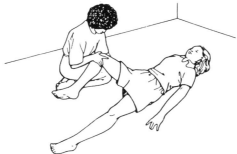

Hip external rotation

Table 8.5.   Example of a motor program for teaching Nick to walk with a rolling walker

Performance Objective:

1.   Nick will walk forward using a rolling walker with assistance for balance a distance of 10′ in 1 minute or less, three out of four trials.

Teaching-Learning Process:

a.   Show Nick his new walker and explain that it will help him walk.
b.   Demonstrate walking using the walker. Help Nick focus on how he will use his arms on the walker for balance and to push his body up so that he can drag his legs under his body.
c.   Place Nick in his walker and cue the key components of the skill. Cue Nick by verbally explaining each component, pointing to walker and body part involved, and then physically assisting him with each component:
    1)   Where to place hands (physically take his hands and place them correctly)
    2)   How to push body up (assist him in pushing off on handles of walker)
    3)   How to lift up his body so that his legs drag under his body
    4)   The recovery position that is achieved by sliding the walker forward
d.   Have Nick practice walking with walker. Provide assistance by standing behind him and supporting him at waist for balance. Also, try to help him maintain proper body alignment (straight up and down).
e.   Help Nick focus on each component of the movement as it is used. For example, cue him to push off and slide his legs under his body once his hands are firmly gripping the walker.
f.   Practice this skill throughout the day when movement from one place to another is needed (e.g., transition between centers, moving from floor to lunch table, and moving from indoors to playground).
g.   Reinforce him for trying as well as for doing the movement correctly, and try to provide specific feedback regarding how he can correct and improve his movements. For example, say, "Nice pushing off, Nick. Next time try to bend your elbows more at the beginning so that you can really push your body up in the air."
h.   When assisting Nick, try to gauge his attitude. If he seems to be getting tired or bored, ask him to do the skill one more time, then put the walker away and carry him the rest of the way. Don't forget to reinforce him for his efforts.

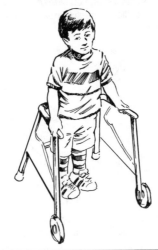

kitchen worker(s), janitor(s), parent volunteers, high school or college volunteers, retired senior citizens (foster grandparents), and older school-age students who stay at the childcare center after school.

   5.   Prepare Staff for Implementation   The next step in the model, and one that is often overlooked, is to prepare and train the staff who will be working with the child who has disabilities. Training can be conducted by the child's special education teacher, parents, and therapists. Whenever possible, training should take place before the child enters the program and should be

	Yes	No	Comments
Does the student have a physical disability that appears to preclude typical performance?	✓		
Is the student having extreme difficulty performing the skill?	✓		*Slow crawling*
Is the student making little to no progress over several months or years despite instruction?	✓		
Does the student seem more comfortable and motivated using a different pattern?	✓		*May be more motivated to walk like peers*
Will an alternative pattern still be useful (i.e., functional) in the targeted environments?	✓		*As he becomes more skilled, will be functional*
Will the alternative pattern increase the student's ability to perform the skill?	✓		

Note: If the answer to some or all of the above questions is yes, the student may need adapted pattern.

Figure 8.2.   Sample form for evaluating if a student needs an alternative way to perform the skill.

supplemented by ongoing training. Childcare staff should have a chance to see the child at his or her home or in the special education placement to gain a better understanding of the child's temperament, behaviors, and interests. Specific handling and behavior techniques as well as methods and materials for adapting typical activities and for conducting ongoing evaluation can be presented during preprogram and ongoing in-services. (See chaps. 3 and 4, this volume, for more detail on the role of specific team members and examples of in-service activities.) For example, Nick will be going to the ABC Childcare Center for the first time in the fall. (Previously he received services in a special preschool class for children with disabilities.) The childcare center director and staff were told about Nick and were given two brief (30–45 minute) in-service sessions in the spring regarding disability in general and describing success stories in including children like Nick in regular childcare centers. Later that spring, the childcare center director and teachers who were scheduled to work with Nick went to Nick's school to visit the program and observe Nick. In addition, these staff members had a chance to talk with Nick's special education teacher. In the summer, Nick came to the childcare center three mornings so that the childcare staff could see him, see how he would fit in, and see what adaptations they might need to make. Nick's mother and special education teacher came with Nick on two visits, and Nick's physical therapist came with Nick on the third visit. Later that summer, Nick's collaborative team was assembled and an IEP was developed. Types of adaptations, schedules of therapies, and extra supports were determined, and ongoing monthly meetings were scheduled. Nick was fully included in the regular childcare center in the fall. (The special education teacher came with Nick the first few days to help in the transition and to answer any questions the regular staff had.) Other than minor problems, he has been doing quite well. The success of the program was due in large part to the preparation given to the regular childcare staff and the teamwork of the regular childcare staff interacting with the special education staff.

    6. Implement Program and Conduct Ongoing Evaluation   Once the staff has been prepared, the child can be included in the childcare program. As suggested above with Nick, special education personnel should try to go to the childcare center as much as possible during the first few days of the transition. In addition, special education staff, including therapists, also should schedule routine visits to the school to work with the child and to talk with the childcare staff. Special education staff also can develop simple checklists for the childcare staff to use to collect ongoing information about the progress the child is making. The checklists should be detailed enough so that specialists can evaluate the progress the student is making in functional activities but not so detailed as to be cumbersome to the regular childcare staff. (See Figures 8.3 and 8.4 for examples of sample data forms for Nick's walking program.) Specialists can come in periodically to verify these reports and to conduct their own, detailed evaluations.

Once the program is successfully under way, special education staff should plan monthly meetings with the childcare staff to evaluate the progress the child is making and to address any concerns the staff might have about the program. Special education staff also should make themselves available for telephone conversations and spot visits when more immediate concerns arise.

Community Movement Programs

1. ***Determine What to Teach*** As was the case above, the first step in the process of including a preschool child with disabilities in a community movement program is to determine the student's specific motor goals. For the sake of this discussion, we will assume that Nick is now going to be included in a community movement program and that the same goals previously outlined are still appropriate for Nick. (See Table 8.3.)

2. ***Analyze Regular Routines*** The next step is to analyze the regular routine and determine where Nick's goals can be embedded. The use of a Daily Routines Chart with the child's goals embedded throughout is the most effective way to determine when specific goals can be taught. (See Table 8.6.) Note how easily Nick's goals are embedded throughout the program during times when these skills are meaningful. For example, warm-up activities are a good time to work on sitting and body management goals while the other students perform different locomotor patterns. Similarly, the reinforcing game at the end of the session can be modified so that Nick can work on his unique goals while participating with peers in the activity. In Nick's case, walking with his walker and manipulation skills are incorporated into games that focus on locomotor and manipulative skills. Finally, the introductory and closing activities are a good place for Nick to work on sitting and body management goals.

Activity: <u>Walking program</u>

Time of day	Number of independent steps	Child's effort
Entrance to room		
To breakfast table		
To circle		
To center		
To playground		
To room		
To lunch table		
To bathroom		

Effort key: + = tries to walk
o = doesn't try, but doesn't resist
− = resists assistance

Figure 8.3. Sample ongoing evaluation form for childcare staff (quantitative analysis).

Activity: Walking program

_____ 1. Place hands correctly on handles of walker
_____ 2. Body in proper, vertical alignment
_____ 3. Flexes then extends arms at elbows to push body up
_____ 4. With body lifted up, drags legs under his body
_____ 5. Slides walker forward to realign body with walker

Key: + = demonstrates component consistently and smoothly (minimum of three out of four trials)
+/− = demonstrates component but not consistently (one out of four to two out of four trials)
+/s = demonstrates component consistently but not smoothly
− = does not demonstrate component

Figure 8.4. Sample ongoing evaluation form for childcare staff (qualitative analysis).

3. Determine Specific Modifications The next step in the process is to specify how each activity is going to be adapted so as to accommodate the unique needs of the chid with disabilities. As was the case above, a specific program including teaching suggestions and suggestions for adapting equipment should be developed by the child's special education teachers and therapists. In addition, suggestions from Chapters 6 and 7 should be presented to the motor program staff. The major questions for Nick include: 1) how will he be prepared for the program? 2) what types of cues or assistance will he need? and 3) what specific adaptations or adapted equipment will he need? In terms of preparation, Nick will probably benefit from the stretching and relaxation program outlined in Figure 8.1. This program can be implemented by Nick's parents just prior to the start of the movement program. In terms of cues, Nick understands verbal cues and demonstra-

Table 8.6. Nick's Daily Routines Chart in a community movement program, with motor goals embedded

Time	Activity	Embedded goals
9:00– 9:03	Introduction	Sitting
9:03– 9:06	Warm-up (moving to music in personal space)	Sitting; body management
9:06– 9:10	Locomotor patterns to music	Walking; body management (tricycle can be substituted for walking)
9:10– 9:20	Skill focus (manipulative patterns, tumbling, movement concepts, climbing, etc.—varies from session to session)	Walking; body management (tricycle can be substituted for walking)
9:20– 9:25	Reinforcing game (application of skill focus into a game)	Walking; body management
9:25– 9:30	Closing circle (review day; move slowly to music)	Sitting; body management

tions quite well, but he still needs physical assistance to participate in most of the motor activities. Such cuing will involve actually physically assisting him in balance and body control so that he can follow the movements as closely as possible. For example, someone will need to help Nick sit with the group so he can move his body parts to various songs and chants. Finally, specific adaptations for Nick can vary from substitutions of one movement for another to adapted equipment. For example, if the group is doing animal walks during warm-ups, Nick can crawl on his stomach, walk with his walker, or use his adapted tricycle. While the other children work on more advanced locomotor patterns such as hopping or skipping, Nick can continue to work on his particular locomotor goals (i.e., walking with his walker). Other adapted equipment besides his walker can be introduced so that Nick receives some variations in his program. (See Figure 8.5 for examples.)

During the skill focus, a variety of adaptations can be made so Nick can be included yet work on meaningful activities geared to his unique goals. For example, if the environment is set up for climbing and exploring equipment, Nick can be assisted by a parent, therapist, or motor program staff member while other children explore the equipment independently. Also, Nick can be allowed to choose what piece of equipment on which he wants to play. Then he and his helper can work on walking while moving to the equipment and a variety of body management/awareness and postural control skills on the equipment. For example, suppose a piece of equipment has a three-rung ladder which leads to a flat platform and then a 3' slide. Nick's assistant can help him walk over to the climber using his walker. Then the assistant can help him climb up the ladder, encouraging Nick to shift weight from one leg to another, to use his hands to pull himself up, and to keep an erect posture while climbing. At the top, the assistant can cue Nick on how to change his body from a hands-and-knees position to a sitting position. Finally, the assistant can cue Nick on how to scoot his body up to the slide and then slide down. Chapter 7 presents other specific suggestions for accommodating children with specific fitness, balance, and coordination problems.

Finally, the motor program culminates with a reinforcing group game. Activities usually include moving and following instructions to music such as "Wheels on the Bus" or "Eensy, Weensy Spider"; playing a fun, low-organized game such as "Ring Around the Rosey" or "Pop Goes the Weasel"; or playing a more active game that reinforces the skill focus of the day such as a throwing/catching relay race to reinforce throwing and catching skills or an obstacle course to reinforce balance and agility skills. Again, Nick can be accommodated by having someone help him sit (work on his sitting goal). For example, Nick's father can assist Nick in sitting (cuing Nick to use proper posture while sitting) so that he can perform the hand movements of "Wheels on the Bus." During a more active game such as "Ring Around the Rosey," Nick's father can help him walk with his walker around the circle, or Nick can just hold onto his peer's hands while his father gives him extra support for balance. The group can be asked to move around the circle a little more slowly to accommodate Nick but, other than that, the game can be played without major changes. Similarly, if a relay race is used as a culminating activity, simple modifications for Nick can be made to make the game fair. Such changes as decreasing the distance Nick must move in his walker, reducing the number of players on Nick's team, or giving Nick assistance when performing a movement such as throwing or catching are just a few suggestions that can easily accommodate Nick while not drastically changing the game for the other children. (See chaps. 6 and 7, this volume, for more suggestions.)

4. ***Determine Support the Student Will Need***   As above, the next step is to determine who will directly implement the program for the child with disabilities. In some cases, the movement program staff may feel comfortable including children with mild disabilities, particularly when there are several staff members for each session. In cases in which a child with more significant disabilities such as Nick is integrated in a community movement program, the staff may request a more knowledgeable person to work with the child. Parents and older siblings can be

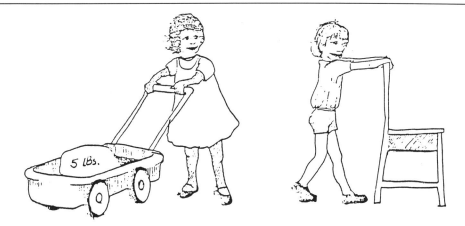

Weighted wagons and chairs can be used as walking aids for some children with cerebral palsy. These are most useful for children who have low muscle tone.

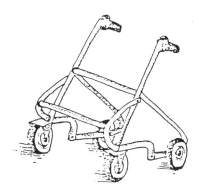

Rolling walkers are used for some school-aged children who have difficulty getting around. Your child's physical therapist can explain how and if these devices would be useful to your child.

Figure 8.5. Example of simple aids to assist in walking. (From Brinson, C.L. [Ed.]. [1982]. *The helping hand: A manual describing methods for handling the young child with cerebral palsy*. Charlottesville, VA: Kluge Children's Rehabilitation Center; reprinted by permission.)

excellent assistants if given some simple guidance from the movement program staff and from the child's teachers and therapists. Guidance can be spending a few minutes with the program staff before each session to discuss the various activities of the day, how the activity area will be utilized, and some possible suggestions for how to include the child with a disability. When possible, the child's teacher and therapist should come to the program at least one time to gain a better understanding of the program. Then these professionals could provide specific programming ideas and suggestions to promote inclusion. In Nick's case, his father brought him to the motor program, and he stayed and assisted Nick throughout. However, Nick's father often "backed-off" to allow Nick to move on his own and interact with his peers. Nick's father always arrived a few minutes early to prepare Nick following a program outlined by Nick's physical therapist. During this time, Nick's father also discussed the plan for the day with the program staff so that they could begin to think of how best to accommodate and include Nick.

   5.   Implement Program and Conduct Ongoing Evaluation   The final step is to implement the program and conduct ongoing evaluation. Again, other persons besides the movement program staff may be needed to assist the child and collect ongoing evaluation data. The program staff should be queried on a regular basis, particularly in the early going, to determine if they feel the child is being successfully included without interfering with the program for the children without disabilities. Changes can be made within the first few sessions if in fact there are problems. Ongoing evaluative data should also be collected regarding how well the child is progressing toward his or her specific goals. The child's special education staff and therapists can help develop a simple checklist and provide suggestions if the child is not making adequate progress. Again, in Nick's case his father assisted him and collected data on Nick's walking skills using the data sheet in Figure 8.4.

Kindergarten Physical Education

As noted earlier in this chapter, many preschool programs for students with disabilities are housed in regular elementary schools, and often older preschool children are included in regular kindergarten physical education. Accommodating a child with disabilities in regular kindergarten physical education poses different problems than the two previous examples. First, only one physical education teacher works with classes as large as 25–30 children. (In some cases two or three kindergarten classes are combined, resulting in class sizes as large as 75 children!) Second, the differences between the skill level of the child with a disability and kindergartners without disabilities can be quite large. Some children with disabilities may be learning how to use wheelchairs or, in Nick's case, still learning how to walk with a walker, while some regular kindergartners may be skipping, jumping rope, and even riding a two-wheel bicycle. Thus, the regular physical education teacher may not be particularly receptive to accepting a child with a disability into his or her regular physical education program. Still, the systematic approach described in Chapter 4 can be applied to kindergarten physical education so that students with disabilities can be safely, successfully, and meaningfully included.

   1.   Determine What to Teach   Again, a systematic approach to inclusion is needed, beginning with identifying the child's strengths and weaknesses and developing specific goals and objectives. In the case of elementary school physical education, a particular child's strengths and weaknesses should be referenced to: 1) skills needed in elementary physical education, 2) skills needed on the playground, and 3) skills needed at home and in the neighborhood. Again, a list of these skills can be developed by the child's parents and the regular physical educator. Then other team members, probably the adapted physical education specialist, the special educator, and the physical therapist (depending on the child's particular disability), can evaluate the child on these functional skills. Table 8.7 provides an example of an evaluation of Rasheed, a kindergartener who is totally blind, and Table 8.8 provides an example of Rasheed's IEP based on the results of this assessment.

   2.   Analyze the Regular Routines   With goals and objectives identified, the team can compare the child's goals to the activities that take place in regular physical education to determine where they might best be embedded. Here is where the regular physical educator can be instrumental to the team in providing general outlines of yearly plans as well as daily routines. While such plans may vary, they can give the team a ballpark idea of the typical routines that take place in kindergarten physical education and what modifications might be needed to include the student with disabilities. Tables 8.9, 8.10, and 8.11 provide examples of yearly, unit, and daily lesson plans for a typical kindergarten physical education program with anticipated modifications for Rasheed.

Table 8.7. Rasheed's present level of performance, referenced to functional activities necessary for him in his kindergarten class

Functional motor skill	Rasheed's present abilities
Demonstrate various locomotor patterns.	Rasheed can run, jump forward on two feet (only 12″), gallop, and slide. He cannot hop on one foot or skip. His locomotor patterns tend to be stiff and jerky, and he moves very slowly and cautiously. His locomotor patterns seem to be affected by limited balance and strength as well as fear from limited vision.
Demonstrate various movement concepts.	Rasheed has good body awareness and understanding of movement concepts such as high/low, forward/backward, fast/slow, and up/down. Again, he is very cautious in his movements and has trouble with space awareness because of his visual impairment, even though he knows how to apply various movement concepts to various movements.
Demonstrate various nonlocomotor skills.	Rasheed can turn, twist, curl, stretch, and jump and land quite well. He does have difficulty with static and dynamic balance, and he often loses balance when performing simple twisting movements or locomotor patterns.
Demonstrate emerging manipulative skills.	Rasheed can throw underhand and overhand, but he does not shift his weight (does not step). His limited vision makes it virtually impossible for him to catch although he will stop a ball that has bells in it that is rolled directly to him. He also can kick a ball that is placed directly in front of him, but he does not use any knee action in the kick or much range of motion in his hips.
Climb up playground structure (stairs and ladder).	Rasheed can climb up the ladder and go down the slide independently. He also can swing if someone pushes him. (He cannot pump.) He does not have the strength to hang on the monkey bars for more than a few seconds.
Ride tricycle.	Rasheed can pedal a two-wheel bike that has training wheels. His parents need to help him with steering, but he can balance himself and pedal the bike on a flat surface. He does not have the strength to pedal uphill.
Play low-organized games.	Rasheed quickly picks up the rules of low-organized games such as dodge ball, tag, and relay races. However, his limited vision prevents him from participating very successfully. For example, he is much slower than his peers in relay races, and he is an easy target in tag and dodge ball.

It should be noted that kindergarten physical education varies from very structured lessons that focus on having children learn how to perform skills in very specific ways (throw overhand using a specific pattern) to movement exploration-based activities that focus on children learning more general movement patterns and movement concepts (e.g., move the ball across the room using your hand). The type of program will no doubt affect how the child's specific goals will be incorporated. Movement exploration programs tend to be more conducive to individual differences. However, in directed programs the physical education teacher may be presenting a skill that focuses on a certain type of performance that is incompatible with the abilities of the child who has a disability. In such a case, the child should be allowed to perform the skill in a way that matches his or her unique abilities.

For example, the class may be learning how to perform an overhand throw by stepping with rotating body, extending arm backward, by rotating body and by shifting weight forward, and stepping with the opposite foot. However, Malcolm, who is being included into the program, has spastic cerebral palsy, uses a wheelchair, and has a goal of improving functional range of motion and control of his arms and hands while performing manipulative activities. A reasonable alternative for this student that matches his specific goal is to allow the child to work on pushing a ball off his lap tray or working on grasping and releasing bean bags while his peers work on the skill of throwing. Specific commands on how to better perform this alternative skill (e.g., lean back, relax arms and slowly flex them toward body, place hands behind ball, lean forward and extend

Table 8.8.   Rasheed's IEP for physical education

LONG-TERM PLAN: By the end of elementary school, Rasheed will demonstrate mastery of a variety of locomotor, nonlocomotor, and manipulative patterns so that he will be able to participate with minimal modifications and assistance in a variety of lead-up sports in middle and high school.

Long-Term Goal 1:   Rasheed will demonstrate all of the components of a mature two-footed horizontal jumping pattern so that he travels a distance of 36" independently, three out of four trials.

Short-Term Instructional Objectives

1. Rasheed will demonstrate the proper leg action of a two-footed horizontal jump independently, four out of five trials.
2. Rasheed will demonstrate the proper arm action of a two-footed horizontal jump independently, four out of five trials.
3. Rasheed will demonstrate the proper landing position when performing a two-footed horizontal jump independently, four out of five trials.
4. Rasheed will demonstrate all the components of a two-footed horizontal jump independently so that his body travels a distance of 30" or more four out of five trials.

Long-Term Goal 2:   Rasheed will demonstrate all of the components of an underhand throw independently so that the ball travels 10' and within 1' of an auditory target, three out of four trials.

Short-Term Instructional Objectives

1. Rasheed will demonstrate the correct arm action of the underhand throw independently, four out of five trials.
2. Rasheed will demonstrate the correct leg action of the underhand throw independently, four out of five trials.
3. Rasheed will demonstrate the correct arm and leg action of the underhand throw independently so that ball travels a distance of 10' toward an auditory wall target, four out of five trials.

Long-Term Goal 3:   Rasheed will demonstrate improved functional balance by exhibiting a variety of locomotor, nonlocomotor, and manipulative patterns without falling.

Short-Term Instructional Objectives

1. Rasheed will shift weight and step when performing the overhand and underhand throw and when planting foot for kicking independently, four out of five trials.
2. Rasheed will perform various nonlocomotor movements (specifically twisting, stretching, bending) during warm-ups, maintaining static balance for up to 10 seconds without falling, four out of five trials.
3. Nick will demonstrate continuous jumping and landing and hopping on one foot for a minimum of five repetitions without losing balance, four out of five trials.

Long-Term Goal 4:   Rasheed will demonstrate an ability to participate in a variety of low-organized games with increasing speed, accuracy, and strength.

Short-Term Instructional Objectives

1. During relay races, Rasheed will run independently toward a peer such that he will need only a 5' head start in relay races of 25' or less to keep up with peers, three out of four trials.
2. During dodge ball games, Rasheed will independently roll a ball toward a peer who is verbally signalling to him from 5' away with enough force and accuracy that he hits the peer, two out of five trials.
3. During games of tag, Rasheed will independently move away from a peer tagger who is clapping his hands and move to a safe area in the playing field so that he will not get tagged more than twice in a 3-minute game of tag.

arms, follow through by pushing ball forward off lap tray) can be developed by an adapted physical education specialist or a physical therapist and carried out by a teacher assistant or older peer tutor. However, the skill can still be practiced and performed in regular physical education.

Usually it is easier to accommodate a child's unique goals in a movement exploration format. In the above example, a teacher might ask the group to get the ball across the gym using a tossing method of their choice. While many children may choose the overhand throw as described above, others may use an underhand throw, a sidearm throw, a two-handed toss, or other patterns. The child whose goal is to push a ball off his or her lap tray can perform the movement any way he or

Table 8.9. Sample yearly plan for kindergarten physical education, with analysis for Rasheed

Month	Focus activities
September	☐ Introduce rules; review body management skills, personal/general space
October	☐ Locomotor and nonlocomotor patterns (focus on proper patterns)
November	☐ Locomotor and nonlocomotor patterns (focus on movement concepts)
December	☐ Underhand roll and trap/catch
January	☐ Locomotor and nonlocomotor patterns (review pattern and concepts)
February	+ Rhythms and dance
March	☐ Tumbling
April	☐ Underhand roll and trap/catch (played in games such as dodge ball)
May	☐ Low-organized games (application of locomotor patterns/movement concepts)
June	☐ Low-organized games (application of locomotor patterns/movement concepts)

Key: + = No modifications needed for Rasheed.

☐ = Some modifications needed for Rasheed.* (Note that modifications can be as simple as a peer assisting Rasheed with adapted equipment and special instruction. These specific decisions are not made at this level in the model.)

■ = Alternative activities needed for Rasheed.

she chooses and still be following directions and participating in regular physical education without the need for any special accommodations.

   3.   *Determine Modifications Needed*   Following the model, the next step in the process is to determine how the child with a disability will perform the targeted skills. The examples of throwing described above are illustrations of how a child might perform a throwing activity. Unfortunately, most regular physical educators do not have the skills nor the time to develop individual plans for each child with a disability who is included in regular physical education. Therefore, an adapted physical education specialist, a special education teacher, or a physical therapist can develop a specific program for the child with a disability. The role of the regular physical educator is to share with these specialists daily, weekly, and monthly lesson plans. This would enable the specialists to mold the child's program to the routines of the regular program. As the regular physical educator learns more about the child, his or her unique needs and goals, and ways to accommodate him or her in regular physical education, the regular physical educator can take a more active role in program development. Again, information on accommodating students with specific disabilities as well as specific ways to modify group activities are contained in Chapters 6 and 7. Questions to answer at this level of the model include: 1) Is special instruction needed? 2) Does the student need special preparation, whether physical or instructional? 3) What types of cues might the student need? and 4) Are specific adaptations needed?

   In Rasheed's case, he will need extra instruction and extra cuing (verbal and physical assistance) if he is going to acquire the skills as well and as quickly as his peers. In fact, he will probably need extra instruction and practice if he is going to achieve his goals. This extra instruction can take place during regular physical education with a different-age peer (older elementary school–age student) or teacher assistant, or outside of class during recess and at home (physical education homework). Adaptations for Rasheed are fairly simple and include giving him a peer to lead him around, trying to keep the environment as clutter-free as possible, and making sure he is made aware of the environment. Again, the team should work together to determine the best

Table 8.10.   Unit plan for locomotor and nonlocomotor patterns, with accommodations for Rasheed

Week 1
 Day 1
  Warm-up (nonlocomotor movements to music in self-space; locomotor movements to music in general space)
  Skill focus (review proper technique for horizontal jump; practice the skill of horizontal jump)
  Reinforcing game ("frog tag")
 Day 2
  Warm-up (same as above)
  Skill focus (review proper technique for horizontal jump; practice the skill of horizontal jump)
  Reinforcing game ("bunny rabbit relay race")
Week 2
 Day 1
  Warm-up (same as above with review of jumping)
  Skill focus (review proper technique for hopping; practice hopping)
  Reinforcing game ("hopping through obstacle course")
 Day 2
  Warm-up (same as above with review of jumping)
  Skill focus (review proper technique for hopping; skill stations working on jumping and hopping)
  Reinforcing game ("hopping tag")
Week 3
 Day 1
  Warm-up (same as above with review of hopping and jumping)
  Skill focus (review proper technique for galloping and sliding; practice skills)
  Reinforcing game ("horse-racing")
 Day 2
  Warm-up (same as above with review of hopping and jumping)
  Skill focus (review proper technique for galloping and sliding; practice skills)
  Reinforcing game ("galloping tag")
Week 4
 Day 1
  Warm-up (same as above)
  Skill focus (review proper technique for jumping, hopping, and galloping; practice skills)
  Reinforcing game (move through obstacle course using these skills)
 Day 2
  Warm-up (same as above)
  Skill focus (review proper technique for jumping, hopping, and galloping; practice)
  Reinforcing game ("animal tag")

General accommodations for Rasheed
 Extra cues for proper positioning during nonlocomotor movement
 Move with peer (holding hands) during warm-up exploration
 Have him near teacher when instruction is given
 Have different-age peer assist him in practicing skills

modifications for Rasheed. In Rasheed's case, his vision therapist and his orientation and mobility specialist will be extremely helpful in developing appropriate modifications.

   4.   Determine and Prepare Support   The next step in the model is to determine who will assist the student while in regular physical education. Again, regular physical educators often have large caseloads, which makes it difficult for them to work one-on-one with children with disabilities. Thus, another person may be needed to assist the student with disabilities in regular physical education. In some cases, the child's peers without disabilities can provide assistance such as retrieving errant balls, helping the child find the correct station, helping the child stay on task, and making the child feel welcome in group activities. The regular physical educator should

Table 8.11. Integrating Rasheed's goals within a regular lesson plan

JUMPING LESSON PLAN

Objective: Students will receive instruction, have an opportunity to practice, and then receive feedback on the essential components of the horizontal jumping pattern.

I.   Introduction
    A. Students come in and sit in assigned squads.
    B. Tell class we are working on the skill of jumping.
    C. Review plan for day (warm-up, skill focus in stations, and reinforcing game).

II. Warm-up
    A. Stand in personal space and move various body parts to music (interject levels [high/low], time [fast/slow], and force [hard/soft]).

head	leg	hips
shoulders	feet	whole body
back	hands	

    B. Find a partner and walk around room at various levels, directions, and speeds.
    C. Perform various locomotor patterns to music around the gym in a scattered pattern (interject directions [forward/backward/sideways] and levels [high/low]).
    *Rasheed's partner should be told to be extra careful guiding Rasheed.
    *Continue to allow Rasheed to have a partner to guide his direction and for safety while other children move independently.

III. Skill focus
    A. Have students sitting facing you, then review the components of a skillful jump (show picture and demonstrate, highlighting key points):
      Preparatory movement includes 90° flexion of both knees with arms extended behind body
      Forceful thrust of both arms and full extension of the legs at the take-off in a forward and upward direction
      Take-off angle (from take-off spot through center of body mass) at approximately *45°*
      Feet make contact with the floor ahead of the body mass
      Thighs near parallel to the floor at touch down
      Simultaneous forward arm action during landing
    B. Have children stand and scatter so that they have adequate space. Break down components of skill and work on each aspect. Give children ample practice of each component. Provide feedback to students.
    C. Put skill together and practice jumping over lines on the floor. Provide feedback.
    D. Give children pieces of paper and have them jump over the paper.
    E. Put hula hoops down on the floor and have children jump over hoops.
    *Match Rasheed up with a peer to give him verbal feedback. Anchor him close to a wall on the side of the gym so that he knows where he is. Have peer watch Rasheed take his turn and give feedback about components. Use different-age peer as needed.

IV. Reinforcing game
    A. "Frog Tag"—Play typical tag game but all participants must jump on two feet. Place several hula hoops on the floor as safe places. If tagged, tagged person becomes another tagger. Remind students to focus on correct pattern to jump farther.
    *Allow Rasheed to jump with partner.
    *When Rasheed is tagger, children must make a sound while jumping so Rasheed knows where they are.
    *When Rasheed is tagger, there are no safe places and only half the gym is available for jumping away.

V.   Concluding activity
    A. Students sit in squads.
    B. Review components of jump and reinforce specific students for doing certain components exceptionally well.
    C. Encourage students to practice jump during recess and at home.
    D. Have students close eyes and take three deep breaths.
    E. Call squads to line up at door and leave with classroom teacher.

direct peers without disabilities in ways to help the child with disabilities. For other children with disabilities, an older peer (different-age peer) or parent volunteer may need to provide assistance. These volunteers should go through training and should be given specific instructions (developed by the child's teacher or therapist) on how to implement the program. (See chap. 4, this volume, for more detail.) In addition, the regular physical educator should help volunteers decide when it is appropriate for the child with disabilities to work on the same skills as the other children or when the child should be working on other skills. For children with more significant disabilities, an adapted physical education specialist, a trained teacher assistant, a teacher, a therapist, or the child's parent may be asked to provide assistance in regular physical education. In Rasheed's case, peers in his class can help him move around the environment safely. For extra instruction, a different-age peer or volunteer may be needed. In addition, Rasheed's orientation and mobility specialist will come into physical education once a week to help Rasheed and to discuss any problems the regular physical educator might have. Again, the team should work together to determine how much support a particular student needs and, once determined, prepare support persons to work with particular students.

5. *Implement Program and Conduct Ongoing Evaluation*   Finally, the program can be implemented and ongoing evaluation conducted. The person who directly implements the program should be responsible for conducting the ongoing evaluation. In the case of a child with a mild disability who comes to physical education without any special support, the regular physical educator can evaluate the progress the student is making in reference to progress and skills of peers without disabilities. That is, the regular physical educator should use the same measurements to assess progress and success with children without disabilities as with the child being included. For example, if a teacher uses a checklist to determine how many components of the underhand throwing pattern her students have achieved at the end of a throwing unit, he or she should use the same assessment for the student with disabilities. If the student appears to be falling behind, then he or she may need more support in regular physical education or some other modifications.

If peer tutors, volunteers, or teacher assistants are responsible for implementation and ongoing evaluation of students with more significant disabilities, they should be given data collection forms and specific instruction on how to collect ongoing data. (See Figure 8.6, as well as Figures 8.3 and 8.4, for examples.) Special education staff should plan on assisting volunteers and assistants early in the program to make sure they are following correct procedures. In addition, the regular physical educator should be asked to provide feedback as to how he or she thinks the program is going and what may need to be changed.

SUMMARY

Regular preschool programs and childcare centers are beginning to work cooperatively with special education programs in an effort to include students with disabilities. While inclusion programs may require some extra staff training, shuffling of schedules, and transfer of adapted equipment from special education classrooms to regular childcare centers, inclusion programs can work. In fact, such programs can be extremely enriching and educational for both regular childcare and special education staff!

Motor aspects of regular childcare programs as well as more-structured community-based motor programs can be modified so that students with disabilities can be accommodated and work on individual goals and objectives without negatively affecting the program for students without disabilities. Again, inclusion programs will only work if a systematic model is followed *prior to* including the student with disabilities. This chapter applied the programming model outlined in Chapter 4 to including preschool students with disabilities in regular childcare centers and com-

Student's name: Malcolm Jones
Task: Pushing ball off tray (increase range of motion and control of arm)
Objective: Push ball off tray in 20 seconds or less independently so that ball travels 2'.
Support: Regular physical education with different-age peer providing assistance

Ball size   **TRIALS**
(t) tennis ball
(s) softball
(8) 8" playground ball

Assistance
(v) verbal cue
(t) touch prompt
(p) partial physical assist
(f) full physical assist

Speed
(4) 40 seconds
(3) 30 seconds
(2) 20 seconds

Figure 8.6. Sample data form to be used by different-age peer for student with significant disabilities.

munity movement programs. This model utilized an ecological approach to program planning in which functional skills and activities that are meaningful to all preschool students are defined and then used as a reference for evaluating the student with disabilities. Information from the ecological assessment can then be used to: 1) write meaningful individualized education programs and 2) analyze regular childcare and movement programs to determine specifically where the student's goals and objectives can be embedded and what modifications and supports are needed for the student to be successful. With systematic planning and implementation, preschool students with disabilities can be successfully and meaningfully included in regular childcare and community-based movement programs.

Chapter 9

Including Elementary School Students with Disabilities in Regular Physical Education

*In order to meet the needs of students with disabilities, the regular physical educa-
tion curriculum needs to be modified. This is particularly true in middle school
and high school, which often follow a sports-based curriculum. Sports training is
not appropriate for many students with disabilities, particularly students with severe disabilities. These students should work on more functional leisure skills,
rather than team sports such as football and field hockey that they will never be
able to play. While inclusion in physical education is important, it does not mean
trying to fit all students into the regular curriculum.*

*Another important point with inclusion in physical education is asking students
with disabilities where they would prefer to be placed. I have found this to be particularly important with children who have normal intelligence but who have some
physical or learning disabilities. These students are well aware of the fact that they
are not as skilled as their peers, and they may feel inadequate or embarrassed
when learning new skills. These students might prefer to work on new skills in private away from the group until they become more proficient. As they gain more
confidence in their abilities, gradually they can be included in the group. The important point is that the student is involved in the decision process, and that his or
her placement is not dictated by those who feel they know what is best for the
student.*

—Joanie Verderber

Sue is a third grader at Jefferson Davis (JD) Elementary School. Her favorite subjects are reading and social studies. She loves music, and she enjoys playing with her friends during recess and
lunch. Sue is paralyzed on one side of her body (hemiparesis) as a result of a car accident 3 years
ago, but she is learning how to push her wheelchair independently. In addition, she is completely
blind in one eye, she has slurred, slow speech that is intelligible only to those who are familiar
with her, and she has difficulty processing information (slow in understanding and following directions). Finally, her accident led to some medical complications that resulted in Sue having a

Joanie Verderber is an APE specialist for the Los Angeles County Office of Education, San Gabriel Unified School
District, San Gabriel, California.

gastrostomy tube for nourishment and a colostomy for the elimination of feces. Nevertheless, Sue is fully included in a regular third-grade class at JD Elementary School in which support services are brought to her rather than having her pulled out for these services.

As one can imagine, the regular physical educator at Davis never worked with a student who had the multitude of disabilities that Sue does. This teacher was initially overwhelmed by the proposition of having Sue in regular physical education, and he even went as far as talking with the directors of physical education and special education for the school district to have a waiver so that Sue could be excused from the mandatory physical education requirement. The directors did not agree with his proposal, but they did assure this teacher that, through collaborative team efforts, adequate support would be provided so that he could accommodate Sue's unique needs yet still provide a comprehensive program to his students without disabilities. How is the team going to help this teacher include Sue in regular physical education? What types of supports and accommodations can be implemented so that Sue is included without negatively affecting the regular physical education program?

While the scenario described above may seem extreme, students like Sue are being fully included in elementary schools across the country. In terms of physical education, regular elementary school physical educators are being asked to work with and accommodate these students (with supports) within the regular program. While including students with disabilities in regular physical education may seem an impossible task to some, elementary school physical education actually offers a easier opportunity for inclusion when compared to middle school and high school programs. First, elementary physical education programs tend to be more developmental than middle school and high school programs. That is, the focus tends to be more on teaching fundamental skills and concepts rather than sports skills. Second, elementary physical education programs tend to be less competitive than middle school and high school programs with a focus on learning how to play low-organized games and lead-up games (i.e., games that have some element of the official sport but focus on only one or two skills and concepts at a time) rather than strictly following the rules of the games. For example, in upper elementary school a lead-up game to basketball might be dribble tag or 2 versus 2 keep-away rather than a regulation 5 versus 5 game of basketball). Third, elementary school physical education tends to be more accommodating to the needs of students with differing abilities. Activities are not so advanced that students who are behind are as noticeable as in middle school and high school physical education. Similarly, instructional activities tend to be easier to modify so as to accommodate the needs of varying skill levels. Finally, preconceived notions of how games and sports "should be" played are not as engraved in the minds of young children as they are in older students, particularly those who have participated in organized sports programs. That is, elementary-age children, with a little guidance from their teachers, tend to be a little more tolerant of peers who may have different abilities than middle school and high school students.

The purpose of this chapter is to suggest specific ways in which children with disabilities can be safely and meaningfully included in regular elementary school physical education programs. The following will be specifically addressed in this chapter: 1) description of typical elementary school physical education programs, 2) application of the model described in Chapter 4 to including elementary-age children with disabilities in regular elementary physical education, and 3) examples of how Sue can be successfully included in regular physical education.

ELEMENTARY SCHOOL PHYSICAL EDUCATION

Main Elements

Implementation of elementary school physical education programs varies from school to school and teacher to teacher. Three major aspects of elementary physical education that tend to vary are:

1) curricular focus or content of the program, 2) teaching approaches, and 3) lesson formats. How best to integrate a student with disabilities will be directly related to how the regular physical educator incorporates these three aspects of the program.

Curricular Focus   Basically, there are two types of curricula that elementary physical education programs follow: 1) programs that focus on the development of movement skills and concepts, and 2) programs that focus on the development of sport-specific skills.

Programs that focus on the development of movement skills focus on the following basic fundamental movement skills: locomotor patterns (running, galloping, jumping, leaping, hopping, skipping, chasing, fleeing); manipulative patterns (throwing, catching, kicking, punting, striking, dribbling, volleying); and nonmanipulative skills (twisting, turning, curling, stretching, transferring weight, landing, rolling). These skills are then applied through the following movement concepts: space awareness (location, levels, directions, pathways, extensions); relationships (of body parts, with objects, with people), and effort (time, force, flow). For example, a teacher might have a unit that focuses on applying effort concepts to locomotor patterns such as running fast/slow, skipping in a stiff/flowing pattern, or hopping hard/light. (See Graham, Holt/Hale, & Parker, 1993, for more detail.)

Programs that focus on sport-specific skills tend to teach skills that are needed for successful participation in a variety of culturally popular sports. Popular team sports include soccer, basketball, softball, and volleyball; popular individual sports include track and field, gymnastics, and racquet sports such as tennis and racquetball. Skills needed for each sport are usually taught in isolation and then applied to lead-up or modified games. For example, a teacher might conduct a basketball unit in which he or she works on basketball skills such as dribbling, passing, shooting, and defense. These skills are then applied to lead-up games of basketball and modified games of basketball such as dribble relay races, line basketball, and zone basketball. (See Nichols, 1990, for more detail.)

It should be noted that both of the above types of programs often include other physical education activities such as rhythms and dance, low-organized games, cooperative/initiative games, and aquatics. What exactly is offered will vary from school to school depending on the facilities/equipment available in the school and/or the interests and abilities of the physical education staff.

Teaching Approaches   Program focus is just one aspect of elementary physical education. In addition, how these programs are presented will vary from teacher to teacher. Recall from Chapter 6 that the the two most common types of teaching approaches are: 1) direct approach (command style), and 2) inquiry approach (movement exploration). In the direct approach, the teacher directly instructs/tells the students exactly what skills to work on, exactly how to perform the skills, and provides specific feedback on their performances. Direct approaches are teacher-centered with students making few decisions themselves. For example, a teacher who wants students to kick a ball using a specific pattern would tell the class that they will be working on kicking, demonstrate the specific components of the kicking pattern, then have equipment and stations set up so that students can practice kicking using the prescribed pattern while she provides specific feedback on performance. In contrast, the inquiry approach allows children to explore their movement abilities and problem-solve different ways to move under different situations rather than to simply copy a teacher's "correct performance." Inquiry approaches are more student-centered than the direct approach, with students making most of the decisions regarding how to move. For example, if a teacher wants her students to learn the concept of over/under, she might set up a rope across the room at a certain height (say head height) and ask students to move to the other side of the rope. Students will discover that they have to move under the rope. The rope gradually can be lowered so that students must adjust their bodies to move under the rope. At a certain point (which will vary from student to student), students will discover that they will want to step over rather than go under the rope. The student learns by doing without any direct instruction from the teacher. In addition, the student makes the decision on when to change from going under to over. Both approaches can be effective in physical education, and in fact many teachers use a direct approach for teaching some skills and an inquiry approach for teaching other skills. (See Mosston, 1981, for a more detailed description of teaching approaches.)

Lesson Format   Lesson format refers to how the content will be presented to the class. Most elementary physical education programs use a lesson format that includes the following three components: 1) warm-up activities, 2) skill focus, and 3) reinforcing group games (Nichols, 1990). Warm-up activities are designed to improve students' overall physical fitness, prepare them physically and mentally for participation in the skill focus of the lesson, and prevent or reduce the chance of injury. Warm-up activities usually include some stretching and strengthening activities followed by aerobic activities such as running laps or moving around the gymnasium to music using different locomotor patterns. Skill focus activities are designed to improve students' abilities in specific skills such as fundamental movement skills, movement concepts, or sports skills. The skill focus can be taught in one large group or in smaller groups or centers. For example, a teacher might arrange the gymnasium into five ball skill stations. Students have specific directions at each station and rotate through each station working on a different ball skill (throwing versus kicking) or a different focus of the same ball skill (throwing for accuracy versus force). Finally, the class concludes with a group activity that reinforces the skill focus of the day. For example, a game of zone basketball could be played that reinforces the skills of passing and defense, or a game of "Clean Up Your Backyard" could be played that reinforces the skill of overhand throwing. How much time a teacher allocates to each portion of the lesson will vary. For example, some teachers spend as much as half the class period on fitness-related warm-up activities such as stretching, calisthenics, strengthening activities, and aerobics while other teachers spend only a few minutes on warm-ups that focus on preparing students for the activities of the day. Similarly, some teachers spend the majority of their class time on skill-building activities, while other teachers spend the majority of their class time on games. Again, specific adaptations for including students with disabilities will vary based on how a teacher organizes his or her lesson.

One final aspect of lesson planning that can affect inclusion is how long a teacher stays with one skill or a group of skills. That is, does a teacher work on a group of skills such as locomotor patterns or basketball skills for several weeks in a row or does he or she teach different skills each day? Most elementary physical education teachers teach in units of 1–6 weeks in length, depending on how often they see each class (i.e., 1–5 days per week). Teaching in units allows students to master skills fully and apply skills to a variety of situations. However, teaching a different activity each day can be confusing for some students (particularly for students with disabilities) and can limit students' skill development and their ability to generalize skills to specific games and sports. Therefore, this chapter presents the ideal situation in which cohesive units of instruction are presented rather than a program that changes from day to day.

A SYSTEMATIC APPROACH TO INCLUDING STUDENTS
WITH DISABILITIES IN REGULAR PHYSICAL EDUCATION

1. Determine Student's Individual Goals and Objectives

Following the steps in the model outlined in Chapter 4, the first step in including students with disabilities in regular physical education is to determine each student's strengths and weaknesses and then to write specific long-term goals and short-term instructional objectives. Ideally, an adapted physical education specialist (with support from other team members) should conduct the motor assessment and write specific goals and objectives. However, other team members (probably the special education teacher, the physical therapist, the regular physical education teacher, and the parent) can work together to assess and plan the program for individual students in the event that the school system does not have an adapted physical education specialist.

Assessment as well as subsequent goals and objectives should be referenced to what skills the student needs to be successful in the present environment (i.e., elementary school physical education, recess, neighborhood) as well as anticipated future environments (Little League sports, Special Olympics, community/neighborhood recreation activities, and so forth). For example, the team utilized the form contained in Figure 9.1 to determine what skills should be prioritized for Sue. Note how Sue's preferences as well as her parents' preferences were considered in the decision process. Similarly, activities in regular physical education (shared by the regular physical educator), activities that are popular with Sue's peers (shared by Sue's friends), and activities that are available in the community for elementary-age children were considered at this level of analysis.

What resulted was a list of targeted activities that are most meaningful to Sue. These targeted activities then become the reference for assessment. That is, a comprehensive evaluation is conducted to determine Sue's abilities and weaknesses referenced to the activities that were determined to be most important for Sue. (See Table 9.1.) Note how many activities that are popular in regular physical education (e.g., tumbling, rhythms, locomotor patterns) and during recess (e.g., bike riding, soccer) are not evaluated since they are not considered priority skills for Sue.

The result of this assessment reveals that Sue has a lot of work ahead of her if she is going to be able to push her wheelchair independently or if she is going to be able to participate in modified lifetime leisure activities independently (i.e., swimming, softball, basketball). In addition, she will need a great deal of assistance climbing up the climbing equipment, but she can swing independently if she is placed on the swing.

Based on this assessment, specific goals and objectives were developed for Sue. (See Table 9.2.) Again, note how the objectives are tied directly to assessment data and thus are meaningful for Sue.

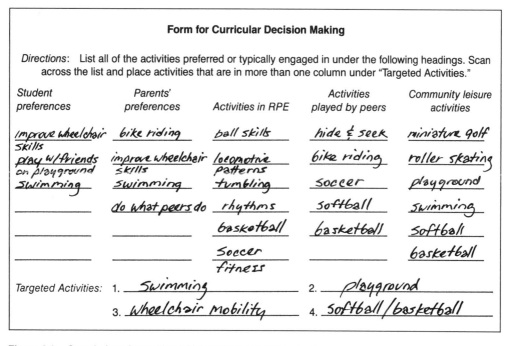

Figure 9.1. Sample form for making initial curricular decisions for Sue.

Table 9.1.   Sue's present level of performance (referenced to functional activities)

Functional motor skill	Sue's present abilities
Swimming	Sue needs assistance to get in the pool. Once in the pool, she can hold onto the side of the pool with one hand, stretch her body out, and kick. She also can move around the pool while holding onto the side. In the water, Sue will float on her back with support from an assistant or with a flotation device for up to 15 seconds. With the flotation device, Sue can swim using a one-arm/one-leg technique such that she can swim 25 yards in 2 minutes. She cannot swim or maintain buoyancy in the water without a flotation device, and she does not have the balance to stand in the pool independently.
Playground (including swings, climbing, and slide)	Sue can sit on a regular saddle swing (once placed on the swing by an assistant) so that she can maintain balance while someone pushes her at a low level. She needs assistance to get off the swing. Sue needs someone to place her up on the platform where the slide is as she does not have the strength or balance to climb the vertical ladder independently. Once up on the platform, Sue can scoot herself over to the slide and slide down while lying on her back. (She does not have the balance to slide down while sitting.)
Wheelchair mobility	Sue can push her wheelchair forward a distance of 20′ (half the length of the gym) in 1 minute. She has the endurance to push her wheelchair around the gym for up to 3 minutes without stopping. She is learning how to move her wheelchair around obstacles, but at present she can only move forward and backward successfully.
Throwing	Sue can hold a regulation softball and, from her wheelchair, throw the ball so that it travels 5′. She can throw a tennis ball slightly farther (7′–8′). Sue is learning how to lean back and twist to improve her throwing distance, but at present she still shows no trunk action when throwing (i.e., all arm).
Catching	Sue can track a balloon and a slow-moving Nerf ball that are tossed directly to her. She can get her hand up to contact the ball, and she can successfully trap the Nerf ball against her body two out of five trials. With a smaller Velcro ball and with a Velcro mitt or paddle, she can catch one of three balls when tossed slowly from 5′ away.
Striking	From her wheelchair, Sue can hold a small plastic bat in one hand and strike a large ball (8″ or larger) that is placed on a tee. She cannot hit smaller balls consistently (one out of five trials) on the tee, and she cannot hit a pitched ball, even when tossed from close range. Sue uses very little trunk action when striking.
Dribbling	Sue can bounce a large (12″ or greater) playground ball three to five times in a row. She has more difficulty with smaller balls (one to two in a row), and she still uses a slapping motion when dribbling. Sue is learning how to use the official "wheelchair dribble" (hold ball on lap while pushing chair forward), and she can now hold the ball on her lap while pushing her chair forward slowly.
Shooting	Sue can toss a Nerf basketball (8″–10″) from her wheelchair into a 4′ high trash can with an opening of 3′ from a distance of 2′–3′ away. She does not have the strength or control to shoot at a higher basket or at a basket farther away. Sue uses an overhand, shot-put type motion when shooting with no trunk action (i.e., all arm action).
Passing/catching	Sue can toss a Nerf basketball (8″–10″) from her wheelchair to a partner 3′ away in the air and 5′ away on a bounce. She can successfully trap the ball against her body two out of five trials when tossed from 3′ away. Sue uses a scooping motion with her arms with her chest as a backstop.

2.   Analyze Regular Physical Education Curriculum

The next step in the model is to determine what specific activities take place in elementary physical education and how (if at all) each of the above goals and objectives can be incorporated into these activities. First, an analysis of the yearly elementary physical education program is needed. As noted earlier, programs implemented in units make it easier to determine which units best

Table 9.2. Sue's IEP including long-term plan, long-term goals, and short-term instructional objectives

LONG-TERM PLAN: Sue will acquire the skills needed to participate with minimal support in a variety of lifetime leisure skills.

Long-Term Goal 1:[a] Sue will demonstrate the ability to swim independently across the pool using a modified sidestroke technique.

Short-Term Instructional Objectives:
1. Sue will demonstrate the modified sidestroke with assistance for technique so that she propels herself forward independently four out of five trials.
2. Sue will demonstrate the modified sidestroke independently so that she maintains buoyancy and propels her body forward in the water for 20 seconds three out of four trials.
3. Sue will swim the width of the pool (15 yards) independently using a modified sidestroke technique in 3 minutes or less three out of four trials.
4. Sue will swim the length of the pool (25 yards) independently using a modified sidestroke technique in 3 minutes or less three out of four trials.

Long-Term Goal 2: Sue will demonstrate the ability to move her wheelchair independently in a variety of directions avoiding obstacles.

Short-Term Instructional Objectives:
1. Sue will demonstrate the ability to push her wheelchair independently around a large circle (20' diameter) so that she is never more than 1' away from the circle four out of five trials.
2. Sue will demonstrate the ability to push her wheelchair independently through a figure-eight obstacle course (obstacles 7'–8' apart) staying within 1' of the obstacle yet not touching the obstacle four out of five trials.
3. Sue will demonstrate the ability to stop her wheelchair independently and make right angle turns around an obstacle staying within 1' of the obstacle without touching the obstacle four out of five trials.
4. Sue will demonstrate the ability to move her wheelchair independently through a variety of randomly placed obstacles and peers placed throughout the gymnasium without touching obstacles or peers four out of five trials.

Long-Term Goal 3: Sue will demonstrate the skills needed to participate with minimal assistance in a lead-up game of softball.

Short-Term Instructional Objectives:
1. Sue will demonstrate the following components of a functional throw from her wheelchair so that the ball travels a minimum of 10' and within 2' of a peer four out of five trials 2 days in a row.
   Throwing components:
   — Rotates body to side by turning shoulder.
   — Extends throwing arm behind body while at the same time pointing nonthrowing arm toward target.
   — Forcefully rotates body forward while lagging throwing arm behind body as long as possible.
   — Forcefully brings arm forward and releases ball.
   — Follows through by leaning body forward and bringing throwing arm down onto lap.
2. Sue will demonstrate the following components of a functional catch from her wheelchair so that she successfully catches a softball-sized Nerf ball four out of five trials 2 days in a row.
   Catching components:
   — Shows ready position by looking at ball and having good hand outstretched at chest height.
   — Opens hand as ball is tossed and leans into ball with chest to intercept ball.
   — Traps ball against body then quickly brings arm around ball to secure it.
3. Sue will independently hit a regulation softball that is placed on a tee using a one-handed striking pattern including body rotation so that ball travels 5' in air and throws another 5'–10' in air four out of five trials.

Long-Term Goal 4: Sue will demonstrate the skills needed to participate with minimal assistance in a lead-up game of basketball.

Short-Term Instructional Objectives:
1. Sue will demonstrate the ability to shoot a Nerf basketball independently using a one-handed push shot technique so that ball hits the rim of a 6' high regulation size basket three out of four trials and ball goes in one out of four trials.
2. Sue will demonstrate the ability to use a wheelchair dribble independently (three strong pushes of chair followed by one dribble) so that she travels a distance of 10' in 30 seconds or less three out of four trials.
3. Sue will demonstrate the ability to trap a bounced playground ball independently against her chest with her hand when ball is bounced to her by a peer from 10' away three out of four trials.

Long-Term Goal 5:[b] Sue will demonstrate ability to participate on playground equipment with peers with minimal assistance.

---

[a]There are no indoor pools available in Sue's community. Sue will practice her swimming with her mother on a daily basis, with an adapted aquatics instructor two times per week, and with her physical therapist at a community swimming pool during the summer months. (This goal will be monitored by Sue's physical therapist.)

[b]Short-term instructional objectives will be developed by the physical therapist and classroom teacher and will be monitored by the physical therapist. This goal will be worked on during regular recess by Sue's physical therapist and fifth-grade peer tutor. (Physical educator has other classes during this time.)

match the goals and objectives of the student with disabilities, which units may be appropriate but require some modification, and which units are incompatible, thus requiring the implementation of alternative activities. However, it becomes much more difficult to determine when activities are appropriate or need modification if activities are different each day.

Using a unit model, Tables 9.3 and 9.4 provide examples of yearly elementary physical education plans for third graders (broken down into months for convenience) following the two basic curricular models described above. A quick glance at the yearly plan in Table 9.3 (basic skills program) suggests that Sue's goals and objectives of throwing and catching match the units on throwing and catching in October and March. Sue should be able to be included in these units with virtually no modification. In addition, Sue should do well in the introductory lesson in September with some minor modifications (e.g., wheelchair mobility rather than locomotor patterns), in January when the class is doing rhythms and dance, and in June when the class is doing cooperative games. Some activities will need modifications if we want Sue to work on specific goals and objectives. For example, Sue can work on throwing as a substitute for kicking and holding the ball on her lap and pushing her wheelchair for dribbling. Finally, gymnastics is incompatible with Sue's goals and objectives and has been determined to be potentially dangerous for Sue. Thus, Sue will work on alternative activities that focus on her individual goals and objectives while her peers do gymnastics.

Examining the units in the sport skills model, Sue should have no problems in September or in June (with some minor modifications to accommodate her needs), nor should she have any problems in May during the t-ball unit when the focus is on throwing and catching. In October (Nerf soccer) and January (Nerf basketball), Sue can participate following the rules of wheelchair basketball. For example, Sue can dribble by keeping the ball on her lap while pushing her wheelchair and shoot at a lower basket. Similarly, Sue can shoot a soccer ball by throwing it rather than kicking it. In both cases, Sue also can work on wheelchair mobility skills. As was the case in the basic skills example, Sue can participate with her peers, with modifications, in badminton/tennis skills (she can practice hitting a pitched ball using a racquet or softball bat) as well as volleyball skills. (Sue can work on catching the ball and shooting it like a basketball to a teammate rather than hitting the ball.) During roller skating, Sue can work on pushing her wheelchair (endurance) while her peers work on skating. Finally, during gymnastics Sue should do alternative activities

Table 9.3. Sample yearly physical education program that follows basic skills content (third-grade focus is on the mastery of manipulative skills)

Month	Focus activities
September	+ introduce rules; review body management skills and locomotor patterns
October	+ throwing and catching
November	■ kicking and dribbling (with feet)
December	☐ striking with a bat and with a racquet
January	+ rhythms and dance
February	■ gymnastics
March	+ throwing and catching
April	■ kicking and dribbling (with feet)
May	■ striking with a bat and with a racquet
June	+ cooperative/initiative games

+ = no modifications needed for Sue.
☐ = some modifications needed for Sue.
■ = alternative activities needed for Sue.

Table 9.4. Sample yearly physical education program that follows sport skills content (third-grade focus is on introduction of and learning basic components of skills needed to participate in individual and team sports)

Month	Focus activities
September	+ introduce rules; review body management skills and locomotor patterns
October	■ Nerf soccer skills (dribbling, passing, shooting)
November	☐ beach ball volleyball skills (setting, bumping, serving)
December	+ badminton/tennis skills (forehand striking, backhand striking, serving)
January	+ Nerf basketball (dribbling, passing, shooting)
February	■ gymnastics
March	☐ roller skating (substitute pushing wheelchair)
April	■ Nerf soccer skills (dribbling, passing, shooting)
May	+ t-ball skills (throwing, catching, striking)
June	+ fun games (relay races, tag)

+ = no modifications needed for Sue.
☐ = some modifications needed for Sue.
■ = alternative activities needed for Sue.

that focus on her fitness goals. It also should be pointed out that wheelchair mobility can be incorporated during warm-up activities throughout the curriculum.

The second level of analysis of the regular physical education curriculum is to determine what happens in each unit and during each lesson. For example, Table 9.5 shows a sample unit plan for a kicking/dribbling unit. A quick analysis of the unit referenced to Sue's individual goals suggests that warm-up activities would be a good time to have Sue work on fitness and wheelchair mobility, throwing could be substituted for kicking, and wheelchair mobility could be substituted for dribbling.

The final step is to analyze a sample lesson plan within each unit to determine exactly where Sue will work on her specific skills. Table 9.6 demonstrates how Sue's goals can be included in a daily lesson plan in which the skill focus is kicking. While at first glance kicking may seem inappropriate for Sue (after all, she cannot move her legs), the modifications needed to include Sue in the lesson and have her work on her individual goals are fairly minimal. During warm-up activities, Sue will get a little more assistance (from teacher or peers) to perform sit-ups, and she will substitute moving in her wheelchair for locomotor patterns. During the skill focus, Sue will substitute throwing for kicking and holding the ball on her lap and pushing her wheelchair for dribbling. During the reinforcing game, Sue will substitute throwing for kicking and her teammates will give her balls. (See Table 9.7.)

Other types of modifications will be needed for other students with disabilities, particularly students with more significant disabilities. In some cases, older peers, teacher assistants, or other support personnel may be needed to assist the student or specialized adapted equipment might be needed. In other cases, an entirely different lesson plan may need to be developed for the student with disabilities. For example, if this was a lesson plan during the gymnastics unit, an alternative lesson plan would have to be developed for Sue that focused on her specific IEP goals and objectives.

It should be noted that the examples here are fairly detailed so as to illustrate exactly how decisions might be made. For more experienced physical education teachers who use previous lesson plans or no longer write detailed lesson plans, the general ideas outlined above can still be used. The important point is that, prior to including the student with a disability, the physical educator should analyze the student's individual goals and objectives as well as the physical edu-

Table 9.5. Unit plan for second-grade kicking/dribbling unit

WEEK 1

Day 1
  Warm-up (nonlocomotor movements to music in self-space; locomotor movements to music in general space)
  Skill focus (introduce proper technique for kicking; practice kicking as group with feedback)
  Reinforcing game ("kick the beach ball tag"—emphasizing kicking techniques)

Day 2
  Warm-up (same as above)
  Skill focus (review proper technique for kicking; skill stations working on kicking)
  Reinforcing game ("Clean Up Your Backyard"—kicking)

WEEK 2

Day 1
  Warm-up (same as above)
  Skill focus (review proper technique for kicking; skill stations working on kicking)
  Reinforcing game ("distance kick relay")

Day 2
  Warm-up (same as above)
  Skill focus (review proper technique for kicking; skill stations working on kicking)
  Reinforcing game ("distance kick relay")

WEEK 3

Day 1
  Warm-up (same as above)
  Skill focus (review proper technique for kicking; introduce dribbling technique; practice dribbling as a group)
  Reinforcing game ("dribble tag")

Day 2
  Warm-up (same as above)
  Skill focus (review proper technique for kicking and dribbling; station work on kicking and dribbling)
  Reinforcing game ("dribble relay races")

WEEK 4

Day 1
  Warm-up (same as above)
  Skill focus (review proper technique for kicking/dribbling; kicking/dribbling stations)
  Reinforcing game ("dribble obstacle course")

Day 2
  Warm-up (same as above)
  Skill focus (review proper technique for kicking/dribbling; kicking/dribbling station)
  Reinforcing game ("1 v. 1 mini soccer games")

General accommodations for Sue include: sit-ups during warm-ups, substitute pushing wheelchair for locomotor patterns, substitute throwing for kicking and pushing wheelchair for dribbling.

cation curriculum to determine where the goals and objectives will be incorporated into the regular program.

3. Determine How Program Will Be Implemented

Now that we have determined where the student's individual goals and objectives will be incorporated into the program, the next step is to determine exactly how the program will be implemented. That is, how will we help the student work on her individual goals and objectives during regular physical education? Recall from Chapter 4 that there are five questions that should be answered by the team to help determine how best to present information and modify activities for students with disabilities. The first question is, how often should the student receive services?

Table 9.6.   Including Sue's goals within a regular lesson plan

KICKING LESSON PLAN

Objective: Students will have an opportunity to practice and receive feedback on the essential components of the kicking pattern.

I.   Introduction

   A.   Students come in and sit in assigned squads.

   B.   Tell class we are working on the skill of kicking.

   C.   Review plan for day (warm-up, skill focus in stations, and reinforcing game).

II.   Warm-up

   A.   Stand in personal space and move various body parts to music (interject levels [high/low], time [fast/slow], and force [hard/soft]).

head	legs	hips
shoulders	feet	whole body
back	hands	

   B.   Find a partner and perform 10 sit-ups each.

   C.   Perform various locomotor patterns to music around the gym in a scattered pattern (interject directions [forward/backward/sideways] and levels [high/low]).

Sue—   Substitute moving arms or twisting wheelchair when action calls for legs.

   —   Have Sue's partner hold her hands to help pull her up for the last few sit-ups.

   —   Sue can push her wheelchair for locomotor patterns. Encourage her to maneuver her wheelchair in different directions and with increasing speed.

III.   Skill focus

   A.   Have students sit facing you, then review the components of a skillful kick: components of kicking (show picture and demonstrate, highlighting key points):

   1.   Look at ball while walking forward toward ball.

   2.   As you get closer to ball, bring arms out to side for balance.

   3.   Last step should be a little leap in which you simultaneously plant nonkicking foot next to ball while swinging lower part of kicking leg backward.

   4.   Forcefully bring kicking leg forward and kick ball with toe or instep.

   5.   Allow kicking leg to follow through up into the air.

   B.   Break into five kicking stations (five students per station) to work on kicking skills. Have a picture of the correct kicking pattern at each station, and emphasize correct pattern to students. Once stations have been set up and students are practicing appropriately, teacher will monitor station #2 below (stations are listed below). Students should stay at each station for 3–5 minutes and move on teacher's command.

   1.   Kicking beach balls as far as possible

   2.   Kicking Nerf balls as hard as possible against a wall (vary distance from wall for each student)

   3.   Kicking and knocking down plastic bowling pins or bottles

   4.   Kicking Nerf balls over small target volleyball net hung low to ground)

   5.   Kicking balloons as far as possible

Sue—   Substitute throwing for kicking at all stations (have a picture of throwing from a wheelchair and make sure she is working on components from her short-term objective).

IV.   Reinforcing game

   A.   "Kicking—Clean Up Your Backyard." Class is divided into two teams with each team standing on either side of a volleyball net hung down to the ground. Each team is given several balloons, beach balls, and Nerf balls. Teacher explains that the purpose of the game is to kick the ball over the net to the other team. At the end of the game, the team that has the *least* number of balls on its side is the winner. Emphasize using proper kicking pattern when kicking the balls and balloons. Begin kicking on teacher's command and play for approximately 2 minutes. Rest, reinforce, and repeat if time permits.

Sue—   Sue is allowed to throw rather than kick.

   —   If she cannot reach balls, make sure her team members continue to give her balls during the game.

V.   Concluding activity

   A.   Students sit in squads.

   B.   Review components of kicking and reinforce specific students for doing certain components exceptionally well.

   C.   Encourage students to practice kicking during recess and at home.

   D.   Have students close eyes and take three deep breaths.

   E.   Call squads to line up at door and leave with classroom teacher.

Table 9.7.   Example of activities to promote the overhand throw

1. Throw over targets.
2. Throw to knock down bowling pins or plastic bottles.
3. Throw to pop balloons taped to the wall.
4. Color-code lines on the floor and encourage student to move to lines farther and farther away from wall.
5. Throw bean bags at wall to see how loud a sound can be made.
6. Throw water balloons against wall (on warm days outside!).
7. Throw balls through a large, suspended hula hoop.
8. Throw bean bags at a large cardboard box, trying to get the box to move.
9. Throw bean bags at a large blow-up toy, trying to knock it over.
10. Use yarn balls and play "throwing dodge ball."
11. Throw at an old screen (screen that is used to show slides or movies) to make a loud noise.
12. Throw chalkboard erasers as far as possible to make chalk marks on the floor.

Important information at this level includes how often the regular students receive physical education, how long it takes the student with disabilities to learn particular skills, how long it takes to prepare particular students, and a student's behaviors. For example, in Sue's school, regular physical education is given twice a week. In addition, some of Sue's goals can be worked on during daily recess (i.e., playground skills) and during other times during the day (i.e., wheelchair mobility). Still, it takes a long time for Sue to acquire skills, and even though she does not have any behavior problems and it does not take much time to prepare her, she will need extra physical education if she is going to achieve her goals. The team decides that Sue can receive adapted physical education twice a week with other students who need work on individual skills, including students without disabilities who are having trouble in regular physical education. During this time Sue can work on throwing, catching, striking, dribbling, and shooting with the help of an older peer tutor. Other students work on individual skills prescribed as needed by the regular physical educator. For example, Bill and Ahmad are third graders who, while not labeled disabled, have problems with endurance. During their individual time they are working on jogging or walking continuously and riding a bicycle around the gym to improve their endurance.

The second question to ask is, where will physical education services and specific goals and objectives be provided? In most cases, physical education services will be provided within the regular setting. For example, Sue's program can be easily incorporated into the regular program, and her individual IEP goals can be embedded throughout the typical lesson plans. (See Figure 9.2 for an example.) In addition, Sue will receive supplementary programming in a remedial/ adapted physical education class that is open to all students at Sue's school, including students without disabilities.

Activities in regular physical education	Sue's IEP objectives					
	Swimming	Wheelchair	Throw	Catch	Strike	Pass
1. Moves from class to gym.		X				
2. Warm-ups		X				
3. Kicking/trapping (instruction and stations)			X	X		X
4. Kicking relays		X	X	X		X

Figure 9.2.   Sue's objectives and where they will be embedded into regular physical education (kicking unit).

It may be appropriate for some students to receive part of their program in an alternative setting. For example, a student with severe autistic-like tendencies who has difficulty in large group settings might receive physical education in the cafeteria, on the stage, or in a large hallway with three or four peers without disabilities. While the program mimics the activities that take place in regular physical education, the setting can be altered to accommodate this student. As the student begins to feel more comfortable with physical education and larger groups, he or she can be gradually included in the larger group. Similarly, older elementary students might participate in a community-based physical education/recreation program in which they go swimming, bowling, skating, or to other community-based recreation facilities to practice functional leisure skills. If, for example, Sue's community had an indoor pool available, she may very well have gone swimming once a week with a small group of peers without disabilities to work on her swimming goals.

The third question to ask is, how much preparation is needed for the student to fully benefit from regular physical education? Recall from Chapter 4 that preparation is usually needed for students with cerebral palsy (stretching, relaxation exercises, positioning) and for students with behavior disorders (transitioning). In Sue's case, no special preparation is needed for her to participate in regular physical education although she is fed through her G-tube just prior to physical education to make sure she has adequate energy.

The fourth question to ask is, what cues and prompts will each student need? Cues vary from verbal prompts to demonstrations and picture cues to varying levels of physical assistance. In Sue's case, she does well with verbal cues and demonstrations, and she does not mind physical assistance to cue her. (See Figure 9.3.) In addition, she can use picture cues to help her see what the correct throwing pattern should look like, she can look in a mirror to get feedback, and she can have peers at her station give her feedback regarding her throwing pattern.

Other students may have difficulty with certain types of cues. For example, a student with a more severe visual impairment than Sue's might need more verbal and physical prompting versus demonstrations, while a student who is deaf will need more demonstrations. Some students with autistic-like tendencies do not like to be touched (i.e., tactually defensive); thus, these students may do better with demonstrations and verbal cues rather than physical prompts. Still others might do well with extra environmental cues such as footprints on the floor or color-coding to

---

Directions: Instruct student in various situations. (See below.) Note how student responds to each type of cue or combination of cues. You may need to repeat in various instructional situations (e.g., outside versus inside; simple skills versus more complex skills).

	Responds correctly	Delayed response (5–10 seconds)	Does not respond
Verbal cues	✓		
Gestures	✓		
Demonstration	✓		
Environmental cues		✓	
Physical assistance	Does not mind if used		

Situations in which this assessment was conducted (whether formally or informally):

✓ Inclusive physical education setting with peers without disabilities (large group)

_____ Inclusive physical education setting with small groups (5–7 students)

_____ Inclusive physical education setting: one-on-one instruction

Figure 9.3. Sample checklist to determine Sue's communication skills.

highlight toward which basket to shoot. The special education teacher and the speech therapist are probably the best resources for determining how best to communicate and cue particular students.

Finally, the last question to ask is, what specific types of modifications and adapted equipment should be implemented to ensure a student's success? Modifications can include teaching methods (direct versus indirect), changes in rules (special zone, no one can steal the ball from student), and changes in requirements (shorter distances to move, more time to throw). Adapted equipment includes any changes in the equipment used by peers without disabilities. Changes can include lighter bats for students who have limited strength, lower baskets and smaller balls for shorter, smaller students, and support aids for students with balance problems. (See chaps. 6 and 7, this volume, for more detail.) The adapted physical education specialist, regular physical educator, physical therapist, special education teacher, and other team members can recommend specific modifications and adapted equipment for each student for developing specific skills.

For example, if Sue is working on throwing, specific curricular adaptations that are appropriate for Sue could be developed by the team. (See Figure 9.4.) Given that Sue has normal intelligence, she can do well with verbal cues, demonstrations, picture cues, and specific feedback. She also should be given a smaller, more graspable ball (e.g., yarn ball) and a shorter distance to throw to accommodate her problems with grip and arm strength. In addition, varying the activities to maintain her motivation should be included in the program. Figure 9.5 provides pictures of how to teach a student who uses a wheelchair to perform an overhand throw. Figure 9.6 provides a list of possible variations to help maintain Sue's interest.

Some students will need more assistance and/or special equipment in order to practice individual goals and objectives during specific activities in regular physical education (i.e., warm-ups, skill focus, and reinforcing game). Again, here is where suggestions described in Chapters 6 and 7 can be applied to specific activities. Utilizing a typical physical education lesson (i.e., warm-up, skill focus, reinforcing game), there are several modifications that can be implemented to accommodate students with varying abilities. For example, a student who has a hearing impairment can copy his peers' performance during warm-ups while a student who has a visual impairment can have a peer provide extra verbal cues plus occasional physical assistance. A student with significant mental retardation can work on learning how to jump while his peers work on applying movement concepts to more advanced locomotor patterns such as hopping and skipping. Similarly, a student with severe cerebral palsy can be assisted in special range-of-motion activities by a physical therapist, teacher, teacher assistant, or parent while the rest of the class works on more traditional warm-up activities.

There are many individual modifications that can be implemented during skill focus. Modifications can range from having peers assist students with disabilities to using adapted equipment or trained assistants. For example, a peer can help a student with muscular dystrophy retrieve balls or help a student with a visual impairment locate the proper station and equipment. For students whose goals are similar to their peers but whose skill level is significantly lower, modifications can include allowing students to work on skills at an appropriate level or making minor adjustments to the requirements of the task. For example, if the class is working on applying movement concepts to skipping, a student with significant mental retardation can be allowed to work on acquiring all the components of a skillful jump. Also, the student can work on a lower level of throwing such as throwing overhand consistently or shifting weight while the class works on applying an already acquired skillful throwing pattern to hitting moving targets. Minor adjustments that accommodate the needs of students with specific disabilities include giving extra verbal cues, demonstrations, or physical assistance to students with mental retardation or learning disabilities, lowering targets or making targets larger for students with problems in strength or accuracy, using slower-moving, lighter balls for catching or striking for students with limited coordination, allowing students with limited strength to stand closer than their peers, allowing

Does the student have limited strength?

Things to consider

Shorten distance to move or project object.

Use lighter equipment (e.g., balls, bats).

Use shorter striking implements.

Allow student to sit or lie down while playing.

Use deflated balls or suspended balls.

Change requirements (a few jumps, then run).

Selected modifications (if any) and Comments

Sit closer for shorter throw.

Lighter, more graspable bat / ball

—

—

Throw 3 balls, rest, then 3 more

Does the student have limited speed?

Things to consider

Shorten distance (or make it longer for others).

Change locomotor pattern (allow running v. walking).

Make safe areas in tag games.

Selected modifications (if any) and Comments

Shorten distance to throw

Can push chair during warm-ups

—

Does the student have limited endurance?

Things to consider

Shorten distance.

Shorten playing field.

Allow "safe" areas in tag games.

Decrease activity time for student.

Allow more rest periods for student.

Allow student to sit while playing.

Selected modifications (if any) and Comments

Shorten distance in warm-ups

—

—

—

Throw a few, then rest

—

Does the student have limited balance?

Things to consider

Provide chair/bar for support.

Teach balance techniques (widen base, extend arms).

Increase width of beams to be walked.

Use carpeted rather than slick surfaces.

Teach student how to fall.

Allow student to sit during activity.

Place student near wall for support.

Allow student to hold peer's hand.

Selected modifications (if any) and Comments

Does student have limited coordination and accuracy?

Things to consider

Use stationary balls for kicking/striking.

Decrease distance for throwing, kicking, and shooting.

Make targets and goals larger.

Use larger balls for kicking and striking.

Increase surface of the striking implements.

Use backstop.

Use softer, slower balls for striking and catching.

In bowling-type games, use lighter, less stable pins.

What can you do to maximize safety?

Selected modifications (if any) and Comments

—

Decrease distance to throw

Larger target, or just throw for distance

—

—

Have peers help retrieve balls

Bean bags or yarn balls

—

—

Note: Some or all of these modifications can be implemented. Also, these modifications can be implemented for one student, for several students, or for the entire class to make the activity more challenging and success-oriented.

Figure 9.4. Checklist to determine curricular adaptations to accommodate individuals with specific limitations (Sue) in throwing activities.

Task Analysis

1. Assume the ready position for the softball throw.
2. Initiate the throw by pushing the left arm slightly to the right, then pulling it back down to the left.
3. Raise the right shoulder as the left shoulder drops, keeping the right arm up.
4. Push the right elbow forward and extend the forearm high over the right leg.
5. Release the ball at a high position, snapping the fingers.
6. Let the right arm follow-through in front of the right shoulder (i.e., in the direction of the throw).
7. Exit the throwing area from the back.

Coaching Suggestions

1. Tell the athlete to use the non-throwing (left) arm as a lever for raising the opposite—or throwing—shoulder.
2. Concentrate on keeping the throwing (right) arm up and releasing the ball at a high position.
3. Have the athlete practice throwing the ball over a high object placed close to him or her (e.g., a volleyball net) in order to work on releasing it at a high position.

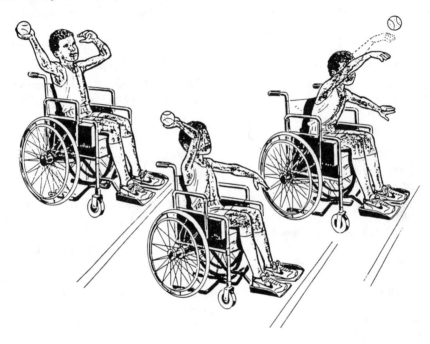

Figure 9.5.   Instructional program to teach throwing from a wheelchair. (From Special Olympics International. [1986]. *Athletics sports skills guide*, p. 50. Washington, DC: Author; reprinted by permission.)

students with limited endurance to practice locomotor patterns for shorter amounts of time, or allowing students with balance difficulties to use a wider balance beam or walk on wide lines on the floor (see chap. 7, this volume, for more detail). Students with more significant disabilities and whose goals and objectives are different than their peers may need more intense accommodations in order to work on their individual goals and objectives. For many, accommodations will include trained assistants and/or special equipment. For example, a student with severe cerebral palsy learning how to walk can practice this skill while his peers work on more advanced locomotor patterns. The student may be assisted by a trained volunteer, teacher assistant, or even a physical therapist and may require special equipment such as canes, crutches, or a walker. Similarly, a student with an upper extremity amputation who is learning how to use a prosthetic device can work on grasping during striking activities, perhaps with the assistance of the occupational therapist.

Modifications to reinforcing games also can vary from providing extra cues, to using adapted equipment, to making changes in the rules of the game for the student or for the entire class. (See Figure 9.6 for suggestions for Sue.) For example, some students may only need a few extra cues to

Things to consider	Selected modifications (if any) and Comments
Can you vary the purpose/goal of the game (e.g., some students play to learn complex strategies, others play to work on simple motor skills)?	Focus on throwing & pushing chair, and bending over to pick up balls
Can you vary number of players (e.g., play small games such as 2 v. 2 basketball)?	—
Can you vary movement requirements (e.g., some students walk, others run; some hit a ball off a tee, others hit pitched ball; skilled students use more complex movements, less skilled use simpler movements)?	She can push chair to get balls
Can you vary the field of play (e.g., special zones for students with less mobility; make the field narrower or wider as needed; shorten the distance for students with movement problems)?	Place Sue closer to net
Can you vary objects used (e.g., some students use lighter bats/larger balls; some use a lower net/basket)?	Sue can use more graspable balls
Can you vary the level of organization (Vary typical organizational patterns; vary where certain students stand; vary the level of structure for certain students.)?	Sue can be closer to net
Can you vary the limits/expectations (Vary the number of turns each student receives; vary the rules regarding how far a student can run, hit, etc.; vary how much you will enforce certain rules for certain players.)?	Give Sue a pile of bean bags that only she can throw; allow her to be closer to throw.

Note: Use these suggestions to modify rules for both students with and without disabilities to make the game challenging, safe, and success-oriented.

Figure 9.6. Checklist to determine curricular modifications for group games and sports for Sue in "Clean Up Your Backyard." (Use these suggestions to modify rules for both students with and without disabilities to make the game challenging, safe, and success-oriented.) (Adapted from Morris and Stiehl [1989].)

understand the rules of the game such as a carpet square or cone to mark key boundaries (e.g., cone marking where to run in a relay race). Other students may need to be positioned so that they get more turns (closer to where the ball usually lands), so that they are in a safer position (farther away from where the ball usually lands), or close to support for balance or stability (near a wall or a bar). Others may be allowed an advantage in relay races (move a shorter distance) or tag games (must be tagged three times before being out). Still other students may need a peer to provide assistance such as having a peer retrieve balls and direct a student with a visual impairment in "Clean Up Your Backyard" or running beside the student during a relay race. Students with more significant disabilities can be given teacher assistants or therapists for partners, can have special zones where they are the only ones allowed to get the ball or object, or can be allowed to use special equipment such as smaller balls, lower baskets, or mobility devices.

The general format of the game also can be changed to allow a student with a disability to safely and meaningfully participate in group games. For example, competitive relay races or games of tag can be changed to cooperative formats (addition tag in which tagged persons hold the hands of the tagger, thus making a large chain of taggers versus sitting out when tagged) or Morris's Games Design Model can be utilized. (See Chapter 6 for more detail.)

In more extreme situations, students can play alternative games with selected peers to the side of the gym. For example, if the class is playing an active lead-up game of soccer, it may be inappropriate and unsafe to include a student with autistic behaviors who is unaware of his surroundings. An alternative game for this student might be passing a ball back and forth with two peers to the side of the gym or in the hallway under the supervision of a trained volunteer or teacher assistant. The student can then be gradually weaned into the more active game for longer and longer periods of time. Peers without disabilities can rotate into the quieter game with this student so that they only miss a few minutes of the more active group game. Similarly, a student with a physical disability can work with one or two peers to the side of the gym on a game using a switch or special piece of equipment as defined in her individual program (e.g., hand-held computer soccer game). Depending on the abilities of the student, peers without disabilities can provide assistance or a trained volunteer or teacher assistant can provide assistance. Again, peers without disabilities can be rotated over to play the adapted game (which may actually be interesting and reinforcing for students without disabilities) so that they only miss a few turns in the regular game.

The above are just a few examples of how typical elementary physical education activities can be modified to accommodate students with disabilities. Information in Chapters 6 and 7 provide many specific examples of modifications that can be applied to elementary physical education. In addition, when a student's goals and objectives are so different from his or her peers or when a particular disability is such that there is a question whether or not certain activities are potentially dangerous, the regular physical educator should consult with members of the PEIT, including the special education teacher, adapted physical education specialist, physical therapist, or parent. (See chap. 3, this volume, for more information on the PEIT.) The important point when making modifications is that the student's individual goals and objectives continue to be the focus. Making modifications so that the student with disabilities can participate with his or her peers is not enough. Modifications should be designed so that the student is working on specific goals and objectives while remaining in the regular setting. In most cases, goals and objectives of elementary school–age students with disabilities will somewhat overlap the general goals and objectives of the class. When the student's goals and objectives do not match, then alternative activities can be implemented within the regular setting so that the student still has an opportunity to work on his or her individual program.

4. Determine Who Will Assist Student

The next step in the model is to determine who will assist the student while he or she is in regular physical education. Some students may not need any extra support, some only need peers for assistance, while still others may need trained volunteers or teacher assistants. For Sue, the regular physical educator and her peers should be able to accommodate some of her needs. (See Figure 9.7.) For example, Sue's peers can help her retrieve balls when she cannot reach them or in other situations as the need arises, and the regular physical educator can provide reinforcement and instructional feedback to Sue throughout each lesson. Still, the regular physical educator will probably need extra assistance if Sue is going to receive needed individual instruction. In Sue's case, a trained, older peer, volunteer, or teacher assistant could help her work on some of her specific goals such as pushing her wheelchair correctly or working on the proper throwing and catching techniques. Specific modifications and teaching techniques (see above) can be developed by an adapted physical education specialist and/or physical therapist, then carried out by these support persons. (See Figure 9.7.) Older peers are often an underutilized resource for physical educators, yet they can be excellent assistants to students with disabilities. Older peers (e.g., upper elementary school–age students) tend to be a little more mature and responsible and can take direction from the regular physical educator or from written instructions prepared by other team members. While the use of peers can be effective, peers should not miss out on their own

	Locker room	Warm-ups	Skills	Games
Can you handle having __Sue__ in these situations without extra support?		No	No	No
If NO, could you handle situation with consultation from specialists? If yes, from which specialists would you like consultative support? (See below.)		APE, PT	APE, PT	APE, PT
Can you handle situation on your own with consultative support?		No	No	No
If NO, could peers in class provide enough extra support (without drastically affecting their program)?		Some	Some	Some
If NO, could an older peer tutor or volunteer provide enough support?		Yes	Yes	Yes
If NO, could a trained teacher assistant provide enough support?		—	—	—
If NO, could a regular visit from a specialist provide enough support? If yes, which specialists would you like for direct support? (See below.)		—	—	—

Comments:

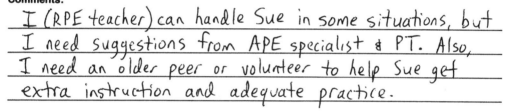

I (RPE teacher) can handle Sue in some situations, but I need suggestions from APE specialist & PT. Also, I need an older peer or volunteer to help Sue get extra instruction and adequate practice.

Key:

APE specialist, Adapted Physical Education Specialist (modifications to physical education).

SE, Special Educator (behavior management, personality, interests).

P, Parent (interests, personality, behaviors, homework).

PT, Physical therapist (gross motor needs, adapted equipment, positioning, contraindicated activities).

OT, Occupational therapist (fine motor skills, adapted equipment).

ST, Speech therapist (communication skills).

VT, Vision therapist (visual skills, adaptations, mobility skills).

Figure 9.7. Checklist for determining general supports in regular physical education for Sue.

physical education programs while they assist a student with disabilities. Peers who are taken from the same physical education class as the student with disabilities should be tutors for only part of the period or for 1 day per month as opposed to working with the student all day every day. Another possibility is to assign two or three peers to work with the student who has disabilities so that they can each take their turn while one of the others works with the student. One final suggestion is to have students who have already mastered targeted skills work with the student who has disabilities. This way, the student will not be missing out on practice of skills he or she has already mastered.

It also is important that peer tutors who will be providing ongoing assistance to particular students go through some formal training. Training can be conducted by members of the PEIT. In addition, the regular physical educator and the adapted physical education specialist should provide peer tutors with ongoing information on how to work with the student. Other PEIT members also can provide specific teaching techniques (including pictures) and behavior management procedures so that the peer can optimize the type of assistance he or she provides.

Volunteers are yet another often untapped resource that can be used to provide extra assistance to students with disabilities in regular physical education. Some schools have a bank of volunteers who can provide assistance to students with disabilities. Volunteers are usually parents of other students in the school, retired persons who live in the community, college students who are majoring in education, or high school students who are required to do some type of public service. As was the case above, it is extremely important that these volunteers go through some formal training program before they assist any student. In addition, volunteers should be given direct instruction from the regular physical educator as well as written instructions from the PEIT on what to do and how to do it, as well as where and when to do it. (See chap. 4, this volume, for more information on how to prepare volunteers, peers, and teacher assistants.)

Choosing the exact person to assist a student should be a thoughtful decision based on the student's abilities and disabilities, the type of regular physical education program that is run (i.e., direct versus indirect instruction), number of children in the class, and type of activity (e.g., gymnastics would require more assistance while rhythms might require less). The important point is that choosing persons to work with students with disabilities as well as the training they go through should be a systematic process that includes input from all team members.

5. Preparing Staff and Students for Inclusion

The next step in the model is to prepare key staff members and students without disabilities for inclusion. Regular physical educators should be briefed by special education staff and other members and how it affects physical education, medical/health concerns, any contraindicated activities, and present level of performance on physical and motor skills. Members of the PEIT can provide this information and, in addition, any other information that can help the regular physical educator present information more effectively and prevent behavior problems. Such information should include how to work with the student, the student's receptive and expressive language ability, the student's ability to follow directions, any inappropriate behaviors the student might have as well as what triggers the behaviors, and things that reinforce the student. (See Table 9.8 for an example.) Ideally, the regular physical educator should go to the student's class to meet the student and get to know his or her abilities, behaviors, and disabilities.

Other staff members and volunteers who will be directly responsible for assisting the student with disabilities in regular physical education also should receive some in-service training. Some of the training will be similar to the types of information given to the regular physical educator. In addition, the regular physical educator should provide information to assistants and volunteers regarding the regular physical education curriculum, normal routines, what he or she expects of the assistant, and any other information that will help the assistant in regular physical education. This information should be presented by the regular physical educator at various times throughout the year.

For example, a gymnastic unit may be run differently than a rhythms and dance unit, which is run differently from a ball skills unit. The regular physical educator should try to keep the assistant informed about the regular physical education at least a few days prior to instruction. Information can be transmitted by a simple note explaining the lesson and if he or she anticipates any special problems for the student. (See Figure 9.8 for an example.)

Table 9.8. Example of general information about a student with mental retardation

1. Communication Skills
   Understands one-word commands; can imitate simple demonstrations (make sure he is looking at you); sometimes responds slowly to verbal directions (takes several seconds for information to sink in); responds well to physical assistance.

2. Behaviors
   Generally well-behaved although he can be very distractible. Has short attention span (maybe 1–2 minutes), and does not sit for very long periods. Can easily be brought back to activity with reminders from peers. Sometimes self-stimulates on balls (likes to spin them in his hand). May hug friends; try to discourage this.

3. Reinforcers
   Loves balls, loves to run, loves to swing, loves to look at bright-colored shirts. Does not like to lie down or sit for long periods.

4. Medical Concerns
   Has a seizure disorder that is controlled with medication (has not had a seizure in 2 years). Wears glasses for looking at books, but will probably not wear them to gym. Doctor said that he has no restrictions in physical activity.

5. Special Friends
   Favorite classmate is Jake, and Jake likes to work with him. He also likes Billy. He does not do well with Terry or Jim.

Finally, students without disabilities should be given information about the student with disabilities. For students with disabilities who have no particular behavior problems, you may only need to inform the class that a student with a disability will be in the class and may need occasional help in certain activities. Students can then be encouraged to ask questions as needed. For a

---

MEMORANDUM

From: Terri Jones, Physical Educator
To: Teacher assistants/volunteers working with students with disabilities

We will be beginning a gymnastics unit next week. Please ask your student's special education teacher to check your student's medical file and, if necessary, call the student's parents to see if he or she can do all of the activities in our unit. Activities I anticipate doing include:

stretching
balance activities
log rolls
egg rolls
forward rolls
backward rolls
cartwheels
round offs
head stands

My tentative lesson format is as follows:

Introduction
Warm-ups (stretching/strengthening activities)
Skill focus (four mats set up with students lined up behind mats taking turns doing various rolls)
Conclusion (cool down with balance activities and simple pyramids)

Thanks! Please contact me if you have any questions. Terri

Figure 9.8. Sample physical educator-to-teacher assistant note.

student with more visible disabilities such as a visual impairment, hearing impairment, or physical disability, you may want to give more specific information about the students, how they will
bers of the PEIT regarding pertinent information about any student with a disability who will be
integrated into their class. Pertinent information includes a description of the student's disability
need certain modifications to be successful, and how other students can help. You may want to do
some role-playing so that students without disabilities gain a better appreciation of the challenges
the students with disabilities face.

6. Implementing the Program

The next step in the model is to implement the program and conduct ongoing evaluation. If available, an adapted physical education specialist should attend as many early class sessions as possible
as well as keep in touch with regular physical educators through telephone conversations and notes.
In addition, key members of the PEIT should be present as much as possible during the first few
times the student is included in regular physical education to give specific information to the regular
physical educator and to make sure initial modifications and teaching techniques are appropriate. For
example, the special education teacher should be there when students with mental retardation or
behavior problems are included, a physical or occupational therapist should be there when students with physical disabilities are included, and a vision therapist should be there when a student
with a visual impairment is being included. PEIT members who do not provide direct instruction
with the student should still check back with the regular physical educator on a regular basis (at
least once a month) to make sure the student is being included safely and successfully. Therapists
also can act as a student's one-on-one assistant in regular physical education once a week or so to
probe how well the student is doing and to provide suggestions to the regular physical educator
and assistants.

Ongoing evaluation of the student's individual goals and objectives is extremely important to
determine the effectiveness of the program. However, collecting evaluation data can be difficult
for the regular physical educator who must monitor all his or her students. Simple data sheets can
be developed by members of the PEIT (ideally, the adapted physical education specialist) that can
help the regular physical educator collect ongoing data. (See Figures 9.9 and 9.10 for examples.)
With training, upper elementary–age peer tutors, volunteers, and teacher assistants can learn
how to evaluate how well a student with disabilities is doing toward achieving his or her goals. At
least one of the PEIT members (ideally, the adapted physical education specialist) should check
the data every few weeks and conduct his or her own assessment to verify the progress each
student is making. While this method may not be perfect, at least there is some effort to measure
student progress. Ongoing evaluation allows the team to make adjustments to the student's program, to the assistants working with him or her, to the setting, and/or to the equipment that the
student is using.

SUMMARY

Since much of what takes place in elementary physical education is appropriate for elementary
school–age students with disabilities, it is relatively easy to modify regular physical education
activities to include students with disabilities. In fact, good elementary physical education programs are already individualized to meet the needs of the range of motor abilities typically found
in any grade level. Including students with disabilities is just extending the range of abilities and
thus the range of pre-existing modifications. In many cases, such modifications are quite simple,
involving such things as allowing students to use different size balls or demonstrate locomotor
patterns different from those of their peers. In other cases, students with disabilities will need
more extensive modifications and support to be meaningfully and successfully included in regular
physical education.

Developmental Sequences for Catching

Directions: Mark the date on the line that best describes the catching pattern exhibited by the child.

Clinician/Semester: _____/_____

Clinician/Semester: _____/_____

Child's name: _____ DOB.: _____   Clinician/Semester: _____/_____

Component	Assessment Dates					
	pre	post	pre	post	pre	post
Body action:						
1. No adjustment of body to flight of ball	____	____	____	____	____	____
2. Arms and trunk begin to move in relation to flight path of ball	____	____	____	____	____	____
3. Feet, arm, and trunk all move to adjust to flight path of ball	____	____	____	____	____	____
Arm action:						
1. Arms remain outstretched and elbows rigid with little "give"	____	____	____	____	____	____
2. Elbows flexed slightly; ball is trapped with arms and chest	____	____	____	____	____	____
3. Initial contact with hands, but child still may need to trap with chest	____	____	____	____	____	____
4. Ball contact is made with hands; elbows and shoulders "give" with ball	____	____	____	____	____	____
Hand action:						
1. Palms of hands face upward	____	____	____	____	____	____
2. Palms of hands face each other; fingers face outward	____	____	____	____	____	____
3. Palms of hands adjust to flight and size of ball (thumbs together for high ball; little fingers together for low ball)	____	____	____	____	____	____

Figure 9.9. Ongoing evaluation form for elementary physical education. (Adapted from Roberton and Halverson [1984].)

Activity: Throwing

Trials	Does student step when throwing?	Student's effort
1.		
2.		
3.		
4.		
5.		
6.		
7.		
8.		
9.		
10.		
11.		
12.		
13.		
14.		

Skill key: +   steps   +v   steps when told   o   does not step
Effort key: +   tries to step   o   doesn't try, but doesn't resist assistance   –   resists assistance

Figure 9.10. Sample ongoing evaluation form for elementary physical education program.

The purpose of this chapter is to present an extended example of how a student with a disability can be included in regular elementary school physical education. It is hoped that this example demonstrates how the concepts and suggestions presented in Chapters 4 through 7 can be applied to elementary school physical education programs.

Chapter 10

Including Middle and High School Students with Disabilities in Regular Physical Education

We started a peer tutoring program in which our juniors and seniors who had completed their physical education requirement and had an interest in special education or one of the therapies assisted our students with moderate and severe disabilities in physical education. Each student without disabilities was trained and then paired up with a student with a disability, and they worked together throughout the year. Later, we opened the program to all students at Lewiston High School, and now we have twice as many students trying to get involved in the program as there are students with disabilities.

Perhaps the greatest effect of this program was on the attitudes of our students without disabilities. Our students without disabilities learned to accept students with disabilities during physical education, and this quickly carried over to other school events. In fact, many of our partners without disabilities befriended their partners, taking them to movies, ball games, and school functions. At the same time, our students with disabilities became more communicative and better behaved when they were with their partners. Even their mannerisms became more 'normal looking.' The interactions between our students with and without disabilities really helped both groups of students.

—Bob Brainerd

INTRODUCTION

Ahmed is a 16-year-old who is a 10th grader at Abraham Lincoln High School. Ahmed loves school, and his favorite subject is physical education. He also enjoys going to Lincoln High football and basketball games with friends, and he especially enjoys going out for pizza or burgers after the game. Ahmed hopes to graduate from Lincoln with his class, then get a job in town. This is Ahmed's second year at Lincoln, but he did not matriculate to Lincoln via Prairie View, Smith, or Southwest Middle School as did most of his classmates. Ahmed spent the previous 9 years of his education at Hope Center, a special school designed for students who have significant disabilities that was closed 2 years ago when the school system decided to move to a full-inclusion model.

Bob Brainerd is director of physical education at Lewiston High School, Lewiston, Maine.

241

Ahmed went to Hope Center because he has mental retardation, the result of prematurity and anoxia (lack of oxygen) at birth. In addition to mental retardation, Ahmed has no intelligible speech, limited understanding of what others say, an inability to read or write, an extremely short attention span, limited functional motor skills (although he can walk and run), and a seizure disorder that is controlled with medication.

Ahmed is one of 15 students from Hope Center who now go to Lincoln. Last year, the first year Ahmed and his classmates from Hope Center were enrolled at Lincoln, the regular physical education staff members were a little nervous about having Ahmed and his classmates in regular physical education. However, the adapted physical education specialist from Hope Center, along with other staff members from Hope Center, gave several in-services to Lincoln staff to help them adjust to having students with significant disabilities in their regular classes. In addition, key staff members from Lincoln, including regular physical education staff, went to Hope Center in the spring to visit and get to know the students who would be enrolled at Lincoln. Through ongoing support by the collaborative team, the regular physical education staff at Lincoln learned how to help Ahmed work on his specific program while being meaningfully included in regular physical education.

Including students with disabilities in regular middle school and high school physical education programs can pose more problems for the regular physical educator than including these same students into elementary school physical education. First, middle school and high school students are typically bigger, stronger, and faster than elementary school–age students. If a middle school or high school student collides with a student with a disability, particularly a frail student who has an orthopedic or health disability, the student with a disability is more likely to get hurt. Related to size and speed, middle school and high school games move much more quickly than elementary physical education games. Differences are immediately evident by comparing a soccer or basketball game played by high school students with one played by elementary school–age students.

Another problem is the skill and knowledge level of middle school and high school students. Many of these students have reached a skillful level of performance where their movements have become quite efficient and automatic, while many students with disabilities may still be learning the fundamental patterns of movements. This discrepancy can make it difficult to equalize games without causing the student with disabilities to fail or without drastically changing the nature of the game for the more skilled students. Similarly, many middle school and high school students understand the rules of various sports along with strategies that can help enhance performance, while many students with disabilities will not have this level of understanding. Again, discrepancies in cognitive abilities make it difficult to equalize games, particularly more complex team sports such as football and basketball.

Finally, the attitudes of middle school and high school students without disabilities toward persons with disabilities can be problematic. While elementary school–age students may be tolerant of students with disabilities, some middle school and high school students fiercely attack (with verbal abuse, teasing, and pranks) persons who are different, including persons with disabilities. Unlike most academic classes in which individual performance is not necessarily known to peers, physical education activities are performed in an open arena in which other members of the class observe individual performances. Thus, a student with a disability who has limited motor skills is more likely to stand out in physical education (and be subject to ridicule) than in other courses.

While the prospects of including students with disabilities in regular middle school and high school physical education seem bleak, it is possible. In fact, depending on the way the regular program is organized, including students with disabilities in regular middle and high school physical education can be as easy as in elementary school. The purpose of this chapter is to suggest specific ways in which children with disabilities can be safely and meaningfully included in regular middle and high school physical education programs. The following will be specifically addressed in this chapter: 1) description of typical middle school and high school physical education programs, 2) application of the planning and programming model outlined in Chapter 4 to high school students with disabilities, and 3) specific examples of how Ahmed can be successfully included in regular physical education programs.

Middle School and High School Physical Education

As was the case with elementary physical education, middle school and high school physical education programs vary from school to school and from teacher to teacher. However, differences are not quite as evident as in elementary school programs. For example, most middle school and high school physical educators use a direct (command) style of teaching in which the teacher directs the students on what skills to perform, how to perform each skill, and where and when to practice the skill. Most middle school and high school physical educators would argue that such an approach provides them with more control of the class and affords them a more efficient way to teach the specific techniques needed for popular sport skills. Similarly, most middle school and high school physical educators follow a format in which a group warm-up is followed by skill work and a group activity. Finally, most programs tend to follow the same general content (i.e., improvement of physical fitness and development of individual and team sport skills). Table 10.1 provides an example of the types of activities that are included in middle school and high school physical education curricula. Note that individual school systems as well as physical education staff will usually present only selected activities from the list. What activities are actually presented will vary based on availability of equipment and facilities, cultural popularity of particular activities, and skills and interests of the physical education staff. For example, many schools in the northeastern United States will offer lacrosse, schools in the midwest may offer ice hockey, and schools in the Rockies may offer skiing. However, the content in most middle school and high school physical education programs across the country will be fairly similar. In addition, some high schools allow their juniors and seniors to choose in what activities they wish to participate. For example, some programs set up 9-week units in which students can choose between tennis, aerobics, weight training, and basketball. Thus, students have an opportunity to choose between team sports, individual sports, and physical fitness. Such programs tend to be more motivating and appealing for students, rather than being told on what they have to work.

What will vary is how much time a physical educator devotes to each activity as well as how much time he or she devotes to actually teaching the skills versus playing the games. Some physical educators prefer to teach skills in extended units of 4–6 weeks or more. This allows students to work on the proper techniques of skills, learn the rules of the various activities, and apply these skills and rules to actual games. However, some physical educators prefer to teach a particular activity for 1–2 week units. (Some even change activities from day to day.) Shorter units limit the

Table 10.1.   Typical content of middle school and high school physical education program

Team sports	Individual sports	Fitness	Dance
Soccer	Tennis	Weight training	Square
Basketball	Golf	Aerobics	Folk
Football	Aquatics		Jazz
Volleyball	Archery		Aerobic
Speedball	Badminton		Modern
Softball	Bowling		
Lacrosse	Roller skating/blading		
Field hockey	Nordic/alpine skiing		
Ice hockey	Wrestling		
	Track and field		

amount of time a student has to learn and practice the various skills. In addition, students rarely have enough time to learn all the rules of the activity nor have a chance to apply their skills to actual games.

Similarly, some physical educators prefer to focus on teaching the critical skills required in each of the various activities while others focus on having students play the sport. Again, by focusing on skills, a physical educator is giving his or her students important instruction and practice time, ensuring that each student has an opportunity to acquire the critical skills for each sport. However, physical educators who allow their students to play games for the majority of the unit tend to limit critical instruction and practice needed by most students to acquire the skills. (See Wessel & Kelly, 1986, for a discussion on teaching skills versus playing games.)

How best to include a student with disabilities will be directly related to how the regular physical educator presents the program. For example, it would be easier to have a student with disabilities work on his or her individual goals in a middle school program that works on a particular unit such as soccer for several weeks versus a program in which units change every week or every other week. Longer units allow the student to work on skill development and begin to understand how to perform the critical skills of the activity as well as the rules of the activity. Similarly, it would be easier to include a student with a disability in a program that focuses on skill development versus a program where students play the games for most of the unit. Understandably, it is easier to work on a student's individual goals and to accommodate individual differences during skill work than in group games.

A SYSTEMATIC APPROACH TO INCLUDING STUDENTS WITH DISABILITIES IN REGULAR MIDDLE SCHOOL AND HIGH SCHOOL PHYSICAL EDUCATION

As was the case with the previous two chapters, the systematic approach outlined here follows the model described in Chapter 4.

1. Determine Student's Individual Goals and Objectives

The first step in including students with disabilities in middle school and high school regular physical education is to determine each student's strengths and weaknesses and then write specific long-term goals and short-term instructional objectives. Strengths and weaknesses should be referenced to real-life activities that are meaningful to the student; that is, skills that the student needs to be successful in his or her present environment (i.e., high school physical education, community-based recreation, special sports programs such as Special Olympics or wheelchair sports) as well as anticipated future environments (e.g., community-based recreation as an adult, special sports programs for adults such as Special Olympics or wheelchair sports). Unlike elementary school students who have several years before they graduate and move into community programs, middle school students, and especially high school students, have only a few years of school remaining. Thus, the majority of targeted activities will be referenced to what lifetime skills they will need upon graduation from school.

Ideally, the team should get together to determine what physical education and recreation activities are most important for each student. For example, Ahmed's team used the Curricular Decision Form in Figure 10.1 to determine which activities seemed most meaningful to Ahmed. Based on input from Ahmed's parents, select peers, the regular physical educator, and several therapists, activities that were targeted for Ahmed included weight training, aerobics, golf, and basketball or softball. These activities were selected because: 1) they were activities that were found in more than one category on the Curricular Decision Form (i.e., functional skill), and 2) the team thought that Ahmed had the greatest likelihood of acquiring the skills needed

---

Form for Curricular Decision Making

Directions: List all of the activities preferred or typically engaged in under the following headings. Scan across the list and place activities that are in more than one column under "Targeted Activities."

Student preferences	Parents' preferences	Activities in RPE	Activities played by peers	Community leisure activities
Enjoys most activities	That Ahmed	Tennis	Baseball	Tennis
	maintains his	Golf	Soccer	Golf/Mini-golf
	health &	Team sports	Riding bikes	Wt. training
	leisure skills	Dance		Softball
	upon	Conditioning/ Aerobics		Bowling
	graduation	Track		Roilerblading
				Karate, Aerobics Special Olympics

Targeted Activities: 1. Weight training   2. Aerobics

3. Golf   4. Basketball or softball
                                    (Also Special Olympics)

Figure 10.1. Sample form for making initial curricular decisions for Ahmed.

to participate in these activities. For example, while bike riding appeared in two categories, Ahmed's skills in bike riding were limited, and the team thought he would never be able to ride a bike independently on the trails that were available in his community.

Once the team has delineated targeted activities, the adapted physical education specialist (with support from other team members) can assess Ahmed on these activities and then write specific goals and objectives. Other team members, such as the student's special education teacher, the regular physical educator, parents, and the physical therapist, can work together to assess and plan the program for individual students in the event that the school system does not have an adapted physical education specialist. In Ahmed's case, the team wanted to assess Ahmed in a variety of physical education and recreation skills because they were not sure how well Ahmed would do in these activities. That is, the team did not know how Ahmed might do in some activities that were not targeted by the team. For example, even though golf was targeted over tennis, they were not sure if Ahmed might do better in tennis. Similarly, the team was not sure with which team sports Ahmed would have the most success, so they evaluated him on all the team sports presented in high school physical education. Results of the assessment suggest that Ahmed's skills are quite limited in most 10th-grade physical education activities, although he does enjoy all activities and did fairly well in hitting a golf ball, walking around the track with a Walkman, weight lifting, and shooting baskets. As suspected, Ahmed did better in golf than in tennis, and his best team sport was basketball. In recreation, Ahmed did best in miniature golf and bowling. (See Tables 10.2 and 10.3 for the results of Ahmed's assessment.) Note that some activities were not assessed in the community since they were already assessed in physical education. Also note that Ahmed's parents conducted the community-based assessment after school over the course of 2 weeks with guidance from the collaborative team (i.e., what specifically to look for).

With the results of the assessment completed, the team can develop an individualized education program (IEP) that includes a long-term plan, long-term goals, and short-term instructional objectives. Again, goals and objectives should be referenced to functional activities that are

Table 10.2.   Present level of performance statement from Ahmed's IEP (referenced to 10th-grade physical education)

Tennis:	Ahmed can hit a suspended tennis ball or a beach ball using a forehand stroke. He cannot hit a tossed or bounced tennis ball. He holds the racquet with two hands and uses his arms for a pushing motion rather than a twisting motion. He cannot hit with a backhand stroke or a serve. He can move toward balls hit to his left and right, but he cannot get his racquet in position quickly enough to hit the ball. He does not understand the rules of tennis. He enjoys chasing down the balls even though he cannot hit them.
Golf:	Ahmed did surprisingly well in hitting with a five iron off a tee. He had a stiff, jerky swing that was generated by arm action rather than trunk and leg action. He hit the ball successfully three out of four times, and one out of four of these hits caused the ball to travel as far as 25 yards. Ahmed really seemed to enjoy hitting the ball off the tee.
Soccer:	Ahmed can kick a stationary soccer ball so that the ball travels approximately 10'. He does plant his opposite foot next to the ball and shows some knee action in the kick but very little follow-through. He can kick a ball that is slowly rolling directly to him three out of four trials, but he has difficulty with faster moving balls. He cannot trap a ball with his feet, nor does he move to balls rolling to his side very well. He does not understand the rules of soccer, but he enjoys chasing the balls.
Volleyball:	Ahmed can set a beach ball or volley-trainer (large, lighter volleyball) when ball is tossed directly to him from 5'–10' away three out of four trials. He uses mostly his arms (very little knee bend), and his accuracy is poor (one out of four back to examiner). He tries to imitate a bump-and-serve pattern, but he is successful only one out of four trials. Again, he enjoys trying to hit the balls and chasing them when he is successful.
Basketball:	Ahmed can dribble a basketball with one hand three to five times in a row. He uses a slapping pattern with the palm of his hands contacting the ball. He cannot walk forward and dribble. Ahmed can demonstrate a chest bounce pass from 10' away and can catch a bounce pass with hands three out of four trials. Ahmed will try to imitate other passes but is less success-ful. Ahmed can shoot a basketball using a two-handed push shot so that the ball will hit the rim three out of four trials and go into the basket one out of four trials from 5' away. Ahmed tries to play defense but cannot keep up with his peers. He tries to rebound, but the ball usu-ally bounces off his hands. Ahmed does not understand the rules of basketball, but he enjoys playing catch and shooting.
Softball:	Ahmed can hit a softball off a tee so that ball travels 7'–10', but he cannot hit a pitched ball. He demonstrates a very stiff swing with mostly arm action. Ahmed can throw overhand so that the ball travels 10' to a teammate. He uses an immature arm action and steps with the same-side foot rather than the opposite foot. Ahmed can pick up grounders that are hit directly to him, and he can catch a softball with a mitt when the ball is tossed directly to him from 5'–7' away. Ahmed can run to first base, but he does not know where the other bases are. Ahmed gets bored when playing softball although he likes to hit the ball off the tee.
Dancing:	Ahmed enjoyed dancing, and he tries to follow the steps to the various dances. However, he usually is off beat and falls behind the class. He does try to imitate dance movements, and he can approximate most simple movements. He enjoys dancing with peers.
Track:	Ahmed will run for approximately 100 meters, but he prefers to walk. He can walk around the track several times if he is walking with a peer or if he has his Walkman on. He seems to enjoy walking, especially with peers.
Conditioning:	Ahmed was able to perform all the various weight lifting activities on the Universal machine in the weight room. He did need assistance to get into the machines and verbal cues to maintain proper cadence. His strength was slightly below his peers but not terribly bad for a 16-year-old. He enjoyed weight lifting and riding the stationary bike if he had his Walkman on.

meaningful for the student. With older students like Ahmed who have only a few years left before they graduate from school, meaningful activities will be lifetime leisure skills that he will need upon graduation. Ahmed's IEP can be found in Table 10.4.

Table 10.3. Present level of performance statement from Ahmed's IEP (referenced to community recreation)

Tennis:	(See previous assessment.)
Golf:	(See previous assessment.)
Aerobics:	(See previous assessment.)
Weight lifting:	(See previous assessment.)
Softball:	(See previous assessment.)
Mini-golf:	Ahmed was able to hold the putter correctly with verbal cues and putt the ball with some accuracy. He had trouble with control (he hit it too hard most of the time), but he seemed to enjoy the game.
Bowling:	Ahmed preferred rolling the ball between his legs, but with verbal cues he was able to place his fingers in the ball and roll the ball from a stationary position so that the ball made it down the lane. The ball went into the gutter four out of five times, but Ahmed did not seem to mind. He seemed to enjoy bowling.
Roller blading:	Ahmed could not stand up on Roller blades, and he seemed nervous on them.
Bike riding:	Ahmed can ride an adult three-wheel bike in an empty parking lot, but he really does not know how to steer or control speed. He can pedal a stationary bike well, and he enjoys riding a stationary bike if he has his Walkman on.
Karate:	Ahmed tried to follow the various stretches and movements, and the instructor was very patient with Ahmed. Still, he had a very hard time keeping up with the other students, and even though he tried to imitate movements, he was rarely close to what was expected of the class. He did not particularly enjoy karate.

Note: Ahmed's parents took Ahmed to the various recreation facilities and reported the results to his special education teacher and other team members at Ahmed's IEP meeting.

2. Analyze Regular Physical Education Curriculum

The next step in the model is to determine what specific activities take place in middle school and high school physical education and how (if at all) each of Ahmed's goals and objectives can be incorporated into these activities. First, an analysis of the yearly middle school and high school physical education program is needed. As was the case with the elementary physical education program, it is easier to determine which activities during the year best match the goals and objectives of the student with disabilities, which may be appropriate but require some modification, and which ones may be incompatible if the program is broken down into units. Table 10.5 provides an example of the yearly physical education plan for the 10th grade at Ahmed's school. Activities in the 10th-grade physical education program are taught in units 5–6 weeks long. Remember, Ahmed only has 5 years of formal schooling remaining, so he is past the point of being exposed to a variety of physical education activities. If he is expected to achieve any competence in the goals that were targeted for him, he will need to work only on those goals for the next 5 years.

A quick glance at the yearly plan shows that the golf, softball, and conditioning units match Ahmed's goals and objectives. While basketball is not part of Ahmed's specific goals, it is an activity that Ahmed enjoys, one he can do well with minor adaptations, and one that is popular in Special Olympics in the community. It is very likely that Ahmed might decide to play Special Olympics basketball, so participating in this activity during regular physical education is deemed appropriate by the team. That leaves soccer and tennis in the fall and volleyball and square dancing in the winter. During soccer and tennis, Ahmed can work on his golf skills with peer tutors his

Table 10.4.   Ahmed's long-term plan with sample of long-term goal with select short-term instructional objectives

---

LONG-TERM PLAN: Ahmed will demonstrate the skills needed to participate independently in three lifetime leisure skills in the community including one fitness-based activity.

Long-Term Goal 1:   Ahmed will demonstrate the ability to get balls and a club independently and then consistently hit golf balls off a tee at a local driving range.

Short-Term Instructional Objectives:

1. Within 30 seconds of entering the driving range shop, Ahmed will independently give the driving range attendant a card that requests a golf club and a small bucket of balls 100% of the time 3 out of 3 days. days.
2. Ahmed will independently give the attendant $3.00 and then independently take the golf club and ball and locate an empty driving tee at the the range 100% of the time 3 out of 3 days.
3. Ahmed will independently hold a golf club using a baseball grip with hands in correct position upon presentation of a golf club with 100% accuracy 5 out of 5 days.
4. Ahmed will independently get into correct start position for hitting a golf ball with 100% accuracy 5 out of 5 days. Correct start position includes:
   a. side orientation to ball with feet approximately 2′ from ball
   b. legs spread shoulder-width apart with slight knee bend
   c. body leaning forward at trunk, both arms straight
5. Ahmed will independently demonstrate the components of a correct golf swing so that he hits the golf ball 80% of the time 3 days in a row. Components include the following:
   a. from correct start position, takes club back by twisting at shoulders and trunk
   b. continues backswing until club is at approximately a 45° angle to ground
   c. downswings by twisting at shoulders and trunk
   d. contacts ball with arms straight
   e. follows through so that chest and stomach face target

Long-Term Goal 2:   Ahmed will independently locate the university recreation center and develop the skills needed to participate in aerobic classes and weight training.

Long-Term Goal 3:   Ahmed will demonstrate the ability to participate safely and follow the rules with verbal reminders from teammates in a class "C" softball team in the community.

Long-Term Goal 4:   Ahmed will independently locate the local bowling alley and develop the skills needed to bowl with peers or join a community bowling league.

---

age either in a field next to the tennis courts or at the local driving range. Ideally, Ahmed and his peer tutor would go to the driving range where he also can work on related objectives of requesting and paying for golf balls. Similarly, during volleyball Ahmed can go to university recreation center with selected peers to work on his weight training and aerobic dance goals and objectives, and during dancing he can work on bowling. This part of the program might be taken over by the special education teacher, teacher assistant, or adapted physical education specialist since the regular physical educator will have to stay at school with his or her classes. The decision as to

Table 10.5.   Tenth-grade physical education program—Yearly plan

---

September–October	■ Soccer (Ahmed will work on golf)
October–November	■ Tennis (Ahmed will work on golf)
November–December	+ Conditioning
January–February	☐ Basketball
February–March	■ Volleyball (Ahmed will work at the recreation center)
March–April	☐ Square/Folk Dancing (Ahmed will go bowling)
April–May	+ Softball
May–June	+ Golf

+ = No modifications needed for Ahmed.

☐ = Some modifications needed for Ahmed.

■ = Alternative activities needed for Ahmed.

which peers go into the community with Ahmed and who is directly in charge of the community recreation aspect of his program should be determined by the team. The important point is that Ahmed should not stay in regular physical education if the activities are not going to help him achieve his long-term goals. Inclusion into community recreation is a fair substitute for inclusion into regular physical education.

The second level of analysis is to determine what happens in each physical education unit. For example, Table 10.6 shows a sample unit plan for basketball. Note how the general activities outlined in the unit plan are examined so that general accommodations for Ahmed can be delineated. At this point, the team, and particularly the regular physical educator, are just making general notes in anticipation of Ahmed participating in the basketball unit. This way he or she can be more prepared to develop specific accommodations for Ahmed. In Ahmed's case, most of the accommodations revolve around peers providing extra assistance and direction, and some minor changes to rules in games. Again, this is not one of Ahmed's goals, so the team is not as concerned that Ahmed learns the rules of basketball. Rather, they hope that he learns some of the basic skills and concepts so that he might choose to participate in Special Olympics basketball in the community.

The next step is to analyze a sample daily lesson plan within each unit to determine exactly where the student will work on specific skills. Table 10.7 demonstrates how activities within the daily lesson plan are modified to accommodate Ahmed. Note how, in many cases, accommodations are fairly simple. For example, at the dribbling station Ahmed does not have to go through cones, he is given a smaller ball for easier grip, and he is given extra practice while he waits his turn. Also note how this accommodation is appropriate for other less-skilled students in the class who may or may not have a specific disability. (See chap. 7, this volume, under basketball modifications for more specific suggestions.)

As was the case with the chapter on elementary physical education, the examples here are fairly detailed to illustrate exactly how decisions might be made. For more experienced middle school and high school physical education teachers who use previous lesson plans or no longer write detailed lesson plans, the general ideas outlined above can still be used. The important point is that, prior to including the student with a disability, the middle school and high school physical educator should analyze the student's individual goals and objectives as well as the physical education curriculum to determine where the goals and objectives will be incorporated in the regular program.

3. Determine How Program Will Be Implemented

Once we establish where to incorporate the student's individual goals and objectives in the regular program, we can determine exactly how the program will be implemented. That is, what will be the specific teaching methods, activities, modifications, and adapted equipment needed to implement the program? Again, the adapted physical education specialist, regular physical educator, physical therapist, special education teacher, and other team members can write specific programs for individual students that can be implemented by support staff or by the regular physical educator. Also, there are prepackaged programs that have excellent teaching outlines that can be used as a guide to develop individual programs.

Many of the assessment forms presented in Chapter 5 can be used at this point to help make proper instructional and curricular decisions. For example, Figure 10.2 presents the checklist for determining instructional modifications filled out for Ahmed. Note how in many cases no special instructional modifications were needed. Ahmed's problems revolve around understanding verbal instructions and staying on task. Therefore, simplifying instructions for Ahmed and having classmates repeat instructions and provide extra demonstrations comprise the instructional modifications needed for Ahmed. Since communication seems to be one of Ahmed's biggest problems, the

Table 10.6.   Unit plan for 10th-grade basketball

WEEK 1

Day 1

Warm-up (daily exercises led by student leader)

Skill focus (review proper technique for dribbling; break into partners and practice dribbling as group with feedback)

Reinforcing game ("dribble keep-away")

Day 2

Warm-up (same as above)

Skill focus (review proper technique for dribbling; dribbling stations)

Reinforcing game ("dribble relay")

Day 3

Warm-up (same as above)

Skill focus (review proper technique for dribbling; dribbling stations)

Reinforcing game ("dribble obstacle course")

Day 4

Warm-up (same as above)

Skill focus (review proper technique for dribbling; dribbling stations; introduce passing)

Reinforcing game ("dribble and pass relay")

Day 5

Warm-up (same as above)

Skill focus (review proper technique for dribbling and passing; dribbling and passing stations)

Reinforcing game ("dribble obstacle course")

WEEK 2

Day 1

Warm-up (same as above)

Skill focus (review proper technique for dribbling and passing; dribbling and passing stations)

Reinforcing game ("dribble/pass keep-away")

Day 2

Warm-up (same as above)

Skill focus (review proper technique for dribbling and passing; dribbling and passing stations; introduce shooting technique)

Reinforcing game ("dribble, stop, and shoot relay")

Day 3

Warm-up (same as above)

Skill focus (review proper technique for dribbling, passing, and shooting; dribbling, passing, and shooting stations)

Reinforcing game ("2 v. 2 games")

Day 4

Warm-up (same as above)

Skill focus (review proper technique for dribbling, passing, and shooting; dribbling, passing, and shooting stations)

Reinforcing game ("2 v. 2 games")

Day 5

Warm-up (same as above)

Skill focus (review proper technique for dribbling, passing, and shooting; dribbling, passing, and shooting stations)

Reinforcing game ("2 v. 2 games")

WEEK 3

Day 1

Warm-up (same as above)

Skill focus (review all skills; introduce defense skills)

Reinforcing game ("3 v. 3 keep-away")

Day 2

Warm-up (same as above)

Skill focus (review all skills; skill stations with all skills)

Reinforcing game ("3 v. 3 half-court basketball")

(continued)

Table 10.6.   *(continued)*

Day 3
 Warm-up (same as above)
 Skill focus (review all skills; skill stations with all skills)
 Reinforcing game ("3 v. 3 half-court basketball")
Day 4
 Warm-up (same as above)
 Skill focus (review all skills; skill stations with all skills)
 Reinforcing game (introduce five-person zone defense)
Day 5
 Warm-up (same as above)
 Skill focus (review all skills; skill stations with all skills; review zone defense)
 Reinforcing game ("5 v. 5 half-court basketball")
WEEK 4
Day 1
 Warm-up (same as above)
 Skill focus (review all skills; skill stations with all skills; review zone defense)
 Reinforcing game (introduce team offense)
Day 2
 Warm-up (same as above)
 Skill focus (review all skills; practice offensive v. zone defense)
 Reinforcing game (controlled 5 v. 5 full-court games)
Day 3
 Warm-up (same as above)
 Skill focus (review all skills; practice offensive v. zone defense)
 Reinforcing game (controlled 5 v. 5 full-court games)
Day 4
 Warm-up (same as above)
 Reinforcing game (split group into teams and play regular 5 v. 5 full-court games)
Day 5
 Warm-up (same as above)
 Reinforcing game (split group into teams and play regular 5 v. 5 full-court games)
 Repeat games during last week of basketball unit.

General accommodations for Ahmed:
1.   Have peers repeat directions and give extra demonstrations and instruction during warm-ups and skill work.
2.   Because of his limited attention span, have a variety of activities at each skill station.
3.   Initially have Ahmed play in smaller games (2 v. 2 and 3 v. 3) rather than full games.
4.   Teach basic concepts such as defense, using extra cues (place a mark on the floor where he is supposed to stand).
5.   Have class create some modified rules for Ahmed such as no stealing, free passes, and free shots.

team fills out the communication skills checklist described in Chapter 5. (See Figure 10.3.) Note how the information from this checklist, while fairly general, helps the regular physical educator understand a little more about Ahmed's communication skills. Based on the results of this assessment, it appears that to understand instruction Ahmed will need extra demonstrations, environmental cues (markings on the floor or wall), and physical assistance provided by the regular physical educator and/or classmates.

The next step is to determine if Ahmed would benefit from any curricular adaptations or adapted equipment. Two checklists can be helpful at this point. These two checklists, "Alternative Way" and "Adapted Equipment," are easy to fill out and should be completed just prior to each unit of instruction. Figures 10.4 and 10.5 show these two checklists filled out for Ahmed in relation to basketball. Ahmed has relatively normal strength and range of motion, so he does not need to perform basketball skills differently than his peers, nor does he need any adapted equipment. However, students who use wheelchairs, who have cerebral palsy, or who have sight im-

Table 10.7. Accommodating Ahmed's goals within a regular lesson plan

BASKETBALL LESSON PLAN

 Objective: Students will have an opportunity to practice and receive feedback on the essential components of proper dribbling and passing techniques.

 I. Introduction
  A. Students come in and sit in assigned squads.
  B. Tell class we are working on basketball skills of dribbling and passing.
 Ahmed usually finds his way to his squad; if not, peers can give extra verbal cues.
 II. Warm-up (led by student leader)
  A. 10 jumping jacks
  B. run in place for 1 minute
  C. 20 sit-ups and 10 push-ups
  D. hamstring stretch
  E. quadricep stretch
  F. Achilles stretch
  G. 3 laps
 Ahmed can do most exercises independently although he usually is off cadence. When he gets confused, his peers in his squad help him with verbal cues. Ahmed can do 20 sit-ups and 10 push-ups, but less skilled students who cannot are given individual goals to work toward that are challenging yet achievable. Some students do 5 sit-ups independently and then are assisted in the remaining 15.)
 III. Skill focus
  A. Have students sit facing you, then review the components of a skillful dribble and skillful chest-and-bounce pass. (Demonstrate skills and have pictures of correct skill on walls at stations.)
  B. Break into two dribbling stations and three passing stations (six students per station) to work on skills. Have a picture of the correct dribbling/passing pattern at each station, and emphasize correct pattern to students. Have students self-evaluate each other's performance. Once stations have been set up and students are practicing appropriately, teacher will monitor station #2 below. (Stations are listed below.) Students should stay at each station for 3–5 minutes and move on teacher's command.
   1. dribbling through cones
   2. dribbling with either hand across the gym
   3. chest-and-bounce passing against wall
   4. chest pass and bounce pass with partner
   5. passing through hoops to partner
 Skilled students—encourage them to increase speed during activities and provide extra assistance to less-skilled students.
 *Ahmed and less-skilled students—work on walking and jogging forward while dribbling without going through cones. Can use smaller basketball if that seems to help. Also, while waiting turn in line, they can practice dribbling in place. (Make sure each student has own ball.)
 IV. Reinforcing game
  A. "Dribble-Pass Relay." Divide class into six relay teams of five per team. Student must dribble forward 15', dribble back 5', stop, and give next person in line a bounce pass. Continue until all students have gone three times.
 Skilled students—must dribble using opposite hand and dribble to outer cone (20' away).
 Ahmed and less-skilled students—evenly distribute less-skilled players in each relay team. Students who are less-skilled dribble to closest cone (10' away).
 V. Concluding activities
  A. Students sit in squads
  B. Review skills covered during day
  C. Review skills to be used tomorrow
  D. Dismissal

pairments might need to perform skills in different ways or use adapted equipment. If these checklists do suggest that adaptations are needed, then refer to specific adaptations in Chapter 7.

  While Ahmed can perform skills like his peers and does not need any adapted equipment, his skill level and general coordination are much lower than those of his peers. Therefore, some curricular adaptations will be needed. To help determine specific curricular adaptations for Ahmed,

Student's name: __Ahmed__   P.E. class/teacher: __10th, Jones__

Who will implement modifications?

(RPE teacher) (Classmates)   Peer tutor   Teacher assistant   Specialist

Instructional component	Things to consider	Selected modifications/Comments
Teaching style	Command, problem-solving, discovery	Use command w/ Ahmed
Class format and size of group	Small/large group; stations/whole class instruction	Small group when possible
Level of methodology	Verbal cues, demonstrations, physical assistance	Extra demonstrations, physical assistance
Starting/stopping signals	Whistle, hand signals, physical assistance	Whistle OK
Time of day	Early A.M., late A.M., early P.M., late P.M.	None
Duration of instruction	How long will student listen to instruction?	Short, may wander; have peer repeat
Duration of expected participation	How long will student stay on task?	Many tasks, short period
Order of learning	In what order will you present instruction?	Same
Instructional setting	Indoors/outdoors; part of gym/whole gym	None
Eliminate distractors	Lighting, temperature, extra equipment	None
Provide structure	Set organization of instruction each day	None
Level of difficulty	Complexity of instructions/organization	Simple; may have peers assist
Levels of motivation	Make setting and activities more motivating	None

Figure 10.2.   Checklist to determine instructional modifications to accommodate Ahmed.

Directions: Instruct student in various situations. (See below.) Note how student responds to each type of cue or combination of cues. You may need to repeat in various instructional situations (e.g., outside versus inside; simple skills versus more complex skills).

	Responds correctly	Delayed response (5–10 seconds)	Does not respond
Verbal cues		✓	✓
Gestures		✓	✓
Demonstration		✓	
Environmental cues	✓ (w/extra cue)		
Physical assistance	✓		

Situations in which this assessment was conducted (whether formally or informally):

__✓__ Inclusive physical education setting with peers without disabilities (large group)

_____ Inclusive physical education setting with small groups (5–7 students)

_____ Inclusive physical education setting: one-on-one instruction

Figure 10.3.   Sample checklist to determine Ahmed's communication skills.

	Yes	No	Comments
Does the student have a physical disability that appears to preclude typical performance?		✓	
Is the student having extreme difficulty performing the skill?		✓	
Is the student making little to no progress over several months or years despite instruction?		✓	
Does the student seem more comfortable and motivated using a different pattern?		✓	
Will an alternative pattern still be useful (i.e., functional) in the targeted environments?		✓	
Will the alternative pattern increase the student's ability to perform the skill?		✓	

Note: If the answer to some or all of the above questions is yes, the student may need an adapted pattern.

Figure 10.4. Does the student (Ahmed) need an alternative way to perform the skill (basketball)?

	Yes	No	Comments
Will adaptation increase the student's participation in the activity?		✓	
Will it allow the student to participate in an activity that is preferred or valued by the student, friends, and family members?		✓	
Will it take less time to teach the student to use the adaptation than to teach the skill directly?		✓	
Will the team have access to the technical expertise to design, construct, adjust, and repair the adaptation?		✓	
Will the adaptation maintain or enhance related motor/communication skills?		✓	

Note: If the answer to most of the above questions is yes, then the student may need adapted equipment.

Figure 10.5. Does the student (Ahmed) need adapted equipment for basketball?

the checklist found in Figure 10.6 was completed. Note that the major modifications are related to Ahmed's problems with coordination. Because strength, speed, and balance are not problems for Ahmed, no modifications were needed. Other students with different abilities and disabilities may need more specific modifications in these areas. If so, specific information found in Chapter 7 could be used. The important point is that you want to implement only those modifications that the student needs to be successful in the activity.

    Since the basketball unit will involve group games, the checklist to help determine curricular modifications for group games and sports also was completed. (See Figure 10.7.) Again, the major modifications for Ahmed revolve around his limited communication skills and coordination. The modifications selected by the team should be shared with nondisabled students to determine if they "buy into" the modifications. They may have other suggestions to help Ahmed participate in the activity. Students with normal to near-normal intelligence should be encouraged to participate in the process as well.

4. Determine Who Will Assist Student

The next step in the model is to determine who will assist the student while he or she is in regular physical education. As noted previously, some students will not need any extra support, some might need extra assistance from peers in the class, and others will need assistance from trained volunteers, teacher assistants, or therapists. In Ahmed's case, he should be able to do well with natural peer support (peers giving him extra cues, peers placing him in correct position, peers telling him where to go and to whom to pass, peers helping him in and out of various equipment). The regular physical educator, with help from the adapted physical education specialist, will have to provide cues to peers on how to assist Ahmed. In some cases, these cues may involve specific teaching techniques and adaptations designed for Ahmed. For example, Ahmed will need physical assistance to get in and out of the weight lifting equipment at his school as well as at a local YMCA, help set the proper weight for each activity, and provide Ahmed with encouragement and feedback on correct technique. With training, his classmates should be able to learn quickly how to provide this type of assistance for Ahmed.

    As noted in Chapter 9, peer tutors, senior citizens, parents from the PTO, and other volunteers can be trained to provide assistance to those students who have more significant disabilities or whose program is vastly different from the regular curriculum. For example, if a student with cerebral palsy is working on bowling while his class is working on soccer, a peer tutor (another student from the school but not necessarily from that physical education class) can assist the student in bowling. Similarly, a senior citizen who enjoys swimming can assist a student with significant disabilities in learning how to swim at a local recreation center. There are many sources of volunteers in every community, and the PEIT should seek these sources to assist in the implementation of the program.

    Choosing the person who will assist a student should be a thoughtful decision that is based on the student's abilities and disabilities, personal characteristics (e.g., age, size, gender), and type of regular physical education activity. For example, it would be inappropriate to have a 100-pound high school girl work with an 18-year-old male student who weighs 200 pounds who needs assistance in dressing and getting in and out of the swimming pool. While it is difficult to be choosy when picking volunteers or paid teacher assistants, all efforts should be made to match the support person to the student's unique needs and characteristics.

    Finally, it is important that any person who provides assistance to students with disabilities be given preservice and ongoing information and training (see below). Members of the PEIT headed up by the adapted physical education specialist can conduct training schools and ongoing seminars. In addition, the adapted physical educator should conduct periodic checks on support staff to make sure they are carrying out the program in the prescribed manner.

5. Preparing Staff/Students for Inclusion

The next step in the model is to prepare key staff members and peers for inclusion. As was the case with the elementary program, regular physical educators should get information from PEIT members regarding any student with a disability who will be included in their classes. Important information includes a description of the student's disability and how it affects physical education, medical/health concerns, any contraindicated activities, and present level of performance on physical and motor skills. In addition, the team should give the regular physical educator information that can help him or her present information more effectively and prevent behavior problems. Such information should include how to work with the student, the student's receptive and expressive language ability, the student's ability to follow directions, any inappropriate behaviors the student might have as well as what triggers the behavior, and things that reinforce the student. (See Table 10.8 for a summary.) Ideally, the regular physical educator should go to the student's class to meet the student and get to know his or her abilities and behaviors.

Does the student have limited strength?

Things to consider	Selected modifications (if any) and Comments
Shorten distance to move or project object.	Closer to help accuracy
Use lighter equipment (e.g., balls, bats).	No
Use shorter striking implements.	No
Allow student to sit or lie down while playing.	No
Use deflated balls or suspended balls.	No
Change requirements (a few jumps, then run).	No

Does the student have limited speed?

Things to consider	Selected modifications (if any) and Comments
Shorten distance (or make it longer for others).	No
Change locomotor pattern (allow running v. walking).	No
Make safe areas in tag games.	No

Does the student have limited endurance?

Things to consider	Selected modifications (if any) and Comments
Shorten distance.	No
Shorten playing field.	No
Allow "safe" areas in tag games.	No
Decrease activity time for student.	No - change activities frequently for behavior
Allow more rest periods for student.	No
Allow student to sit while playing.	No

Does the student have limited balance?

Things to consider	Selected modifications (if any) and Comments
Provide chair/bar for support.	No
Teach balance techniques (widen base, extend arms).	No
Increase width of beams to be walked.	No
Use carpeted rather than slick surfaces.	No
Teach student how to fall.	No
Allow student to sit during activity.	No
Place student near wall for support.	No
Allow student to hold peer's hand.	No

Does student have limited coordination and accuracy?

Things to consider	Selected modifications (if any) and Comments
Use stationary balls for kicking/striking.	No
Decrease distance for throwing, kicking, and shooting.	Closer for shooting & passing
Make targets and goals larger.	Give point for hitting rim
Use larger balls for kicking and striking.	No
Increase surface of the striking implements.	No
Use backstop.	Can practice shooting against wall
Use softer, slower balls for striking and catching.	Bounce pass for catching
In bowling-type games, use lighter, less stable pins.	No
What can you do to maximize safety?	Teach safety rules, have Ahmed play defense away from basket.

Note: Some or all of these modifications can be implemented. Also, these modifications can be implemented for one student, for several students, or for the entire class to make the activity more challenging and success-oriented.

Figure 10.6.   Checklist to determine curricular adaptations to accommodate Ahmed (basketball).

Things to consider	Selected modifications (if any) and Comments
Can you vary the purpose/goal of the game (e.g., some students play to learn complex strategies, others play to work on simple motor skills)?	Focus on skills and general rules for Ahmed
Can you vary number of players (e.g., play small games such as 2 v. 2 basketball)?	Start w/smaller 2 v 2 or 3v.3 games
Can you vary movement requirements (e.g., some students walk, others run; some hit a ball off a tee, others hit pitched ball; skilled students use more complex movements, less skilled use simpler movements)?	Ahmed can walk & dribble, can shoot & pass w/out anyone stealing
Can you vary the field of play (e.g., special zones for students with less mobility; make the field narrower or wider as needed; shorten the distance for students with movement problems)?	No
Can you vary objects used (e.g., some students use lighter bats/larger balls; some use a lower net/basket)?	No
Can you vary the level of organization (Vary typical organizational patterns; vary where certain students stand; vary the level of structure for certain students.)?	Have marker on floor for Ahmed's defensive & offensive positions.
Can you vary the limits/expectations (Vary the number of turns each student receives; vary the rules regarding how far a student can run, hit, etc.; vary how much you will enforce certain rules for certain players.)?	Do not enforce travelling & double-dribbling rules; relax defense against him.

Note: Use these suggestions to modify rules for both students with and without disabilities to make the game challenging, safe, and success-oriented.

Figure 10.7. Checklist to determine curricular modifications for Ahmed for group games and sports (basketball).

Table 10.8. Example of general information about Ahmed

1. Communication skills
   Understands one-word commands; can imitate simple demonstrations (make sure he is looking at you); sometimes responds to verbal directions (takes several seconds for information to sink in); responds well to physical assistance. You will probably need to demonstrate skills first, then provide physical assistance.

2. Behaviors
   Generally well-behaved although he can be very distractible. Has short attention span (maybe 1–2 minutes), and does not sit for very long periods. Can easily be brought back to activity with reminders from peers. Sometimes self-stimulates on balls (likes to spin them in his hand). May hug friends (especially girls). Try to discourage this and help him learn appropriate behaviors (e.g., shake hands, wave hi).

3. Reinforcers
   Loves balls, loves to run, loves to look at bright-colored shirts. Likes to hug peers (do not let him do this; rather, make him shake hands). Doesn't like to sit for very long (maybe just 3–4 minutes).

4. Medical concerns
   Has a seizure disorder that is controlled with medication (has not had a seizure in 2 years). Doctor said that he has no restrictions in physical activity.

5. Special friends
   None really; he likes all the kids in his class.

Other staff members and volunteers who will be directly responsible for assisting the student with disabilities in regular physical education also should receive some in-service training. Some of the training will be similar to the types of information given to the regular physical educator. In addition, the regular physical educator should provide information to assistants and volunteers regarding the regular physical education curriculum, normal routines, what he or she expects of the assistant, and any other information that will help the assistant in regular physical education. This information should be presented by the regular physical educator at various times throughout the year. For example, a basketball unit may be run differently than a tennis unit, which is run differently from a dance unit. The regular physical educator should try to keep the assistant informed about the regular physical education program at least a few days prior to instruction. (See Figure 10.8 for an example.)

Finally, peers should be given information about the student with disabilities. For students with disabilities and no particular behavior problems, you may only need to inform the class that a student with a disability will be in the class and may need occasional help in certain activities. Students can then be encouraged to ask questions as needed. For students with more visible disabilities such as a visual impairment, hearing impairment, or physical disability, you may want to give more specific information about the student, how he or she will need certain modifications to be successful, and how you (the students) can help.[1] You may want to do some role-playing so that peers gain a better appreciation of the challenges the student will face. Also, explain to students that they will be asked throughout the year to think of ways to modify activities and games so that the student can be meaningfully included in the regular program.

6. Implementing the Program

The next step is to implement the program and continuously assess students to determine if they are making adequate progress. If the regular physical educator is responsible for implementing the

---

MEMORANDUM

From: Pat Smith, Physical Educator
To: Teacher assistants/volunteers working with students with disabilities

We will be beginning a 5-week basketball unit next week. Please ask your student's special education teacher to check your student's medical file and, if necessary, call the student's parents to see if he or she can do all of the activities in our unit. Activities I anticipate doing include:

Usual warm-ups   Shooting (lay-ups, jump shots)
Dribbling   Rebounding
Passing/catching (chest, bounce, overhead)   Defense
Lead-up games   Regulation games

My tentative lesson format is as follows:

  Introduction
  Warm-ups (usual)
  Basketball skill (demonstration followed by stations)
  Games (begin with skill games, then lead-up games, and finally full-court games the last week)

Thanks! Please contact me if you have any questions.   Pat

Figure 10.8. Sample memorandum from physical educator to teacher assistants.

---

[1]Note that some personal and medical information may be inappropriate to give to students without disabilities. For example, it would not be appropriate to discuss specific medication a student takes. It also is illegal to identify which students have AIDS. For more information, talk with special education personnel or the building principal.

program, support personnel such as the adapted physical education specialist, special education teacher, and/or therapists should try to visit the regular physical educator during the first few classes. Support personnel can provide direct assistance to the student, model strategies for the regular physical educator, and discuss how to include the student with disabilities successfully and meaningfully. As the regular physical educator feels more comfortable with the situation, these support persons can begin to back off and take on a more consultative role (perhaps checking back with the regular physical educator three to four times per month).

For example, a student with cerebral palsy who uses a walker to locomote will be included in regular physical education. The regular physical educator has seen the student and has been briefed on her IEP. The adapted physical education specialist has outlined specific modifications for this student so that she can be safely, successfully, and meaningfully included during the first unit of physical education. In addition, the physical therapist has developed an individual stretching program for the student to do while other students do more traditional stretches. Still, the regular physical educator is a little nervous about having this student in regular physical education. During the first week of regular physical education, the student's physical therapist might assist this student in regular physical education two times per week and the adapted physical education specialist can assist the student three times per week. They can model appropriate modifications and talk with the regular physical educator. As the regular physical educator begins to feel more comfortable with this student and how to provide appropriate modifications, he can back off to a more consultative role, perhaps visiting the class two to three times per month.

Ongoing evaluation of a student's individual goals and objectives is extremely important to determine the effectiveness of the program. However, collecting ongoing evaluation data can be difficult for the regular physical educator who must monitor all his or her students. Simple data sheets can be developed by members of the PEIT (ideally, an adapted physical education specialist) that can help the regular physical educator collect ongoing data. (See Figures 10.9, 10.10, and 10.11 for examples.) In addition, classmates without disabilities can learn how to evaluate each other including evaluating how well a student with disabilities is doing toward achieving his or her goals. These forms could be used by peer tutors, volunteers, and teachers assistants. Ideally, the adapted physical education specialist should check the data every few weeks and conduct his or her own assessment to verify the progress each student is making. While this method may not be perfect, at least there is some effort to measure the progress the student is making. Ongoing evaluation allows the team to make adjustments to the student's program, to the assistants working with him or her, to the setting, and/or to the equipment that the student is using.

SUMMARY

The purpose of this chapter is to apply the model described in Chapter 4 to including a high school student with disabilities in regular physical education. An ongoing example of Ahmed, a 10th grader with severe mental retardation and a seizure disorder, was used throughout this chapter to highlight how the process outlined in Chapter 4 and specific assessment procedures described in Chapter 5 can be applied in including a middle school or high school student with disabilities in regular physical education.

As seen through this example, middle school and high school students with disabilities like Ahmed can be successfully included in regular physical education programs. However, inclusion at the high school level will work only if the physical education inclusion team (PEIT) works together prior to inclusion to determine: 1) what skills are important for the student, 2) what happens in regular high school physical education, 3) what modifications are needed to accommodate the student in regular high school physical education, and 4) what support staff does the student need to be successful in regular high school physical education. If such an approach is

Activity: Dribbling a basketball

Trials	Can student walk forward and dribble? (Note how far he dribbles.)	Student's effort
1. 2.		
3. 4.		
5. 6.		
7. 8.		
9. 10.		
11. 12.		
13. 14.		

Skill key: + = steps,   +v = steps when told,   o = does not step.
Effort key: + = tries to step, o = doesn't try, but doesn't resist assistance, − = resists assistance.

Figure 10.9.   Sample ongoing evaluation form for high school physical education program.

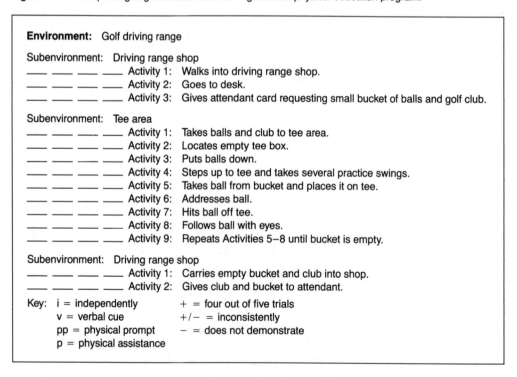

Environment: Golf driving range

Subenvironment: Driving range shop
—— —— —— —— Activity 1:   Walks into driving range shop.
—— —— —— —— Activity 2:   Goes to desk.
—— —— —— —— Activity 3:   Gives attendant card requesting small bucket of balls and golf club.

Subenvironment: Tee area
—— —— —— —— Activity 1:   Takes balls and club to tee area.
—— —— —— —— Activity 2:   Locates empty tee box.
—— —— —— —— Activity 3:   Puts balls down.
—— —— —— —— Activity 4:   Steps up to tee and takes several practice swings.
—— —— —— —— Activity 5:   Takes ball from bucket and places it on tee.
—— —— —— —— Activity 6:   Addresses ball.
—— —— —— —— Activity 7:   Hits ball off tee.
—— —— —— —— Activity 8:   Follows ball with eyes.
—— —— —— —— Activity 9:   Repeats Activities 5–8 until bucket is empty.

Subenvironment: Driving range shop
—— —— —— —— Activity 1:   Carries empty bucket and club into shop.
—— —— —— —— Activity 2:   Gives club and bucket to attendant.

Key: i = independently   + = four out of five trials
      v = verbal cue   +/− = inconsistently
      pp = physical prompt   − = does not demonstrate
      p = physical assistance

Figure 10.10.   Ongoing assessment form for golf (based on ecological inventory).

Student's name: Jason Jones

Task: Pushing ball down ramp (increase range of motion and control of arm)

Context: Bowling at local bowling alley

Objective: Push ball off tray in 20 seconds or less independently so that ball travels down ramp toward bowling pins

Support: Peer tutor providing assistance

Ball size
(r) regulation bowling ball
(f) rubber bowling ball

Assistance
(v) verbal cue
(t) touch prompt
(p) partial physical assist
(f) full physical assist

Speed (time to do skill)
(4) within 40 seconds of cue
(3) within 30 seconds of cue
(2) within 20 seconds of cue
(1) within 10 seconds of cue

TRIALS

Figure 10.11. Sample data form to be used by peer for student with more significant disabilities.

followed, students with a variety of abilities, including students with more significant disabilities, can have meaningful, beneficial, and successful experiences in regular high school physical education.

References

Adams, R., & McCubbin, J. (1991). *Games, sports and exercises for the physically disabled* (4th ed.). Philadelphia: Lea & Febiger.

Arbogast, G., & Lavay, B. (1986). Combining students with different ability levels in games and sports. *Physical Educator, 44*, 255–259.

Aufderheide, S. (1983). ALT-PE in mainstreamed physical education classes. *Journal of Teaching in Physical Education* [Summer Monograph], *1*, 22–26.

Aufsesser, P.M. (1991). Mainstreaming and the least restrictive environment. How do they differ? *Palaestra, 7*(2), 31–34.

Auxter, D., & Pyfer, J. (1989). *Principles and methods of adapted physical education.* St. Louis: Times Mirror/Mosby College Publishing.

Bayley, N. (1969). Manual for the *Bayley Scales of Infant Development.* New York: The Psychological Corporation.

Beuter, A. (1983). Effects of mainstreaming on motor performance of intellectually normal and trainable mentally retarded students. *American Corrective Therapy Journal, 37*(2), 48–52.

Block, M.E. (1992). What is appropriate physical education for students with profound disabilities? *Adapted Physical Activity Quarterly, 9*, 197–213.

Block, M.E. (1994). All kids can have physical education the regular way. In M.S. Moon (Ed.), *Making school and community recreation fun for everyone: Places and ways to integrate.* Baltimore: Paul H. Brookes Publishing Co.

Block, M.E. (in press). Why all students with disabilities should be included in regular physical education. *Palaestra.*

Block, M.E., & Krebs, P.L. (1992). An alternative to least restrictive environments: A continuum of support to regular physical education. *Adapted Physical Activity Quarterly, 9*, 97–113.

Block, M.E., & Provis, S. (1992, October). *Effects of ball size on throwing patterns in children with Down Syndrome.* Paper presented at the North American Federation of Adapted Physical Activity Symposium. Montreal.

Block, M.E., Provis, S., & Nelson, E. (1994). Accommodating students with severe disabilities in regular physical education: Extending traditional skill stations. *Palaestra, 10*(1), 32–35.

Bricker, D., & Cripe, J.J.W. (1992). *An activity-based approach to early intervention.* Baltimore: Paul H. Brookes Publishing Co.

Brinson, C.L. (Ed.). (1982). *The helping hand: A manual describing methods for handling the young child with cerebral palsy.* Charlottesville, VA: Kluge Children's Rehabilitation Center.

Brown, L., Branston, M.B., Hamre-Nietupski, S., Pumpian, I., Certo, N., & Gruenewald, L. (1979). A strategy for developing chronological age-appropriate and functional curricular content for severely handicapped adolescents and young adults. *Journal of Special Education, 13*, 81–90.

Brown, L., Schwarz, P., Udvari-Solner, A., Kampschroer-Frattura, E., Johnson, F., Jorgensen, J., & Gruenewald, L. (1991). How much time should students with severe intellectual disabilities spend in regular education classrooms or elsewhere? *Journal of The Association for Persons with Severe Handicaps, 16*, 39–47.

Bruininks, R.H. (1978). *Bruininks-Oseretsky Test of Motor Proficiency—Manual* (pp. 82–85). Circle Pines, MN: American Guidance Service.

Burton, A.W., Greer, N.L., & Wiese, D.M. (1992). *Variations in the components of the one-hand overhand throw as a function of ball diameter*. Paper submitted for publication.

Carnine, D. (1991). Direct instruction applied to mathematics for the general education classroom. In J.W. Lloyd, N.N. Singh, & A.C. Repp (Eds.), *The regular education initiative: Alternative perspectives on concepts, issues, and models* (pp. 163–176). Sycamore, IL: Sycamore Press.

Chadsey-Rusch, J. (1990). Social interactions of secondary-aged students with severe handicaps: Implications for facilitating the transition from school to work. *Journal of The Association for Persons with Severe Handicaps, 15*, 69–78.

Clark, G., French, R., & Henderson, H. (1985). Teaching techniques that develop positive attitudes. *Palaestra, 5*(3), 14–17.

Council for Exceptional Children. (1975). What is mainstreaming? *Exceptional Children. 42*, 174.

Council on Physical Education for Children. (1992). *Developmentally appropriate physical education practices for children*. Reston, VA: Author.

Cowden, J.E., & Eason, R.L. (1991). Legislative terminology affecting adapted physical education. *Journal of Physical Education, Recreation, and Dance, 62*(8), 34.

Dattilo, J. (1991). Recreation and leisure: A review of the literature and recommendations for future directions. In L.H. Meyer, C.A. Peck, & L Brown (Eds.), *Critical issues in the lives of people with severe disabilities* (pp. 171–194). Baltimore: Paul H. Brookes Publishing Co.

Davis, W.E. (1984). Motor ability assessment of populations with handicapping conditions: Challenging basic assumptions. *Adapted Physical Activity Quarterly, 1*, 125–140.

Davis, W.E., & Burton, A.W. (1991). Ecological task analysis: Translating movement behavior theory into practice. *Adapted Physical Activity Quarterly, 8*, 154–177.

DePaepe, J. (1985). The influence of three least restrictive environments on the content, motor-ALT and performance of moderately mentally retarded students. *Journal of Teaching in Physical Education, 5*, 34–41.

Deschler, D.D., & Schumaker, J.B. (1986). Learning strategies: An instructional alternative for low-achieving adolescents. *Exceptional Children, 52*, 583–590.

Dunn, J., & Fait, H. (1989). *Special physical education*. Dubuque, IA: William C. Brown.

Dunn, S.E., & Wilson, R. (1991). Cooperative learning in the physical education classroom. *Journal of Physical Education, Recreation, and Dance, 62*(6), 22–28.

Eichstaedt, C.B., & Lavay, B.W. (1992). *Physical activity for individuals with mental retardation*. Champaign, IL: Human Kinetics.

Federal Register. (1977, Aug. 23). Education of Handicapped Children: Implementation of Part B of the Education of the Handicapped Act, Vol. 42, No. 163, Part II, 42474-42518.

Florida Department of Education. (1982). *Comprehensive Physical Activity Curriculum* (Project COMPAC). Miami: Dade County Public Schools.

Fluegelman, A. (1976). *New games book*. New York: Doubleday & Co.

Fluegelman, A. (1980). *More new games*. New York: Doubleday & Co.

Folio, M., & DuBose, R.F. (1974). *Peabody Developmental Motor Scales*. Nashville, TN: George Peabody College for Teachers.

Folsom-Meeks, S.L. (1984). Parents: Forgotten teacher aides in adapted physical education. *Adapted Physical Activity Quarterly, 1*, 275–281.

Folsom-Meeks, S.L. (1992, April). *Moving together: A model for integrating preschoolers with disabilities in movement activities*. Paper presented at the National Convention of the American Alliance for Health, Physical Education, Recreation, and Dance. Indianapolis, IN.

Forest, M., & Lusthaus, E. (1989). Promoting educational equality for all students: Circles and maps. In S. Stainback, W. Stainback, & M. Forest (Eds.), *Educating all students in the mainstream of regular education* (pp. 43–58). Baltimore: Paul H. Brookes Publishing Co.

French, C., Gonzalez, R.T., & Tronson-Simpson, J. (1991). *Caring for people with multiple disabilities: An interdisciplinary guide for caregivers*. Tucson, AZ: Therapy Skill Builders.

Gabbard, C. (1992). *Lifelong motor development*. Madison, WI: William C. Brown.

Giangreco, M.F., & Putnam, J.W. (1991). Supporting the education of students with severe disabilities in regular education environments. In L.H. Meyer, C.A. Peck, & L. Brown (Eds.), *Critical issues in the lives of people with severe disabilities* (pp. 245–270). Baltimore: Paul H. Brookes Publishing Co.

Giangreco, M.F., York, J., & Rainforth, B. (1989). Providing related services to learners with severe handicaps in educational settings: Pursuing the least restrictive option. *Pediatric Physical Therapy, 1*(2), 55–63.

Graham, G., Holt/Hale, S., & Parker, M. (1993). *Children moving: A reflective approach to teaching physical education* (3rd ed.). Mountain View, CA: Mayfield.

Hastad, D.N., & Lacy, A.C. (1989). *Measurement and evaluation in contemporary physical education*. Scottsdale, AZ: Gorsuch, Scarisbrick.

Helmstetter, E. (1989). Curriculum for school-age students: The ecological model. In F. Brown & D.H. Lehr (Eds.), *Persons with profound disabilities: Issues and practices* (pp. 239–264). Baltimore: Paul H. Brookes Publishing Co.

Herkowitz, J. (1978). Developmental task analysis: The design of movement experiences and evaluation of motor development status. In M. Ridenour (Ed.), *Motor development: Issues and applications* (pp. 139–164). Pennington, NJ: Princeton Book Co.

Individuals with Disabilities Education Act of 1990 (IDEA), PL 101-476 (October 30, 1990). Title 20, U.S.C. 1400 et seq: *U.S. Statutes at Large, 104*, 1103–1151.

Jansma, P., Decker, J., Ersing, W., McCubbin, J., & Combs, S. (1988). A fitness assessment system for individuals with severe disabilities. *Adapted Physical Activity Quarterly, 5*, 223–231.

Johnson, D.W., & Johnson, R.T. (1989). Cooperative learning and mainstreaming. In R. Gaylord-Ross (Ed.), *Integration strategies for students with handicaps* (pp. 233–248). Baltimore: Paul H. Brookes Publishing Co.

Karper, W.B., & Martinek, T.J. (1983). Motor performance and self-concepts of handicapped and nonhandicapped children in integrated physical education classes. *American Corrective Therapy Journal, 37*(3), 91–95.

Kelly, L.E., et al. (1991). *Achievement-based curriculum: Teaching manual.* Charlottesville: University of Virginia.

Kirchner, G. (1992). *Physical education for elementary school children* (8th ed.). Madison, WI: W.C. Brown & Benchmark

Krebs, P.L. (1990). Rhythms and dance. In J.P. Winnick (Ed.), *Adapted physical education and sport* (pp. 379–390). Champaign, IL: Human Kinetics.

Madden, N.M., & Slavin, R.E., (1983). Mainstreaming students with mild handicaps: Academic and social outcomes. *Reviews of Educational Research, 53*, 519–569.

Marsallo, M., & Vacante, D. (1983). *Adapted games and developmental motor activities for children.* Annandale, VA: Marsallo/Vacante.

Minner, S.H., & Knutson, R. (1982). Mainstreaming handicapped students into physical education: Initial considerations and needs. *Physical Educator, 39*, 13–15.

Mizen, D.W., & Linton, N. (1983). Guess who's coming to P.E.: Six steps to more effective mainstreaming. *Journal of Health, Physical Education, Recreation, and Dance, 54*(8), 63–65.

Moon, M.S., & Bunker, L. (1987). Recreation and motor skills programming. In M.E. Snell (Ed.), *Systematic instruction of persons with severe handicaps* (pp. 214–244). Columbus, OH: Charles E. Merrill.

Morris, G.S.D., & Stiehl, J. (1989). *Changing kids' games.* Champaign, IL: Human Kinetics.

Mosston, M. (1981). *Teaching physical education.* Columbus, OH: Charles E. Merrill.

National Association for Sport and Physical Education. (1992). *The physically educated person.* Reston, VA: Author.

Nichols, B. (1990). *Moving and learning: The elementary school physical education experience.* St. Louis: Times Mirror/Mosby College Publishing.

Orlick, T. (1978). *The cooperative sports and games book.* New York: Pantheon Press.

Orlick, T. (1982). *The second cooperative sports and games book.* New York: Pantheon Press.

Pangrazi, R.P., & Dauer, V.P. (1992). *Dynamic physical education for elementary school children* (10th ed.). New York: Macmillan.

Peck, C.A., Donaldson, J., & Pezzoli, M. (1990). Some benefits nonhandicapped adolescents perceive for themselves from their social relationships with peers who have severe handicaps. *Journal of The Association for Persons with Severe Handicaps, 15*, 211–230.

Priest, E.L. (1990). Aquatics. In J.P. Winnick (Ed.), *Adapted physical education and sport* (pp. 391–408). Champaign, IL: Human Kinetics.

Putnam, J., Rynders, J., Johnson, R., & Johnson, D. (1989). Collaborative skill instruction for promoting positive interactions between mentally handicapped and nonhandicapped children. *Exceptional Children, 55*(6), 550–558.

Rainforth, B., York, J., & Macdonald, C. (1992). *Collaborative teams for students with severe disabilities: Integrating therapy and educational services.* Baltimore: Paul H. Brookes Publishing Co.

Rizzo, T.L. (1984). Attitudes of physical educators towards teaching handicapped pupils. *Adapted Physical Activity Quarterly, 1*, 267–274.

Rizzo, T.L., & Vispoel, W.P. (1992). Changing attitudes about teaching students with handicaps. *Adapted Physical Activity Quarterly, 9*, 54–63.

Roberton, M.A., & Halverson, L.E. (1984). *Developing children: Their changing movements.* Philadelphia: Lea & Febiger.

Rohnke, K. (1977). *Cowtails and cobras: A guide to ropes courses, initiative games, and other adventure activities.* Hamilton, MA: Project Adventure.

Safrit, M.J. (1990). *Introduction to measurement in physical education and exercise science* (2nd ed.). St. Louis: Times Mirror/Mosby College Publishing.

Sailor, W., Gee, K., & Karasoff, P. (1983). Full inclusion and school restructuring. In M.E. Snell (Ed.), *Instruction of students with severe disabilities* (4th ed.) (pp. 1–30). New York: Merrill.

Santomier, J. (1985). Physical educators, attitudes and the mainstream: Suggestions for teacher trainers. *Adapted Physical Activity Quarterly, 2,* 328–337.

Santomier, J., & Kopczuk, W. (1981). Facilitation of interactions between retarded and nonretarded students in a physical education setting. *Education and Training of the Mentally Retarded, 16,* 20–23.

Schnorr, R.F. (1990). Peter? He comes and goes . . ." First graders' perspective on a part-time mainstreamed student. *Journal of The Association for Persons with Severe Handicaps, 15,* 231–240.

Seaman, J.A., & DePauw, K.P. (1989). *The new adapted physical education: A developmental approach.* Mountain View, CA: Mayfield.

Semmel, M.I., Gottlieb, J., & Robinson, N.M. (1979). Mainstreaming: Perspectives on educating handicapped children in the public school. *Review of Research in Education, 7,* 223–279.

Sherrill, C. (1993). *Adapted physical activity, recreation, and sport: Crossdisciplinary and lifespan* (4th ed.). Madison, WI: W.C. Brown & Benchmark.

Silverman, S., Dodds, P., Placek, J., Shute, S., & Rife, F. (1984). Academic learning time in elementary school physical education (ALT-PE) for student subgroups and instructional activity units. *Research Quarterly for Exercise and Sport, 55,* 365–370.

Slavin, R.E., & Stevens, R.J. (1991). Cooperative learning and mainstreaming. In J.W. Lloyd, N.N. Singh, & A.C. Repp (Eds.), *The regular education initiative: Alternative perspectives on concepts, issues, and models* (pp. 177–192). Sycamore, IL: Sycamore Press.

Snell, M.E. (1988). Gartner and Lipsky's "Beyond special education: Toward a quality system for all students," Messages for TASH. *Journal of The Association for Persons with Severe Handicaps, 13,* 137–140.

Snell, M.E., & Eichner, S.J. (1989). Integration for students with profound disabilities. In F. Brown & D.H. Lehr (Eds.), *Persons with profound disabilities: Issues and practices* (pp. 109–138). Baltimore: Paul H. Brookes Publishing Co.

Snell, M.E., & Janney, R. (1993). Including and supporting students with disabilities within general education. In B.S. Billingsley (Ed.), *Program leadership in special education manual* (pp. 244–282). Blacksburg: Virginia Polytechnic Institute and State University.

Snell, M.E., & Zirpoli, T.J. (1987). Intervention strategies. In M.E. Snell (Ed.), *Systematic instruction of persons with severe handicaps* (pp. 110–150). Columbus, OH: Charles E. Merrill.

Special Olympics International. (1986). *Athletics sports skills guide.* Washington, DC: Author.

Stainback, S., & Stainback, W. (1985). *Integration of students with severe handicaps into regular schools.* Reston, VA: Council for Exceptional Children.

Stainback, W., & Stainback, S. (Eds.). (1990). *Support networks for inclusive schooling: Interdependent integrated education.* Baltimore: Paul H. Brookes Publishing Co.

Stainback, W., Stainback, S., & Bunch, G. (1989). A rationale for the merger of regular and special education. In W. Stainback, S. Stainback, & Forest, M. (Eds.), *Educating all students in the mainstream of regular education* (pp. 15–28). Baltimore: Paul H. Brookes Publishing Co.

Stainback, S., Stainback, W., & Forest, M. (Eds.). (1989). *Educating all students in the mainstream of regular education.* Baltimore: Paul H. Brookes Publishing Co.

Stainback, S., Stainback, W., & Jackson, H.J. (1992). Towards inclusive classrooms. In S. Stainback & W. Stainback (Eds.), *Curriculum considerations in inclusive classrooms: Facilitating learning for all students* (pp. 3–18). Baltimore: Paul H. Brookes Publishing Co.

Strain, P.S. (1991). Ensuring quality of early intervention for children with severe disabilities. In L.H. Meyer, C.A. Peck, & L. Brown (Eds.), *Critical issues in the lives of people with severe disabilities* (pp. 479–484). Baltimore: Paul H. Brookes Publishing Co.

Taylor, S.J. (1988). Caught in the continuum: A critical analysis of the principle of the least restrictive environment. *Journal of The Association for Persons with Severe Handicaps, 13,* 41–53.

Turnbull, H.R. (1990). *Free appropriate public education: The law and children with disabilities* (3rd ed.). Denver: Love Publishing Co.

Ulrich, D.A. (1985, August). *Current assessment practices in adapted physical education: Implications for future training and research activities.* Paper presented at the annual meeting of the National Consortium on Physical Education and Recreation for the Handicapped, New Carollton, MD.

Vandercook, T., & York, J. (1990). A team approach to program development and support. In W. Stainback & S. Stainback (Eds.), *Support networks for inclusive schooling: Interdependent integrated education* (pp. 95–122). Baltimore: Paul H. Brookes Publishing Co.

Vergason, G.A., & Anderegg, M.L. (1991). Beyond the regular education initiative and the resource room controversy. *Focus on Exceptional Children, 23,* 1–7.

Voeltz, L.M. (1980). Children's attitudes toward handicapped peers. *American Journal of Mental Deficiency, 84*(5), 455–464.

Voeltz, L.M. (1982). Effects of structured interactions with severely handicapped peers on children's attitudes. *American Journal of Mental Deficiency, 86,* 380–390.

Voeltz, L.M., Wuerch, B.B., & Bockhaut, C.H. (1982). Social validation of leisure activities training with severely handicapped youth. *Journal of The Association for the Severely Handicapped. 7*(4), 3–13.

Wang, M.C., & Baker, E.T. (1986). Mainstreamed programs: Design features and effects. *The Journal of Special Education, 19,* 503–521.

Wang, M.C., Peverly, S.T., & Randolph, R. (1984). An investigation of implementation and effects of a full-time mainstreamed program. *Remedial and Special Education, 5,* 21–32.

Wang, M.C., Reynolds, M.C., & Walberg, H.J. (1987). Rethinking special education. *Journal of Learning Disabilities, 20,* 290–293.

Wessel, J.A. (1976). *ICAN Lifetime Leisure Skills.* Northbrook, IL: Hubbard.

Wessel, J.A., & Curtis-Pierce, E. (1990). *Ballhandling activities: Meeting special needs of children.* Belmont, CA: Fearon Teacher Aids.

Wessel, J.A., & Kelly, L. (1986). *Achievement-based curriculum development in physical education.* Philadelphia: Lea & Febiger.

Wickstrom, R.L. (1983). *Fundamental motor patterns* (3rd ed.). Philadelphia: Lea & Febiger.

Will, M.C. (1986). Educating children with learning problems: A shared responsibility. *Exceptional Children, 52,* 411–416.

Winnick, J.P. (1991). Program organization and management. In J.P. Winnick (Ed.), *Adapted physical education and sport* (pp. 19–36). Champaign, IL: Human Kinetics.

Woodruff, G., & McGonigel, M.J. (1988). Early intervention team approaches: The transdisciplinary model. In J.B. Jordan, J.J. Gallagher, P.L. Hutinger, & M.B. Karnes (Eds.), *Early childhood special education: Birth to three* (pp. 163–182). Reston, VA: Council for Exceptional Children.

York, J., Giangreco, M.F., Vandercook, T., & Macdonald, C. (1992). Integrating support personnel in the inclusive classroom. In S. Stainback & W. Stainback (Eds.), *Curricular considerations in inclusive classrooms: Facilitating learning for all students* (pp. 101–116). Baltimore: Paul H. Brookes Publishing Co.

York, J., & Rainforth, B. (1991). Developing individualized adaptations. In F.P. Orelove & D.J. Sobsey (Eds.), *Educating children with multiple disabilities: A transdisciplinary approach* (2nd ed.) (pp. 259–295). Baltimore: Paul H. Brookes Publishing Co.

Index

Page numbers followed by t *and* f *denote tables and figures, respectively.*